SPRING

PRESCR

POCKET GUIDE
TO COMMON
DRUGS

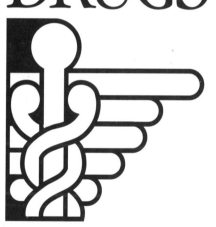

SPRINGHOUSE

PRESCRIBER'S
POCKET GUIDE
TO COMMON
DRUGS

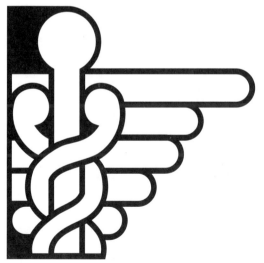

Springhouse Corporation
Springhouse, Pennsylvania

The clinical procedures described and recommended in this publication are based on research and consultation with nursing, medical, and legal authorities. To the best of our knowledge, these procedures reflect currently accepted practice; nevertheless, they can't be considered absolute and universal recommendations. For individual application, all recommendations must be considered in light of the patient's clinical condition and, before the administration of new or infrequently used drugs, in light of the latest package-insert information. The authors and publisher disclaim responsibility for adverse effects resulting directly or indirectly from the suggested procedures, from undetected errors, or from the reader's misunderstanding of the text.

Printed in the United States of America
PPG-010398

A member of the Reed Elsevier plc group

ISBN: 0-87434-948-6
ISSN: 1096-3885

Contents

Clinical reviewers and consultants

Deborah Becker, MSN, RN, CCRN, Clinical Site Coordinator for Adult Critical Care, Nurse Practitioner Program, University of Pennsylvania, Philadelphia

Daniel A. Behrens, RPh, PharmD, Medical Information Projects Manager, Zeneca Pharmaceuticals, Wilmington, Del.

James Camamo, PharmD, Clinical Pharmacist, University Medical Center, Tucson, Ariz.

James H. Cook, RN, MD, Resident Physician, Temple University Hospital, Philadelphia

Teresa S. Dunsworth, PharmD, BCPS, Clinical Associate Professor of Clinical Pharmacy, West Virginia University School of Pharmacy, Morgantown

Dan J. Halberstadt, RPh, Director, Department of Pharmacy Services, Allegheny University Hospital, Philadelphia

Lori Ann Hytrek, PharmD, Specialty Resident in Pharmacy Administration, University of California School of Pharmacy, San Francisco

James A. Koestner, PharmD, Clinical Pharmacist-Trauma, Vanderbilt University Medical Center, Nashville, Tenn.

Randall A. Lynch, RPh, PharmD, Assistant Director of Pharmacy Services, Presbyterian Medical-Center, University of Pennsylvania Health System, Philadelphia

Marie Maloney, PharmD, Clinical Pharmacist, University Medical Center, Tucson, Ariz.

Jan E. Markind, RPh, PharmD, Drug Information Specialist, Clinical Assistant Professor, University of Illinois at Chicago

Michael K. McGuire, PharmD, Network Clinical Coordinator, Albert Einstein Healthcare Network, Philadelphia

Steven B. Meisel, PharmD, Assistant Director of Pharmacy, Fairview Southdale Hospital, Edina, Minn.

George Melko, PharmD, Clinical Pharmacist, Home Infusion, Thomas Jefferson University, Philadelphia

Andrew M. Peterson, PharmD, Assistant Professor of Pharmacy, Philadelphia College of Pharmacy, Philadelphia

David Pipher, RPh, PharmD, Director of Pharmacy, Forbes Regional Hospital, Monroeville, Pa.

Joel Shuster, PharmD, Clinical Associate Professor, School of Pharmacy, Temple University; Clinical Pharmacist, Medical College of Pennsylvania, Philadelphia

Kenneth Weiland, RPh, PharmD, Clinical Coordinator, Chestnut Hill Hospital, Philadelphia

Foreword

By putting up-to-date prescribing information at your fingertips, *Prescriber's Pocket Guide to Common Drugs* can improve therapeutic outcomes for your patients. Tailored to busy prescribers like you, this compact, quick-reference resource provides essential information on nearly 900 of today's most commonly prescribed drugs.

As you're undoubtedly aware, new drugs are approved every year, and some existing ones receive approval for new indications or precautions. For many prescribers, staying abreast of these changes is a major challenge.

This book helps you meet that challenge. The authors, contributors, and editors at Springhouse have streamlined a massive pharmacology database down to the most important facts for daily practice. Everything about the book — from its size and shape to its organization and content — is designed to promote fast, easy access to information. Compact and lightweight, it fits easily into your pocket, so you can use it in any practice setting. It's comprehensive enough to include virtually all the drugs you would typically prescribe in an average day.

Drugs are arranged alphabetically. Shaded letter tabs help you zero in on the specific drug you're looking for. Individual drug entries are pared down to the indispensable facts you need to make prescribing decisions with confidence:
- generic and trade names
- pharmacologic and therapeutic classes
- pregnancy risk category
- controlled substance schedule (if any)
- currently available dosage forms
- currently approved indications with specific dosages
- critical precautions.

To help you avoid medication errors — a major cause of medical liability lawsuits nowadays — appendices detail the components of a properly written prescription and identify abbreviations to avoid when writing prescriptions.

A separate appendix lists therapeutic classifications of selected drugs so you can quickly compare drugs within a specific class. Another lists unlabeled and unusual uses of common drugs, such as atenolol, verapamil, and valproic acid. Why is it important to know about such uses? By one estimate, about 40% to 60% of all prescriptions written today are for uses that are not approved but are recognized and accepted by most prescribers.

Most important, you can rely on *Prescriber's Pocket Guide to Common Drugs* for accuracy. Each entry has been thoroughly reviewed by a team of clinical specialists, the same team that brings you *Physician's Drug Handbook* and *Nurse Practitioner's Drug Handbook*. In short, this powerful little book helps you make well-informed and fully appropriate use of drugs in your practice. It's a valuable resource for meeting the precise needs of the modern prescriber.

Carol Warfield, MD
Associate Professor of Anesthesia
Harvard Medical School
Chief, Division of Pain Medicine
Beth Israel Deaconess Medical Center
Boston, Massachusetts

The *Prescriber's Pocket Guide to Common Drugs* offers comprehensive dosage information in a unique, quick-scan format. The book opens with a list of abbreviations used in the book. Then, organized alphabetically by generic name, each drug entry covers generic and common trade names, pharmacologic and therapeutic class, pregnancy risk category, controlled substance schedule (where appropriate), common dosage forms and strengths, common indications and dosages, and key precautions. Information is divided into columns for quick reference.

The first column shows the generic name in boldface, followed by trade names. (Trade names are not available for some generic drug names.) Canadian and Australian brand-name drugs are denoted by a dagger (†) or double-dagger (‡), respectively. Below the list of trade names are the drug's pharmacologic class and then its therapeutic class. Pregnancy risk category and, where applicable, controlled substance schedule are listed next.

Pregnancy risk categories parallel those assigned by the FDA to reflect a drug's potential to cause birth defects:
A: Adequate studies in pregnant women have failed to show a risk to the fetus.
B: Animal studies have not shown a risk to the fetus, but controlled studies have not been conducted in pregnant women; or animal studies have shown an adverse effect on the fetus, but adequate studies in pregnant women have not shown a fetal risk.
C: Animal studies have shown an adverse effect on the fetus, but adequate studies have not been conducted in humans. The benefits may be acceptable despite potential risks.

D: The drug may pose risks to the human fetus, but potential benefits may be acceptable despite the risks.
X: Studies in animals or humans show fetal abnormalities, or reports of adverse reactions indicate evidence of fetal risk. The risks involved clearly outweigh the potential benefits.
NR: Not rated.

Drugs regulated under the Controlled Substances Act of 1970 are divided into the following schedules:
I: high abuse potential, no accepted medical use
II: high abuse potential, severe dependence liability
III: less abuse potential than schedule II drugs, moderate dependence liability
IV: less abuse potential than schedule III drugs, limited dependence liability
V: limited abuse potential.

The second column lists common dosage forms and strengths. The third column covers major indications and the most common dosages ordered for a particular drug. The final column lists the more important precautions applicable for the drug.

Appendices include an example of a properly written prescription, common pharmacologic abbreviations to avoid, a list of common drugs classified according to their clinical use or therapeutic class, and unusual and unlabeled uses of common drugs. The index is organized by generic name, trade name, and disease.

Abbreviations used in this book

ABG	arterial blood gas	IPPB	intermittent positive-pressure breathing
ACE	angiotensin-converting enzyme	INR	international normalized ratio
ADH	antidiuretic hormone	IOP	intraocular pressure
ALT	alanine aminotransferase	LDL	low-density lipoprotein
AST	aspartate aminotransferase	liq	liquid
		MAO	monoamine oxidase
AVM	arteriovenous malformation	MI	myocardial infarction
buff	buffered	mo	month
CABG	coronary artery bypass graft	NG	nasogastric
		NSAID	nonsteroidal anti-inflammatory drug
CAD	coronary artery disease	O_2 sat, SaO_2	oxygen saturation
cap	capsule	oint	ointment
CDC	Centers for Disease Control and Prevention	PABA	para-aminobenzoic acid
		PCWP	pulmonary capillary wedge pressure
chew	chewable	ped	pediatric
CK	creatine kinase	periop	perioperative
CMV	cytomegalovirus	pharm	pharmacologic
conc	concentration, concentrated	pkg	package
		pkt	packet
contr-release	controlled-release	PSVT	paroxysmal supraventricular tachycardia
COPD	chronic obstructive pulmonary disease		
		PT	prothrombin time
CSF	cerebrospinal fluid	PTT	partial thromboplastin time
CV	central venous		
CVP	central venous pressure	PVD	peripheral vascular disease
ECG	electrocardiogram		
EEG	electroencephalogram	REM	rapid eye movement
equiv	equivalent	SA	sinoatrial
ET	endotracheal	SIADH	syndrome of inappropriate antidiuretic hormone
ext-release	extended-release		
G	gauge	supp	suppository
gram-neg	gram-negative	susp	suspension
gram-pos	gram-positive	sust-release	sustained-release
gyn	gynecologic	tab	tablet
Hct	hematocrit	T_3	triiodothyronine
HDL	high-density lipoprotein	T_4	thyroxine
Hgb	hemoglobin	TB	tuberculosis
HR	heart rate	TIA	transient ischemic attack
H_1, H_2	histamine-1, histamine-2	UCE	urea cycle enzymopathy
I&O	intake and output	USP	United States Pharmacopeia
ICP	intracranial pressure		
IND	investigational new drug	UTI	urinary tract infection
inf	infusion	vag	vaginal, vaginally
inh	inhaled or inhalation		
inj	injection		

DRUG/CLASS/CATEGORY	DOSAGE FORMS	INDICATIONS/DOSAGES	KEY PRECAUTIONS
abciximab ReoPro *Antiplatelet aggregate* *Platelet aggregation inhibitor* Preg. Risk Category: C	**inj:** 2 mg/ml	*Adjunct to PTCA or atherectomy to prevent acute cardiac ischemic complications in patients at high risk for abrupt closure of treated coronary vessel* — **Adults:** 0.25 mg/kg IV bolus 10 to 60 min before start of PTCA or atherectomy, then continuous IV infusion of 10 mcg/min for 12 hr.	▪ Use cautiously in increased risk for bleeding; in patients < 75 kg or > age 65; history of GI disease; prolonged or failed PTCA; and concomitant heparin anticoagulation. ▪ Contraindicated in hypersensitivity to drug component or to murine proteins, active internal bleeding, recent GI or GU bleeding of clinical significance, history of CVA within past 2 yr or CVA with significant residual neurologic deficit, bleeding diathesis, thrombocytopenia, recent major surgery or trauma, intracranial neoplasm, intracranial arteriovenous malformation, intracranial aneurysm, severe uncontrolled hypertension, or history of vasculitis; within 7 days of oral anticoagulant therapy (unless PT ≤ 1.2 times control); or with use of IV dextran before PTCA or intent to use it during PTCA.
acarbose Precose *Alpha-glucosidase inhibitor* *Antidiabetic* Preg. Risk Category: B	**tab:** 50, 100 mg	*Adjunct to diet to lower blood glucose in non-insulin-dependent diabetes mellitus when hyperglycemia can't be managed by diet alone or by diet and sulfonylureas* — **Adults:** Individualized. Initially, 25 mg PO tid at start of main meals; then adjust q 4 to 8 wk. Maintenance: 50 to 100 mg PO tid; don't exceed 50 mg tid in patients < 60 kg.	▪ Use cautiously in renal impairment and in patients receiving sulfonylureas or insulin. ▪ Contraindicated in hypersensitivity, diabetic ketoacidosis, cirrhosis, inflammatory bowel disease, colonic ulcers, partial intestinal obstruction, chronic intestinal disease associated with marked digestive or absorptive disorders, and conditions that may worsen with increased intestinal gas formation. ▪ Not recommended for creatinine > 2 mg/dl or in pregnant or breast-feeding patients.

Drug	Forms	Indications & Dosage	Cautions & Contraindications
acebutolol, acebutolol hydrochloride Monitan†, Sectral *Beta-adrenergic blocker* *Antihypertensive/antiarrhythmic* Preg. Risk Category: B	*cap:* 200, 400 mg	*Hypertension* — **Adults:** 400 mg PO as 1 daily dose or in divided doses bid to max 1,200 mg qd. *Ventricular arrhythmias* — **Adults:** 400 mg PO daily divided bid; increase prn for adequate response. Usual dosage 600 to 1,200 mg.	• Use cautiously in heart failure, peripheral vascular disease, bronchospastic disease, hyperthyroidism, and diabetes. • Contraindicated in persistent severe bradycardia, second- and third-degree heart block, overt cardiac failure, and cardiogenic shock.
acetazolamide Acetazolam†, AK-Zol, Dazamide, Diamox **acetazolamide sodium** Diamox Parenteral *Carbonic anhydrase inhibitor* *Antiglaucoma agent/diuretic* Preg. Risk Category: C	*tab:* 125, 250 mg; *cap:* 500 mg; *inj:* 500 mg	*Secondary glaucoma and preop treatment of acute angle-closure glaucoma* — **Adults:** 250 mg PO q 4 hr; or 250 mg PO bid for short-term therapy. To rapidly lower IOP, initially, 500 mg IV, then 125 to 250 mg IV q 4 hr. *Edema in heart failure* — **Adults:** 250 to 375 mg PO or IV qd in morning. *Chronic open-angle glaucoma* — **Adults:** 250 mg to 1 g PO daily in divided doses qid, or 500 mg (ext-release) PO bid.	• Use cautiously in respiratory acidosis, emphysema, or diabetes and in patients receiving other diuretics. • Contraindicated in hypersensitivity to drug; in long-term therapy for chronic noncongestive angle-closure glaucoma; and in hyponatremia, hypokalemia, renal or hepatic disease or dysfunction, adrenal gland failure, and hyperchloremic acidosis.
acetic acid Domeboro Otic, VoSol Otic Acid *Antibacterial/antifungal* Preg. Risk Category: NR	*otic sol:* 2% in aluminum acetate sol (Domeboro Otic), 2% in 3% propylene glycol diacetate (VoSol Otic)	*External ear canal infection* — **Adults and children:** 4 to 6 drops into ear canal q 2 to 3 hr; or insert saturated ear wick for 1st 24 hr, then continue with instillations.	• Contraindicated in patient with perforated eardrum.
acetohydroxamic acid Lithostat *Urease inhibitor* *Antiurolithic/adjunctive agent in treatment of UTI* Preg. Risk Category: X	*tab:* 250 mg	*UTI caused by kidney stones* — **Adults:** 250 mg PO q 6 to 8 hr on empty stomach. Max 1.5 g daily. **Children:** 10 mg/kg/day PO in 2 or 3 divided doses.	• Contraindicated if physical state and disease amenable to surgery and appropriate antibiotics, when urine infected by nonurease-producing organisms, during pregnancy, and in poor renal function.

DRUG/CLASS/ CATEGORY	DOSAGE FORMS	INDICATIONS/ DOSAGES	KEY PRECAUTIONS
acetylcholine chloride Miochol *Cholinergic agonist* *Miotic* Preg. Risk Category: NR	*ophth sol:* 1%	*Anterior segment surgery —* **Adults and children:** during surgery, 0.5 to 2 ml instilled gently into anterior or chamber.	• Contraindicated in hypersensitivity to drug or its components.
acetylcysteine Airbron†, Mucomyst, Mucomyst-10, Mucosil-10, Mucosil-20, Parvolex†‡ *Amino acid (L-cysteine) derivative* *Mucolytic agent/antidote for acetaminophen overdose* Preg. Risk Category: B	*sol:* 10%, 20%; *inj:* 200 mg/ml‡	*Adjuvant therapy for abnormal viscid or inspissated mucus secretions in pneumonia, bronchitis, TB, cystic fibrosis, emphysema, atelectasis (adjunct), pulmonary complications of thoracic and CV surgery —* **Adults and children:** 1 to 2 ml 10% or 20% sol by direct instillation into trachea up to q hr; or 1 to 10 ml of 20% solution or 2 to 20 ml of 10% sol by nebulization q 2 to 6 hr, prn. *Acetaminophen toxicity —* **Adults and children:** initially, 140 mg/kg PO, then 70 mg/kg PO q 4 hr for 17 doses.	• Use cautiously in elderly or debilitated patients with severe respiratory insufficiency. • Contraindicated in hypersensitivity to drug.
activated charcoal Actidose, Actidose-Aqua, Charcoaid, Charcocaps, Liqui-Char *Adsorbent* *Antidote/antiflatulent* Preg. Risk Category: C	*tab:* 200, 300, 325, 650 mg; *cap:* 260 mg; *powder:* 30, 50 g; *oral susp:* 0.625, 0.83 mg and 1 g, 1.25 g/5 ml	*Flatulence or dyspepsia —* **Adults:** 600 mg to 5 g PO as single dose or 0.975 g to 3.9 g PO tid after meals. *Poisoning —* **Adults and children:** initially, 1 to 2 g/ kg (30 to 100 g) PO or 10 times amount of poison ingested, given as susp in 120 to 240 ml of water. Check with poison control center for specific uses in poisonings or overdoses.	• Most effective if used within 30 min of toxic ingestion.
acyclovir Zovirax *Synthetic purine nucleoside* *Antiviral agent* Preg. Risk Category: C	*oint:* 5%	*Initial herpes genitalis; limited, non-life-threatening mucocutaneous herpes simplex virus infections in immunocompromised patients —* **Adults and children:** cover all lesions q 3 hr, 6 times daily for 7 days.	• Contraindicated in hypersensitivity or chemical intolerance to drug.

acyclovir sodium
Avirax†, Zovirax
Synthetic purine nucleoside
Antiviral agent
Preg. Risk Category: C

cap: 200 mg; *tab:* 400, 800 mg; *susp:* 200 mg/5 ml; *inj:* 500 mg/vial, 1 g/vial

Mucocutaneous herpes simplex virus (HSV-1 and HSV-2) infections in immunocompromised patients, genital herpes in immunocompetent patients —
Adults and children ≥ 12 yr: 5 mg/kg IV at constant rate over 1 hr q 8 hr for 7 to 14 days (5 to 7 days for severe initial episode of genital herpes). **Children < 12 yr:** 250 mg/m² IV at constant rate over 1 hr by IV q 8 hr for 7 days.
Initial genital herpes — **Adults:** 200 mg PO q 4 hr while awake (total 5 caps daily); or 400 mg PO q 8 hr. Continue 7 to 10 days.
Varicella (chickenpox) infections in immunocompromised patients — **Adults and children ≥ 12 yr:** 10 mg/kg IV infused at constant rate over 1 hr q 8 hr for 7 days. **Children < 12 yr:** 500 mg/m² IV infused at constant rate over 1 hr q 8 hr for 7 to 10 days.
Acute herpes zoster infection in immunocompetent patients — **Adults and children ≥ 12 yr:** 800 mg PO q 4 hr 5 times daily for 5 to 10 days.

- Use cautiously in underlying neurologic disorders, renal disease, or dehydration and in patients receiving other nephrotoxic drugs.
- Contraindicated in hypersensitivity to drug.

---

albumin 5%
Albuminar 5%, Albutein 5%
albumin 25%
Albuminar 25%, Albutein 25%
Blood derivative
Plasma protein
Preg. Risk Category: C

albumin 5% — *sol:*
50-, 250-, 500-, 1,000-ml vials.
albumin 25% — *sol:*
10-, 20-, 50-, 100-ml vials

Hypovolemic shock — **Adults:** initially, 500 to 750 ml 5% sol by IV infusion, repeated q 30 min, prn. Alternatively, 100 to 200 ml IV of 25% sol, repeat in 10 to 30 min, if needed. **Children:** 12 to 20 ml 5% sol/kg by IV infusion, repeat in 15 to 30 min if response inadequate. Or, 2.5 to 5 ml IV of 25% sol/kg, repeat in 10 to 30 min if needed.
Hypoproteinemia — **Adults:** 200 to 300 ml of 25% albumin.
Hyperbilirubinemia — **Infants:** 1 g albumin (4 ml 25%)/kg during or 1 to 2 hr before exchange transfusion.

- Use cautiously in hypertension, cardiac disease, severe pulmonary infection, or hypoalbuminemia with peripheral edema.
- Contraindicated in hypersensitivity to drug, severe anemia, or cardiac failure.

DRUG / CLASS / CATEGORY	DOSAGE FORMS	INDICATIONS / DOSAGES	KEY PRECAUTIONS
albuterol (salbutamol) Asmol‡, Proventil, Ventolin **albuterol sulfate (salbutamol sulfate)** Proventil, Proventil Repetabs, Respolin Inhaler‡, Respolin Respirator Solution‡, Ventolin *Adrenergic* *Bronchodilator* Preg. Risk Category: C	*aerosol inhaler:* 90 mcg/metered spray, 100 mcg/metered spray‡; *caps for inh:* 200 mcg; *tab:* 2, 4 mg; *tab (ext-release):* 4, 8 mg; *syrup:* 2 mg/5 ml; *sol for inh:* 0.083, 0.5%	*To prevent or treat bronchospasm in reversible obstructive airway disease or to prevent exercise-induced bronchospasm —* **Adults and children ≥ 12 yr:** dosage and frequency vary with dosage form. *Aerosol inh:* 1 to 2 inh q 4 to 6 hr. *Sol for inh:* 2.5 mg tid or qid by nebulizer. *Caps for inh:* 200 mcg inh q 4 to 6 hr using Rotahaler. Some patients may need 400 mcg q 4 to 6 hr. *Oral tab:* 2 to 4 mg PO tid or qid; max 8 mg qid. *Ext-release tab:* 4 to 8 mg PO q 12 hr; max 16 mg bid. **Children 6 to 13 yr:** 2 mg (1 tsp) PO t d or qid. **Children 2 to 5 yr:** 0.1 mg/kg PO tid; max 2 mg (1 tsp) tid. **Adults > 65 yr:** 2 mg PO tid or qid.	▪ Use cautiously in CV disorders, hyperthyroidism, diabetes mellitus, and unusual responsiveness to adrenergics. ▪ Contraindicated in hypersensitivity to drug or any drug component.
aldesleukin (interleukin-2, IL-2) Proleukin *Lymphokine* *Immunoregulatory agent* Preg. Risk Category: C	*powder for inj:* 22 million IU/ vial	*Metastatic renal cell carcinoma —* **Adults:** 600,000 IU/kg (0.037 mg/kg) IV q 8 hr for 5 days (total of 14 doses). After 9-day rest, repeat sequence for another 14 doses. May give repeat courses after rest period of ≥ 7 wk.	▪ Use cautiously in cardiac or pulmonary disease or seizure disorders. ▪ Contraindicated in hypersensitivity to drug component, abnormal cardiac (thallium) stress test or pulmonary function tests, and organ allografts. ▪ Retreatment contraindicated in pericardial tamponade; arrhythmias uncontrolled or unresponsive to intervention; sustained ventricular tachycardia; chest pain accompanied by ECG changes, indicating MI or angina pectoris; renal dysfunction requiring dialysis for ≥ 72 hr; coma or toxic psychosis lasting ≥ 48 hr; repetitive or hard-to-control seizures; bowel ischemia or perforation; and GI bleeding requiring surgery.

Drug	Forms	Indications & Dosage	Contraindications & Precautions
alendronate sodium Fosamax *Osteoclast-mediated bone resorption inhibitor* *Anti-osteoporotic agent* Preg. Risk Category: C	**tab:** 10, 40 mg	*Osteoporosis in postmenopausal women* — **Adults:** 10 mg PO daily, taken with plain water only, ≥ 30 min before 1st food, beverage, or medication of day. *Paget's disease of bone* — **Adults:** 40 mg PO daily for 6 mo, taken with plain water only, ≥ 30 min before 1st food, beverage, or medication of day.	■ Use cautiously in dysphagia, symptomatic esophageal disease, gastritis, duodenitis, ulcers, or mild to moderate renal insufficiency. ■ Contraindicated in hypersensitivity to drug, hypocalcemia, or severe renal insufficiency.
alfentanil hydrochloride Alfenta *Opioid* *Analgesic/adjunct to anesthesia/anesthetic* Preg. Risk Category: C Controlled Sub. Sched.: II	**inj:** 500 mcg/ml	*Adjunct to general anesthetic* — **Adults:** initially, 8 to 50 mcg/kg IV; then increments of 3 to 15 mcg/kg IV q 5 to 20 min. *As primary anesthetic* — **Adults:** initially, 130 to 245 mcg/kg IV; then 0.5 to 1.5 mcg/kg/min IV.	■ Use cautiously in head injury, pulmonary disease, decreased respiratory reserve, and hepatic or renal impairment. ■ Contraindicated in hypersensitivity to drug.
allopurinol Alloremed‡, Lopurin‡, Purinol†, Zyloprim *Xanthine oxidase inhibitor* *Antigout* Preg. Risk Category: C	**tab:** 100, 300 mg; **cap:** 100, 300 mg	*Gout, primary or secondary to hyperuricemia; secondary to certain diseases* — dosage varies with disease severity; doses > 300 mg should be divided. **Adults:** mild gout, 200 to 300 mg PO qd; severe gout with large tophi, 400 to 600 mg PO qd. Same for maint. in secondary hyperuricemia. Max 800 mg/day. *Hyperuricemia secondary to malignancies* — **Children < 6 yr:** 50 mg PO tid. **Children 6 to 10 yr:** 300 mg PO daily or divided tid. *Prevention of acute gouty attacks* — **Adults:** 100 mg PO daily; increase weekly by 100 mg without exceeding max (800 mg), until uric acid 6 mg/dl or less.	■ Contraindicated in hypersensitivity to drug and idiopathic hemochromatosis.
alpha₁ proteinase inhibitor (human) Prolastin *Enzyme inhibitor* *Replacement protein* Preg. Risk Category: C	**inj:** 500, 1,000 mg/vial	*Chronic replacement therapy in congenital alpha₁-antitrypsin deficiency and demonstrable panacinar emphysema* — **Adults:** 60 mg/kg IV q wk. May give at 0.08 ml/kg/min rate or greater.	■ Use cautiously in risk for circulatory overload. ■ Contraindicated in selective IgA deficiency with known antibodies against IgA.

†Canadian ‡Australian

DRUG / CLASS / CATEGORY	DOSAGE FORMS	INDICATIONS / DOSAGES	KEY PRECAUTIONS
alprazolam Apo-Alpraz†, Novo-Alprazol†, Nu-Alpraz†, Xanax *Benzodiazepine* *Antianxiety agent* Preg. Risk Category: D Controlled Sub. Sched.: IV	**tab:** 0.25, 0.5, 1, 2 mg; ***oral*** **sol:** 0.5 mg/5 ml, 1 mg/ml (concentrate)	*Anxiety* — **Adults:** usual initial dose 0.25 to 0.5 mg PO tid, to max 4 mg daily in divided doses. For elderly or debilitated patients or those with advanced liver disease, usual initial dose 0.25 mg PO bid or tid, to max 4 mg daily in divided doses. *Panic disorders* — **Adults:** 0.5 mg PO tid, increased q 3 to 4 days in increments of no more than 1 mg. Max 10 mg qd in divided doses.	▪ Use cautiously in hepatic, renal, or pulmonary disease. ▪ Contraindicated in hypersensitivity to drug or other benzodiazepines and in acute angle-closure glaucoma.
alprostadil Caverject *Prostaglandin* *Corrective agent for impotence* Preg. Risk Category: NR	**inj:** 10, 20 mcg/vial	*Erectile dysfunction due to vasculogenic, psychogenic, or mixed etiology* — **Adults:** dosages highly individualized, with initial dose of 2.5 mcg intracavernously. If partial response occurs, give 2nd dose of 2.5 mcg, then increase in increments of 5 to 10 mcg until suitable erection. If no response, may increase 2nd dose to 7.5 mcg within 1 hr, then increase in increments of 5 to 10 mcg until suitable erection. *Erectile dysfunction of neurologic etiology (spinal cord injury)* — **Adults:** dosages highly individualized, with initial dose of 1.25 mcg intracavernously. If partial response occurs, give 2nd dose of 1.25 mcg, followed by increments of 2.5 mcg, to dose of 5 mcg, and then in increments of 5 mcg until suitable erection. If no response, may give next higher dose within 1 hr.	▪ Contraindicated in hypersensitivity to drug, conditions associated with predisposition to priapism (sickle cell anemia or trait, multiple myeloma, leukemia), and penile deformation (angulation, cavernosal fibrosis, Peyronie's disease). ▪ Don't use in men with penile implants or if sexual activity is inadvisable or contraindicated. ▪ Don't give to women or children.
alprostadil Prostin VR Pediatric *Prostaglandin* *Ductus arteriosus patency adjunct* Preg. Risk Category: NR	**inj:** 500 mcg/ ml	*Palliative therapy for temporary maintenance of patency of ductus arteriosus until surgery* — **Infants:** 0.05 to 0.1 mcg/kg/min IV infusion. When therapeutic response achieved, reduce infusion rate to lowest cosage that will maintain response; max 0.4 mcg/kg/ min. Alternatively, give through umbilical artery catheter placed at ductal opening.	▪ Use cautiously in neonates with bleeding disorders. ▪ Contraindicated in neonatal respiratory distress syndrome.

alteplase (tissue plasminogen activator, recombinant; tPA)
Actilyse‡, Activase
Enzyme
Thrombolytic enzyme
Preg. Risk Category: C

inj: 50-mg (29 million-IU), 100-mg (58 million-IU) vials

Lysis of thrombi obstructing coronary arteries in acute MI — **Adults:** 100 mg IV infusion over 3 hr as follows: 60 mg in 1st hr, of which 6 to 10 mg given as bolus over 1st 1 to 2 min. Then 20 mg/hr infusion for 2 hr. Smaller adults (< 65 kg) should receive 1.25 mg/kg in similar fashion (60% in 1st hr, 10% as bolus; then 20% of total dose per hr for 2 hr).
Management of acute massive pulmonary embolism — **Adults:** 100 mg IV infusion over 2 hr. Begin heparin at end of infusion when PTT or thrombin time returns to twice normal or less. Don't exceed 100-mg dose.
Acute ischemic stroke — **Adults:** 0.9 mg/kg IV infusion over 1 hr with 10% of total dose given as initial IV bolus over 1 min. Max 90 mg total. *Note:* Give within 3 hr after symptoms occur and only when intracranial bleed has been ruled out.

- Use cautiously within 10 days of major surgery; in pregnancy and 1st 10 days postpartum; in organ biopsy, trauma, GI or GU bleeding, cerebrovascular disease, hypertension, likelihood of left heart thrombus, hemostatic defects, hepatic dysfunction, occluded AV cannula, severe neurologic deficit, mitral stenosis, atrial fibrillation, acute pericarditis or subacute bacterial endocarditis, septic thrombophlebitis, and diabetic hemorrhagic retinopathy; in patients receiving anticoagulants; and in patients > 75 yr.
- Contraindicated in active internal bleeding, intracranial neoplasm, arteriovenous malformation, aneurysm, severe uncontrolled hypertension, history of CVA, recent intraspinal or intracranial trauma or surgery, known bleeding diathesis, history or current intracranial hemorrhage, suspicion of subarachnoid hemorrhage, and seizure at onset of stroke when used for acute ischemic stroke.

altretamine (hexamethylmelamine; HMM)
Hexalen, Hexastat‡
Alkylating agent
Antineoplastic
Preg. Risk Category: D

cap: 50 mg

Palliative treatment of persistent or recurrent ovarian cancer after 1st-line therapy with cisplatin or alkylating agent–based combination therapy — **Adults:** 260 mg/m² PO daily in 4 divided doses with meals and hs for 14 or 21 consecutive days in 28-day cycle.

- Contraindicated in hypersensitivity to drug and in preexisting severe bone marrow suppression or severe neurotoxicity.

aluminum carbonate
Basaljel
Inorganic aluminum salt
Antacid/hypophosphatemic
Preg. Risk Category: B

equiv to alum. hydroxide — *tab, cap:* 500 mg; *oral susp:* 400 mg/5 ml

Antacid — **Adults:** 5 to 10 ml of oral susp PO q 2 hr, prn; or 1 to 2 tabs or caps PO q 2 hr, prn. Max 24 caps, tabs, or tsp/24 hr.
To prevent urinary phosphate stones (with low-phosphate diet) — **Adults:** 15 to 30 ml oral susp in water or juice PO 1 hr after meals and hs; or 2 to 6 tabs or caps 1 hr after meals and hs.

- Use cautiously in chronic renal disease.

ALUMINUM CARBONATE   9

†Canadian †Australian

DRUG/CLASS/CATEGORY	DOSAGE FORMS	INDICATIONS/DOSAGES	KEY PRECAUTIONS
aluminum hydroxide AlternaGEL, Alu-Cap, Amphojel, Dialume, Nephrox *Aluminum salt* *Antacid* Preg. Risk Category: C	*tab:* 300, 600 mg; *cap:* 475, 500 mg; *oral susp:* 320, 450, 600, 675 mg/5ml	*Antacid* — **Adults:** 500 to 1,500 mg PO (5 to 30 ml of most susp products) 1 hr after meals and hs; alternatively, 300-mg tab or 600-mg tab (chewed before swallowing) taken with milk or water 5 to 6 times daily after meals and hs.	■ Use cautiously in chronic renal disease.
aluminum phosphate Phosphaljel *Aluminum salt* *Phosphate replacement* Preg. Risk Category: NR	*oral susp:* 233 mg/5 ml	*To reduce fecal elimination of phosphorus* — **Adults:** 15 to 30 ml undiluted PO q 2 hr between meals and hs.	■ Use cautiously in chronic renal disease.
amantadine hydrochloride Antadine†, Symadine, Symmetrel *Synthetic cyclic primary amine* *Antiviral* Preg. Risk Category: C	*cap:* 100 mg; *syrup:* 50 mg/5 ml	*Prophylaxis or symptomatic treatment of influenza type A virus, or symptomatic treatment of respiratory tract illnesses* — **Adults < 65 yr with normal renal function and children > 9 yr weighing > 45 kg:** 200 mg PO daily in single dose. **Children 1 to 9 yr or < 45 kg:** 4.4 to 8.8 mg/kg PO daily, as single dose or divided bid. Max 150 mg daily. **Adults ≥ 65 yr with normal renal function:** 100 mg PO qd. Start treatment within 24 to 48 hr after symptoms appear and continue for 24 to 48 hr after they disappear. Start prophylaxis as soon as possible after initial exposure.	■ Use cautiously in seizure disorders, heart failure, peripheral edema, hepatic disease, mental illness, eczematoid rash, renal impairment, orthostatic hypotension, and CV disease and in elderly patients. ■ Contraindicated in hypersensitivity to drug.
ambenonium chloride Mytelase Caplets *Cholinesterase inhibitor* *Antimyasthenic* Preg. Risk Category: NR	*tab:* 10 mg	*Symptomatic treatment of myasthenia gravis in patients who can't take neostigmine bromide or pyridostigmine bromide* — **Adults:** individualized; usual range 5 to 25 mg PO tid or qid. Usual starting dose 5 mg PO tid or qid, increased and adjusted at 1- to 2-day intervals. Usual dosage range 5 to 25 mg PO tid	■ Use very cautiously in asthma. Use cautiously in seizure disorders, bradycardia, recent coronary occlusion, vagotonia, peptic ulcer, hyperthyroidism, arrhythmias, postop atelectasis, and pneumonia.

	or qid (some patients may require up to 75 mg bid to qid).	▪ Contraindicated in hypersensitivity to anticholinesterase agents or mechanical obstruction of intestine or urinary tract and in patients receiving ganglionic blockers.
amcinonide Cyclocort *Topical adrenocorticoid* *Anti-inflammatory* Preg. Risk Category: C	**cream:** 0.1%; **lotion:** 0.1%; **oint:** 0.1%	*Inflammation associated with corticosteroid-responsive dermatoses* — **Adults and children:** apply light film to affected areas bid or tid. Rub in gently until medication disappears.	▪ Contraindicated in hypersensitivity to drug.
amifostine Ethyol *Organic thiophosphate* *Cytoprotective* Preg. Risk Category: C	**inj:** 500 mg anhydrous base and 500 mg mannitol in 10-ml vial	*Reduction of cumulative renal toxicity associated with repeated cisplatin administration in patients with advanced ovarian cancer or non-small-cell lung cancer* — **Adults:** 910 mg/m² daily as 15-min IV infusion, starting 30 min before chemotherapy. If hypotension occurs and BP doesn't return to normal within 5 min after treatment stops, use dose of 740 mg/m² for subsequent cycles.	▪ Use cautiously in elderly patients and in ischemic heart disease, arrhythmias, heart failure, or history of CVA or TIA. ▪ Contraindicated in hypersensitivity to aminothiol compounds or mannitol, hypotension, dehydration, and patients on antihypertensives not stopped during 24 hr before amifostine. Don't use in chemotherapy for curable malignancies, unless enrolled in studies.
amikacin sulfate Amikin *Aminoglycoside* *Antibiotic* Preg. Risk Category: D	**inj:** 50, 250 mg/ml	*Serious infections caused by susceptible organisms* — **Adults and children:** 15 mg/kg/day divided q 8 to 12 hr by IM or IV infusion (in 100 to 200 ml D₅W or 0.9% NaCl sol run in over 30 to 60 min). **Neonates:** loading dose of 10 mg/kg IV, then 7.5 mg/kg q 12 hr. *Uncomplicated UTI* — **Adults:** 250 mg IM or IV bid.	▪ Use cautiously in impaired renal function or neuromuscular disorders and in neonates, infants, and elderly patients. ▪ Contraindicated in hypersensitivity to drug or other aminoglycosides.
amiloride hydrochloride Kalurit‡, Midamor *Potassium-sparing diuretic* *Diuretic/antihypertensive* Preg. Risk Category: B	**tab:** 5 mg	*Hypertension; edema associated with heart failure, usually in patients also taking thiazide or other potassium-wasting diuretics* — **Adults:** usual dosage 5 mg PO daily. Increase to 10 mg daily, if necessary. Max 20 mg daily.	▪ Use cautiously in diabetes, cardiopulmonary disease, severe hepatic insufficiency and in elderly or debilitated patients. ▪ Contraindicated in anuria, renal insufficiency, diabetic nephropathy, hypersensitivity, hyperkalemia, and patients on other potassium-sparing diuretics.

DRUG / CLASS / CATEGORY	DOSAGE FORMS	INDICATIONS / DOSAGES	KEY PRECAUTIONS
aminocaproic acid Amicar *Carboxylic acid derivative* *Fibrinolysis inhibitor* Preg. Risk Category: C	**tab:** 500 mg; **syrup:** 250 mg/ml; **inj:** 250 mg/ml	*Excessive bleeding resulting from hyperfibrinolysis* — **Adults:** initially, 5 g PO or slow IV infusion, then 1 to 1.25 g hourly until bleeding controlled. Max 30 g daily.	■ Use cautiously in cardiac, renal, or hepatic disease. ■ Contraindicated in active intravascular clotting or DIC unless heparin used concomitantly. Inj form contraindicated in neonates.
aminoglutethimide Cytadren *Antiadrenal hormone* *Antineoplastic* Preg. Risk Category: D	**tab:** 250 mg	*Suppression of adrenal function in Cushing's syndrome and adrenal cancer* — **Adults:** 250 mg q 6 hr. May increase in increments of 250 mg daily q 1 to 2 wk; max 2 g qd.	■ Contraindicated in hypersensitivity to drug or to glutethimide.
aminophylline (theophylline ethylenediamine) Aminophyllin, Cardophyllin‡, Corophyllin†, Phyllocontin, Somophyllin, Truphylline *Xanthine derivative* *Bronchodilator* Preg. Risk Category: C	**tab:** 100, 200 mg; **tab (ext-release):** 225, 350 mg‡; **oral liq:** 105 mg/5 ml; **inj:** 250 mg/10 ml, 500 mg/20 ml, 100 mg/100 ml in 0.45% NaCl, 200 mg/100 ml in 0.45% NaCl; **rectal supp:** 250, 500 mg; **rectal sol:** 300 mg/5 ml	*Symptomatic relief of bronchospasm* — **Patients not taking theophylline who need rapid relief:** loading dose 6 mg/kg (equiv to 4.7 mg/kg anhydrous theophylline) IV, then maintenance infusion. **Adults (nonsmokers):** 0.7 mg/kg/hr IV for 12 hr; then 0.5 mg/kg/hr IV for 12 hr. **Otherwise healthy adult smokers:** 1 mg/kg/hr IV for 12 hr; then 0.8 mg/kg/hr. **Children 9 to 16 yr:** 1 mg/kg/hr IV for 12 hr; then 0.8 mg/kg/hr. **Children 6 mo to 9 yr:** 1.2 mg/kg/hr for 12 hr; then 1 mg/kg/hr. **Patients taking theophylline:** Determine time, amount, route, and dosage form of last dose. Infusions of 0.63 mg/kg (0.5 mg/kg anhydrous theophylline) increase plasma drug level by 1 mcg/ml. If no obvious signs of toxicity, give 3.1 mg/kg (2.5 mg/kg anhydrous theophylline). *Chronic bronchial asthma* — **Adults and children:** 16 mg/kg or 400 mg (whichever is less) PO qd in divided doses q 6 to 8 hr if using rapidly absorbed forms. May increase in increments of 25% q 2 to 3 days. Or,	■ Use cautiously in neonates and infants < 1 yr, young children, and elderly patients; and in heart failure or other cardiac or circulatory impairment, COPD, cor pulmonale, renal or hepatic disease, hyperthyroidism, diabetes mellitus, peptic ulcer, severe hypoxemia, and hypertension. ■ Contraindicated in hypersensitivity to xanthine compounds and ethylenediamine and in active peptic ulcer disease and seizure disorders (unless adequate anticonvulsant therapy given). Rectal suppositories contraindicated in irritation or infection of rectum or lower colon. ■ Before loading dose, ensure that patient hasn't had recent theophylline therapy.

12 mg/kg or 400 mg (whichever is less) PO qd in divided doses q 8 to 12 hr if using ext-release. May increase by 2 to 3 mg/kg daily q 3 days. *Note:* Rectal dosage same as oral dosage.

---

amiodarone hydrochloride
Aratac‡, Cordarone, Cordarone X‡
Benzofuran derivative
Ventricular and supraventricular antiarrhythmic
Preg. Risk Category: D

tab: 100, 200 mg; *inj:* 50 mg/ml

Recurrent ventricular fibrillation and recurrent hemodynamically unstable ventricular tachycardia refractory to other antiarrhythmics — **Adults:** loading dose 800 to 1,600 mg PO daily for 1 to 3 wk until initial therapeutic response, then 600 to 800 mg/day PO for 1 mo and maintenance of 200 to 600 mg PO daily. Or, loading dose 150 mg IV over 10 min (15 mg/min); then 360 mg IV over next 6 hr (1 mg/min); then 540 mg IV over next 18 hr (0.5 mg/min). After first 24 hr, continue maintenance infusion of 720 mg/24 hr (0.5 mg/min).

- Use cautiously in patients receiving other antiarrhythmics, beta blockers, or calcium channel blockers.
- Contraindicated in hypersensitivity to drug and in severe SA node disease resulting in preexisting bradycardia. Unless artificial pacemaker present, also contraindicated in cardiogenic shock or second- or third-degree AV block and in bradycardia that has caused syncope.

---

amitriptyline hydrochloride
Apo-Amitriptyline†, Elavil
amitriptyline pamoate
Elavil†
Tricyclic antidepressant
Antidepressant
Preg. Risk Category: NR

hydrochloride — tab: 10, 25, 50, 75, 100, 150 mg; *inj:* 10 mg/ml.
pamoate — syrup: 10 mg/5 ml

Depression — **Adults:** initially, 50 to 100 mg PO hs, increased to 150 mg daily; max 300 mg daily, if needed. Maint: 50 to 100 mg/day PO or 20 to 30 mg IM qid. **Elderly patients and adolescents:** 10 mg PO tid and 20 mg hs daily.

- Use cautiously in history of seizures, in urine retention, angle-closure glaucoma, increased IOP, hyperthyroidism, CV disease (recent MI), diabetes, impaired liver or renal function, and patients receiving thyroid medications.
- Contraindicated during acute recovery phase of MI, in hypersensitivity, and within 14 days of MAO inhibitor therapy.

---

amlodipine besylate
Norvasc
Dyhydropyridine calcium channel blocker
Antianginal/antihypertensive
Preg. Risk Category: C

tab: 2.5, 5, 10 mg

Chronic stable angina, vasospastic angina (Prinzmetal's [variant] angina) — **Adults:** initially, 5 to 10 mg PO daily.
Hypertension — **Adults:** initially, 2.5 to 5 mg PO daily. With small, frail, or elderly patients, those taking other antihypertensives, or those with hepatic insufficiency, begin at 2.5 mg daily. Adjust according to response and tolerance. Max 10 mg/day.

- Use cautiously in patients receiving other peripheral vasodilators and in severe aortic stenosis, heart failure, or severe hepatic disease.
- Contraindicated in hypersensitivity to drug.

AMLODIPINE BESYLATE   13

DRUG/CLASS/ CATEGORY	DOSAGE FORMS	INDICATIONS/ DOSAGES	KEY PRECAUTIONS
ammonium chloride *Acid-forming salt* *Acidifying agent* Preg. Risk Category: C	**tab:** 500, 1,000 mg; **inj:** 2.14% (0.4 mEq/ml), 26.75% (5 mEq/ml)	*Metabolic alkalosis; chloride replacement* — **Adults and children:** IV dose (in mEq) equal to chloride deficit (in mEq/L) multiplied by extracellular fluid volume (20% of body weight in kg). Give half of calculated volume, then reassess patient. *Acidifier* — **Adults:** 4 to 12 g PO qd in divided doses q 4 to 6 hr. **Children:** 75 mg/kg PO qd in 4 divided doses.	▪ Use cautiously in pulmonary insufficiency or in infants with cardiac edema. ▪ Contraindicated in primary respiratory acidosis and high total CO_2 and buffer base and in severe hepatic or renal dysfunction (as self-medication).
amoxapine Asendin *Dibenzoxazepine* *Tricyclic antidepressant* Preg. Risk Category: C	**tab:** 25, 50, 100, 150 mg	*Depression* — **Adults:** initially, 50 mg PO bid or tid, increased to 100 mg bid or tid by end of first wk if tolerated. Make increases > 300 mg daily only if this dose ineffective during trial of at least 2 wk. Max recommended for outpatients 400 mg daily. When effective dosage established, entire dosage (not to exceed 300 mg) may be given hs. **Elderly patients:** initially, 25 mg bid or tid. If tolerated by end of 1st wk, increase to 50 mg bid or tid. Carefully increase up to 300 mg daily.	▪ Use cautiously in CV disease and in history of urine retention, angle-closure glaucoma, or increased IOP. Use with extreme caution in history of seizure disorders. ▪ Contraindicated in hypersensitivity, during acute recovery phase of MI, and within 14 days of MAO inhibitor therapy.
amoxicillin/clavulanate potassium (amoxycillin/ clavulanate potassium) Augmentin, Clavulin† *Aminopenicillin and beta-lactamase inhibitor* *Antibiotic* Preg. Risk Category: B	**tab (chew), oral susp:** 125 mg amox/ 31.25 mg clav acid; 250 mg amox/62.5 mg clav acid; **tab (film-coated):** 250 mg amox/ 125 mg clav acid; 500 mg amox/125 mg	*Lower respiratory infections, otitis media, sinusitis, skin and skin-structure infections, and UTI caused by susceptible strains of gram-pos and gram-neg organisms* — **Adults and children ≥ 40 kg:** 250 mg (based on amoxicillin component) PO q 8 hr. For more severe infections, 500 mg q 8 hr. **Children < 40 kg:** 20 to 40 mg/kg (based on amoxicillin component) PO daily in divided doses q 8 hr.	▪ Use cautiously in mononucleosis and in patients with other drug allergies, especially to cephalosporins. ▪ Contraindicated in hypersensitivity to drug or other penicillins and in previous history of amoxicillin-associated cholestatic jaundice or hepatic dysfunction.

amoxicillin trihydrate (amoxycillin trihydrate†)
Amoxil, Cilamox‡, Larotid, Polymox, Trimox, Wymox
Aminopenicillin
Antibiotic
Preg. Risk Category: NR

clav acid; 875 mg amox/125 mg clav acid

tab (chew): 125, 250, 500 mg; *cap:* 250, 500 mg; *oral susp:* 50 mg/ml (ped drops), 125, 250 mg/5 ml (after reconstitution)

Systemic infections, acute and chronic UTI caused by susceptible strains of gram-pos and gram-neg organisms — **Adults and children ≥ 20 kg:** 250 to 500 mg PO q 8 hr. **Children < 20 kg:** 20 mg/kg PO daily in divided doses q 8 hr; in severe infection, 40 mg/kg PO daily in divided doses q 8 hr or 500 mg to 1 g/m² PO in divided doses q 8 hr.

Uncomplicated gonorrhea — **Adults and children > 45 kg:** 3 g PO with 1 g probenecid given as single dose. Don't give to children < 2 yr.

Endocarditis prophylaxis for dental procedures — **Adults:** initially, 3 g PO 1 hr before procedure; then 1.5 g 6 hr later. **Children:** initially, 50 mg/kg PO 1 hr before procedure; then half of initial dose 6 hr later.

- Use cautiously in mononucleosis (high incidence of maculopapular rash) and in other drug allergies, especially to cephalosporins (possible cross-sensitivity).
- Contraindicated in hypersensitivity to drug or other penicillins.

amphetamine sulfate
Amphetamine
CNS stimulant/short-term adjunctive anorexigenic/sympathomimetic amine
Preg. Risk Category: C
Controlled Sub. Sched.: II

tab: 5, 10 mg

Attention deficit disorder with hyperactivity — **Children 3 to 5 yr:** 2.5 mg PO daily, increased at 2.5-mg increments weekly, prn. **Children ≥ 6 yr:** 5 mg PO daily to bid, increased in 5-mg increments weekly, prn. Give first dose on awakening; add. doses (one or two) at intervals of 4 to 6 hr. Dosage rarely exceeds 40 mg/day.
Narcolepsy — **Adults and children ≥ 12 yr:** 10 mg PO daily. Increase in 10-mg increments weekly, prn. May divide daily dosage, giving first dose on awakening. **Children 6 to 12 yr:** 5 mg PO daily. Increase in 5-mg increments weekly, prn. May divide daily dosage, giving first dose on awakening, additional doses at intervals of 4 to 6 hr. *Short-term adjunct in exogenous obesity —* **Adults:** 5 to 30 mg PO daily in divided doses 30 to 60 min before meals.

- Use cautiously in elderly, debilitated, or hyperexcitable patients, in history of suicidal or homicidal tendencies, or in patients with psychopathic personalities.
- Contraindicated in agitation, hypersensitivity or idiosyncrasy to sympathomimetic amines, symptomatic CV disease, hyperthyroidism, moderate to severe hypertension, glaucoma, advanced arteriosclerosis, and history of drug abuse or within 14 days of MAO inhibitor therapy.

AMPHETAMINE SULFATE 15

DRUG/CLASS/ CATEGORY	DOSAGE FORMS	INDICATIONS/ DOSAGES	KEY PRECAUTIONS
amphotericin B Amphocin, Amphotericin B for Injection, Fungilin Oral‡, Fungizone Intravenous *Polyene macrolide* *Antifungal* Preg. Risk Category: B	**tab:** 100 mg†; **oral susp:** 100 mg/ml†; **lozenges:** 10 mg/ml†; **inj:** 50-mg lyophilized cake	*Systemic fungal infections (histoplasmosis, coccidioidomycosis, blastomycosis, cryptococcosis, disseminated moniliasis, aspergillosis, phycomycosis), meningitis —* **Adults:** initially, test dose of 1 mg in 20 ml D₅W infused IV over 20 to 30 min may be recommended. If tolerated, initiate daily dosage as 0.25 to 0.3 mg/kg by slow IV infusion (0.1 mg/ml) over 2 to 6 hr. Increase dosage gradually to max 1 mg/kg daily. If discontinued for 1 wk or more, resume drug with initial dose and increase gradually. *GI tract infections caused by Candida albicans —* **Adults:** 100 mg PO qid for 2 wk. *Oral and perioral candidal infections —* **Adults:** 1 lozenge (dissolved slowly) qid for 7 to 14 days.	▪ Use cautiously in impaired renal function. ▪ Contraindicated in hypersensitivity to drug.
amphotericin B Fungizone, Abelcet *Polyene macrolide* *Antifungal* Preg. Risk Category: B	**cream:** 3%; **lotion:** 3%; **oint:** 3%	*Cutaneous or mucocutaneous candidal infections —* **Adults and children:** apply liberally bid to qid for 1 to 3 wk; treat interdigital lesions and paronychias for 2 to 4 wk and onychomycoses for several months (relapses common).	▪ Contraindicated in hypersensitivity to drug.
ampicillin Apo-Ampi†, Novo Ampicillin†, Nu-Ampi†, Omnipen, Principen **ampicillin sodium** Ampicin†, Ampicyn Injection‡, Omnipen-N, Penbritin†, Polycillin-N, Totacillin-N **ampicillin trihydrate** Omnipen, Penbritin‡, Polycillin, Principen, Totacillin	**cap:** 250, 500 mg; **oral susp:** 100 mg/ml (ped drops), 125, 250, 500 mg/5 ml (after reconstitution); **inj:** 125, 250, 500 mg, 1, 2 g; **infusion:** 500	*Systemic infections and acute and chronic UTI caused by susceptible strains of gram-pos and gram-neg organisms —* **Adults and children ≥ 20 kg:** 250 to 500 mg PO q 6 hr, or 2 to 12 g IM or IV daily, in divided doses q 4 to 6 hr. **Children < 20 kg:** 50 to 100 mg/kg PO daily in divided doses q 6 hr; or 100 to 200 mg/kg IM or IV daily in divided doses q 6 hr. *Meningitis —* **Adults:** 8 to 14 g IV daily in divided doses q 3 to 4 hr. **Children:** up to 300 mg/kg IV daily in divided doses q 3 to 4 hr.	▪ Use cautiously in other drug allergies and in mononucleosis. ▪ Contraindicated in hypersensitivity to drug or other penicillins.

Aminopenicillin *Antibiotic* Preg. Risk Category: B	mg, 1, 2 g; ***pharm bulk*** ***pkg:*** 10-g vial	*Uncomplicated gonorrhea* — **Adults and children** **> 45 kg:** 3.5 g PO with 1 g probenecid given as single dose.	■ Use cautiously in other drug allergies and in mononucleosis. ■ Contraindicated in hypersensitivity to drug or other penicillins.
ampicillin sodium/ sulbactam sodium Unasyn *Aminopenicillin/beta-lactamase* *inhibitor combination* *Antibiotic* Preg. Risk Category: B	**inj:** vials and piggyback vials containing 1.5 and 3 g; ***pharm bulk pkg:*** 15 g	*Intra-abdominal, gyn, and skin-structure infections caused by susceptible strains* — **Adults:** dosage expressed as total drug (each 1.5-g vial contains 1 g ampicillin sodium and 0.5 g sulbactam sodium) — 1.5 to 3 g IM or IV q 6 hr. Max daily dosage 4 g sulbactam and 8 g ampicillin (12 g of combined drugs).	
amrinone lactate Inocor *Bipyridine derivative* *Inotropic/vasodilator* Preg. Risk Category: C	**inj:** 5 mg/ml in 20-ml ampules	*Short-term management of heart failure* — **Adults:** initially, 0.75 mg/kg IV bolus over 2 to 3 min. Then start maintenance infusion of 5 to 10 mcg/kg/min. May give additional bolus of 0.75 mg/kg 30 min after therapy starts. Don't exceed 10 mg/kg total daily dosage. Dosage depends on clinical response.	■ Use cautiously in hypertrophic cardiomyopathy. ■ Don't use in severe aortic or pulmonic valvular disease or in place of surgical correction of obstruction or during acute phase of MI. Contraindicated in hypersensitivity to amrinone or bisulfites.
amyl nitrite *Nitrate* *Vasodilator/cyanide poisoning* *adjunct* Preg. Risk Category: X	**amp *(crush- able)*:** 0.3 ml	*Relief of angina pectoris* — **Adults and children:** 0.3 ml by inhalation (1 glass ampule), prn. *Antidote for cyanide poisoning* — **Adults and children:** 0.3 ml by inhalation for 15 to 60 seconds q 5 min until conscious.	■ Use cautiously in glaucoma (except angle-closure type, a contraindication), volume depletion, or hypotension. ■ Contraindicated in angle-closure glaucoma, hypersensitivity to nitrates, severe anemia, postural hypotension, early MI, increased ICP, and pregnancy.
anastrozole Arimidex *Nonsteroidal aromatase inhibitor* *Antineoplastic* Preg. Risk Category: D	***tab:*** 1 mg	*Treatment of advanced breast cancer in post-menopausal women with disease progression after tamoxifen therapy* — **Adults:** 1 mg PO daily.	■ No known contraindications. ■ Pregnancy must be ruled out before treatment.

DRUG/CLASS/ CATEGORY	DOSAGE FORMS	INDICATIONS/ DOSAGES	KEY PRECAUTIONS
anistreplase (anisoylated plasminogen-streptokinase activator complex; APSAC) Eminase *Thrombolytic enzyme* *Thrombolytic enzyme* Preg. Risk Category: C	*inj:* 30 units/vial	*Lysis of coronary artery thrombi following acute MI* — **Adults:** 30 units IV over 2 to 5 min. Give by direct inj.	▪ Use cautiously < 10 days of surgery and in trauma, GI or GU bleeding, cerebrovascular disease, hypertension, mitral stenosis, atrial fibrillation, acute pericarditis, subacute bacterial endocarditis, septic thrombophlebitis, diabetic hemorrhagic retinopathy, pregnancy and postpartum, anticoagulation therapy, and patients > 75 yr. ▪ Contraindicated in history of severe allergic reaction to anistreplase or streptokinase, internal bleeding, CVA, recent intraspinal or intracranial surgery or trauma, aneurysm, AVM, intracranial neoplasm, uncontrolled hypertension, and known bleeding diathesis.
antihemophilic factor (AHF) Hemofil M, Humate-P, Hyate:C, Koate-HP, Koate-HS *Blood derivative* *Antihemophilic* Preg. Risk Category: C	*inj:* vials with diluent. Units specified on label.	*Spontaneous hemorrhage with hemophilia A* — **Adults and children:** calculate dosage using this formula: *AHF required (IU) = body weight (kg) × desired factor VIII increase (% of normal) × 0.5.* To prevent spontaneous hemorrhage, desired level of factor VIII is 5% of normal; for mild hemorrhage, 30% of normal; for moderate hemorrhage and minor surgery, 30% to 50% of normal; for severe hemorrhage, 80% to 100% of normal. *Treatment of bleeding in hemophilia A* — **Adults and children:** for minor hemorrhage into muscle and joints, 8 to 10 IU/kg IV (or raise plasma factor VIII levels to 20% to 40% of normal) q 8 to 12 hr for 1 to 3 days, prn. For overt bleeding, 15 to 25 IU/kg IV, then 8 to 15 IU/kg q 8 to 12 hr for 3 to 4 days. To treat massive bleeding or hemorrhage involving	▪ Use cautiously in neonates and infants and in hepatic disease. ▪ Contraindicated in hypersensitivity to murine (mouse) protein or to drug.

anti-inhibitor coagulant complex

Autoplex T, Feiba VH Immuno

Activated prothrombin complex

Hemostatic agent

Preg. Risk Category: C

inj: number of units of factor VIII correctional activity indicated on label of vial

major organs, 40 to 50 IU/kg IV, followed by 20 to 25 IU/kg IV q 8 to 12 hr.

Prevention of bleeding in hemophilic patients requiring surgery — **Adults:** 25 to 30 IU/kg IV 1 hr before surgery, then half of initial dosage 5 hr later. Adjust to AHF 80% to 100% of normal during surgery and 30% to 60% of normal for ≥ 10 to 14 days postop.

Prevention and control of hemorrhagic episodes in certain patients with hemophilia A who have developed inhibitor antibodies to antihemophilic factor; management of bleeding in patients with acquired hemophilia who have spontaneously acquired inhibitors to factor VIII — **Adults and children:** highly individualized and varies among manufacturers. For Autoplex T, 25 to 100 units/kg IV, depending on hemorrhage severity. If no hemostatic improvement within 6 hr after initial administration, repeat dosage. For Feiba VH Immuno, 50 to 100 units/kg IV q 6 to 12 hr until clear signs of improvement. Max 200 units/kg daily.

- Use cautiously in liver disease.
- Contraindicated in DIC, in signs of fibrinolysis, and in patients with normal coagulation mechanism.

---

antithrombin III, human (AT-III, heparin cofactor I)

ATnativ, Thrombate III

Glycoprotein

Anticoagulant/antithrombotic

Preg. Risk Category: C

inj: 500 IU

Thromboembolism associated with hereditary AT-III deficiency — **Adults and children:** initial dose individualized to increase AT-III activity to 120% of normal as determined 30 min after administration. Usual dose 50 to 100 IU/min IV, max 100 IU/min. Dose based on anticipated 1% increase in plasma AT-III activity produced by 1 IU/kg of body weight using the formula: *Dose required (IU) = (desired activity [%] – baseline activity [%]) × weight (kg) ÷ 1.4.* Maint. dosage to increase AT-III activity to 80% of normal and given at 24-hr intervals. To calculate subsequent dosages, multiply desired AT-III activity (as % of normal) minus baseline AT-III activity (as % of normal) by body weight (in kg). Divide by actual increase in AT-III activity (as %)

- Use cautiously in neonates and children.
- Not recommended for long-term prophylaxis of thrombotic episodes.

(continued)

DRUG/CLASS/CATEGORY	DOSAGE FORMS	INDICATIONS/DOSAGES	KEY PRECAUTIONS
antithrombin III, human *(continued)*		produced by 1 IU/kg as determined 30 min after initial dose. Treatment continues 2 to 8 days; may be longer in pregnancy or with surgery or immobilization.	
apraclonidine hydrochloride Iopidine *Alpha-adrenergic agonist* *Ocular hypotensive agent* Preg. Risk Category: C	*ophth sol:* 0.5%, 1%	*Prevention or control of elevated IOP before and after ocular laser surgery —* **Adults:** 1 drop 1% sol instilled 1 hr before start of laser surgery on anterior segment, then 1 drop immediately after surgery. *Short-term adjunct therapy in patients who require additional IOP reduction —* **Adults:** 1 or 2 drops of 0.5% sol instilled into affected eye tid.	• Use cautiously in cardiac disease, hypertension, and vasovagal attacks. • Contraindicated in hypersensitivity to apraclonidine or clonidine or with concurrent MAO inhibitor therapy.
aprotinin Trasylol *Naturally occurring protease inhibitor* *Systemic hemostatic agent* Preg. Risk Category: B	*inj:* 10,000 KIU (kallikrein inactivator units)/ml (1.4 mg/ml) in 100- and 200-ml vials	*To reduce blood loss or need for transfusion in patients undergoing CABG —* **Adults:** start with 10,000 units (1 ml) test dose ≥ 10 min before loading dose. If no allergic reaction, anesthesia may be induced while loading dose of 2 million units given slowly over 20 to 30 min. When loading dose complete, sternotomy may be performed. Before bypass initiated, cardiopulmonary bypass circuit primed with 2 million units by replacing aliquot of priming fluid with drug. Continuous inf at 500,000 units/hr given until patient leaves OR. This is known as *regimen A*. Or, *regimen B:* give half dosage of *regimen A*, except for test dose.	• Contraindicated in hypersensitivity to beef (drug prepared from bovine lung).
asparaginase (L-asparaginase) Elspar, Kidrolase† *Enzyme* *Antineoplastic* Preg. Risk Category: C	*inj:* 10,000-unit vial	*Acute lymphocytic leukemia (in combination with other drugs) —* **Adults and children:** 1,000 IU/kg IV qd for 10 days, injected over 30 min; or 6,000 IU/m² IM at intervals specified in protocol. *Sole induction agent for acute lymphocytic leukemia —* **Adults:** 200 IU/kg IV daily for 28 days.	• Use cautiously in hepatic dysfunction. • Contraindicated in pancreatitis or history of pancreatitis and in previous hypersensitivity to drug (unless desensitized).

astemizole Hismanal *Histamine$_1$-receptor antagonist* *Antiallergy agent* Preg. Risk Category: C	***tab:*** 10 mg; ***oral susp:*** 2 mg/ml‡	*Relief of symptoms associated with chronic idiopathic urticaria and seasonal allergic rhinitis* — **Adults and children > 12 yr:** 10 mg PO daily.	▪ Use cautiously in hepatic, renal, or lower respiratory tract disease, especially asthma. ▪ Contraindicated in hepatic failure or hypersensitivity to drug and in patients taking itraconazole, ketoconazole, or macrolide antibiotics.
atenolol Apo-Atenolol†, Noten‡, Nu-Atenolol†, Tenormin *Beta-adrenergic blocker* *Antihypertensive/antianginal* Preg. Risk Category: D	***tab:*** 25, 50, 100 mg; ***inj:*** 5 mg/10 ml	*Hypertension* — **Adults:** initially, 50 mg PO daily as single dose, increased to 100 mg once daily after 7 to 14 days. Dosages > 100 mg unlikely to bring further benefit. *Angina pectoris* — **Adults:** 50 mg PO once daily, increased to 100 mg daily after 7 days for optimal effect. Max 200 mg daily. *To reduce CV mortality and risk of reinfarction in acute MI* — **Adults:** 5 mg IV, repeat in 10 min. After add. 10 min, 50 mg PO, then 50 mg PO in 12 hr. Then 100 mg PO qd (or 50 mg bid) for ≥ 7 days.	▪ Use cautiously in patients at risk for heart failure and in bronchospastic disease, diabetes, and hyperthyroidism. ▪ Contraindicated in sinus bradycardia, > first-degree heart block, overt cardiac failure, or cardiogenic shock.
atorvastatin calcium Lipitor *Hydroxymethylglutaryl-coenzyme A (HMG-COA) reductase inhibitor* *Antilipemic* Preg. Risk Category: X	***tab:*** 10, 20, 40 mg	*Adjunct to diet in primary hypercholesterolemia and mixed dyslipidemia* — **Adults:** 10 mg PO qd; increase prn to max 80 mg qd. Dosage based on lipid levels drawn 2 to 4 wk after therapy starts. *Alone or as adjunct to lipid-lowering treatments in homozygous familial hypercholesterolemia* — **Adults:** 10 to 80 mg PO qd.	▪ Use cautiously in history of liver disease or heavy alcohol use. ▪ Contraindicated in hypersensitivity to drug, active liver disease, unexplained persistent serum transaminase elevations, pregnancy, breast-feeding, and women of childbearing age (except those not at risk for becoming pregnant) ▪ Withhold or discontinue in serious, acute conditions that suggest myopathy; patients at risk for renal failure secondary to rhabdomyolysis due to trauma; major surgery; severe metabolic, endocrine, or electrolyte disorders; severe acute infection; hypotension; and uncontrolled seizures.

†Canadian ‡Australian

DRUG/CLASS/CATEGORY	DOSAGE FORMS	INDICATIONS/DOSAGES	KEY PRECAUTIONS
atovaquone Mepron *Ubiquinone analogue* *Antiprotozoal* Preg. Risk Category: C	*susp:* 750 mg/5 ml	*Acute, mild to moderate* Pneumocystis carinii *pneumonia in patients who can't tolerate co-trimoxazole* — **Adults:** 750 mg PO bid with food for 21 days.	▪ Use cautiously in breast-feeding patients. ▪ Contraindicated in hypersensitivity to drug.
atracurium besylate Tracrium *Nondepolarizing neuromuscular blocker* *Skeletal muscle relaxant* Preg. Risk Category: C	*inj:* 10 mg/ml	*Adjunct to general anesthesia to promote endotracheal intubation and provide skeletal muscle relaxation during surgery or mechanical ventilation —* dosage depends on anesthetic used, individual needs, and response. Representative doses given here. **Adults and children > 2 yr:** 0.4 to 0.5 mg/kg IV bolus. During prolonged surgery, give maintenance 0.08 to 0.10 mg/kg within 20 to 45 min. May give maintenance dosages q 12 to 25 min in patients receiving balanced anesthesia. During prolonged procedures, may use constant infusion of 5 to 9 mcg/kg/min. **Children 1 mo to 2 yr:** initial dose 0.3 to 0.4 mg/kg. Frequent maintenance doses may be needed.	▪ Use cautiously in CV disease, severe electrolyte disorders; bronchogenic carcinoma; hepatic, renal, or pulmonary impairment; neuromuscular disease; or myasthenia gravis and in elderly or debilitated patients. ▪ Contraindicated in hypersensitivity to drug.
atropine sulfate *Anticholinergic/belladonna alkaloid* *Antiarrhythmic/vagolytic* Preg. Risk Category: C	*tab:* 0.4, 0.6 mg; *inj:* 0.05, 0.1, 0.3, 0.4, 0.5, 0.6, 0.8, 1, 1.2 mg/ml	*Symptomatic bradycardia, brad/arrhythmia (junctional or escape rhythm)* — **Adults:** usually 0.5 to 1 mg IV push; repeat q 3 to 5 min to max 2 mg as needed. **Children:** 0.01 mg/kg IV; may repeat q 4 to 6 hr; max 0.4 mg or 0.3 mg/m². *Preop to diminish secretions and block cardiac vagal reflexes* — **Adults and children ≥ 20 kg:** 0.4 to 0.6 mg IM or SC 30 to 60 min before anesthesia. **Children < 20 kg:** 0.01 mg/kg IM or SC up to max 0.4 mg 30 to 60 min before anesthesia.	▪ Use cautiously in patients with Down syndrome. ▪ Contraindicated in hypersensitivity to drug or sodium metabisulfite, acute angle-closure glaucoma, obstructive uropathy, obstructive disease of GI tract, paralytic ileus, toxic megacolon, intestinal atony, unstable CV status in acute hemorrhage, tachycardia, myocardial ischemia, asthma, and myasthenia gravis.

atropine sulfate
Atropisol, Atropt†, BufOpto
Atropine, Isopto Atropine
Anticholinergic/belladonna alkaloid
Cycloplegic/mydriatic
Preg. Risk Category: C

ophth oint:
0.5%, 1%;
ophth sol:
0.5%, 1%, 2%

Acute iritis; uveitis — **Adults:** 1 to 2 drops instilled into eyes qid, or small strip of oint applied to conjunctival sac tid. **Children:** 1 to 2 drops of 0.5% sol instilled into eyes tid, or small strip of oint applied to conjunctival sac tid.

Cycloplegic refraction — **Adults:** 1 to 2 drops of 1% sol instilled 1 hr before refraction. **Children:** 1 to 2 drops of 0.5% sol instilled in each eye bid for 1 to 3 days before eye exam and 1 hr before refraction.

- Use cautiously in increased IOP and in elderly patients.
- Contraindicated in glaucoma, hypersensitivity to drug or belladonna alkaloids, or adhesions between iris and lens.
- Don't give to infants < 3 mo.

attapulgite
Children's Kaopectate, Diasorb, Donnagel, Fowler's†, Rheaban Maximum Strength
Hydrated magnesium aluminum silicate
Antidiarrheal agent
Preg. Risk Category: NR

tab: 300, 600†, 630†; 750 mg;
tab (chew): 300, 600 mg;
oral susp: 600 mg/15 ml, 750 ml/5 ml; 750 mg/15 ml†, 900 mg/15 ml†

Acute, nonspecific diarrhea — **Adults and adolescents:** 1.2 to 1.5 g (up to 3 g of Diasorb) PO after each loose bowel movement, not to exceed 9 g in 24 hr. **Children 6 to 12 yr:** 600 mg (susp) or 750 mg (tab) PO after each loose bowel movement, not to exceed 4.2 g (susp) or 4.5 g (tab) in 24 hr. **Children 3 to 6 yr:** 300 mg PO after each loose bowel movement, not to exceed 2.1 g in 24 hr.

- Use cautiously in dehydration. Promote adequate fluid intake.
- Contraindicated in dysentery or suspected bowel obstruction.

auranofin
Ridaura
Gold salt
Antiarthritic
Preg. Risk Category: C

cap: 3 mg

Rheumatoid arthritis — **Adults:** 6 mg PO daily, either as 3 mg bid or 6 mg qd. After 6 mo, may increase to 9 mg daily.

- Use cautiously with other drugs that cause blood dyscrasias or in renal, hepatic, or inflammatory bowel disease; rash; or bone marrow depression.
- Not recommended in pregnant women.
- Contraindicated in history of severe gold toxicity or that caused by previous exposure to other heavy metals, in necrotizing enterocolitis, pulmonary fibrosis, exfoliative dermatitis, bone marrow aplasia, severe hematologic disorders, urticaria, eczema, colitis, severe debilitation, hemorrhagic conditions, and systemic lupus erythematosus or after recent radiation therapy.

DRUG/CLASS/ CATEGORY	DOSAGE FORMS	INDICATIONS/ DOSAGES	KEY PRECAUTIONS
aurothioglucose Gold-50‡, Solganal **gold sodium thiomalate** Myochrysine *Gold salt* *Antiarthritic* Preg. Risk Category: C	**aurothioglucose — inj:** 50 mg/ml in sesame oil in 10-ml vial; **gold sodium thiomalate — inj:** 25, 50 mg/ml with benzyl alcohol	*Rheumatoid arthritis —* **aurothioglucose — Adults:** 10 mg IM, then 25 mg for 2nd and 3rd doses at weekly intervals. Then, 50 mg q wk until 800 mg to 1 g given. If improvement without toxicity, 25 to 50 mg continued at 3- to 4-wk intervals indefinitely. **Children 6 to 12 yr:** ¼ usual adult dosage. Don't exceed 25 mg per dose. **gold sodium thiomalate — Adults:** 10 mg IM, then 25 mg in 1 wk. Then 25 to 50 mg q wk to total dose of 1 g. If improvement without toxicity, 25 to 50 mg q 2 wk for 2 to 20 wk; then 25 to 50 mg q 3 to 4 wk as maintenance. If relapse, resume inj at weekly intervals. **Children:** 10 mg IM, then 1 mg/kg IM weekly. Follow adult spacing of doses.	▪ Use cautiously in rash, hypertension, compromised cerebral or CV circulation, renal or hepatic disorders, or blood dyscrasias (or family history of above). ▪ Contraindicated in hypersensitivity to drug, severe uncontrollable diabetes, renal disease, hepatic dysfunction, uncontrolled heart failure, systemic lupus erythematosus, colitis, Sjögren's syndrome, urticaria, eczema, hemorrhagic conditions, severe hematologic disorders, recent radiation therapy, or history of severe toxicity from previous exposure to gold or other heavy metals, hepatitis, or exfoliative dermatitis.
azathioprine Imuran, Thioprine‡ *Purine antagonist* *Immunosuppressive* Preg. Risk Category: D	**tab:** 50 mg; **powder for inj:** 100 mg	*Immunosuppression in kidney transplantation —* **Adults and children:** 3 to 5 mg/kg PO or IV qd, starting on day of transplantation. Maintain at 1 to 3 mg/kg qd (dosage varies per patient response). *Severe, refractory rheumatoid arthritis —* **Adults:** 1 mg/kg PO as 1 or 2 doses. If response unsatisfactory after 6 to 8 wk, may increase by 0.5 mg/kg daily (to max 2.5 mg/kg daily) at 4-wk intervals.	▪ Use cautiously in hepatic or renal dysfunction. ▪ Contraindicated in hypersensitivity to drug and in pregnant patients.
azelastine hydrochloride Astelin *Histamine₁-receptor antagonist* *Antihistamine* Preg. Risk Category: C	**nasal spray:** 137 mcg/metered spray	*Seasonal allergic rhinitis —* **Adults and children ≥ 12 yr:** 2 sprays per nostril bid.	▪ Contraindicated in hypersensitivity. ▪ Use in pregnancy only if benefit justifies potential risk to fetus. Don't give to breast-feeding patients. Safety and effectiveness in children < 12 yr not established.

azithromycin

Zithromax

Azalide macrolide

Macrolide anti-infective

Preg. Risk Category: B

cap: 250 mg; Z-pak (contains 5 days of therapy); **oral susp:** 100, 200 mg/5 ml; **single-dose powder for oral susp:** 1 g; **tab:** 250, 600 mg

Acute bacterial exacerbations of COPD, uncomplicated skin-structure infections, mild community-acquired pneumonia, or second-line therapy of pharyngitis or tonsillitis caused by susceptible organisms— **Adults and ≥ 16 yr:** 500 mg PO as 1 dose on day 1, then 250 mg qd on days 2 through 5. Total 1.5 g.

Nongonococcal urethritis or cervicitis caused by C. trachomatis— **Adults and ≥ 16 yr:** 1 g PO as 1 dose.

Prevention of disseminated M. avium complex disease in adv. HIV infection— **Adults:** 1,200 mg PO q wk.

- Use cautiously in impaired hepatic function.
- Contraindicated in hypersensitivity to macrolides.

aztreonam

Azactam

Monobactam

Antibiotic

Preg. Risk Category: B

inj: 500-mg, 1- and 2-g vials

UTI, lower respiratory tract infections, septicemia, skin and skin-structure infections, intra-abdominal infections, surgical infections, and gyn infections caused by susceptible strains of gram-neg aerobic organisms; also respiratory infections caused by H. influenzae— **Adults:** 500 mg to 2 g IV or IM q 8 to 12 hr. For severe systemic or life-threatening infections, may give 2 g q 6 to 8 hr. Max 8 g daily.

- Use cautiously in elderly patients and in impaired renal function.
- Contraindicated in hypersensitivity to drug.

b

bacampicillin hydrochloride

Penglobe, Spectrobid

Aminopenicillin

Antibiotic

Preg. Risk Category: B

tab: 400 mg

Upper respiratory tract infections and otitis media caused by streptococci, pneumococci; staphylococci, and H. influenzae; UTI caused by E. coli, P. mirabilis, and E. faecalis; skin infections caused by streptococci and susceptible staphylococci— **Adults and children ≤ 25 kg:** 25 mg/kg/day PO q 12 hr. **Children > 25 kg:** 400 mg PO q 12 hr. **Children ≤ 25 kg:** 25 mg/kg/day PO in divided doses q 12 hr.

Lower respiratory tract infections; other severe infections— **Adults and children > 25 kg:** 800 mg PO q 12 hr. **Children ≤ 25 kg:** 50 mg/kg/day PO in divided doses q 12 hr.

Gonorrhea— **Adults:** 1.6 g PO with 1 g probenecid, given as single dose.

- Use cautiously in mononucleosis and in patients with other drug allergies.
- Contraindicated in hypersensitivity to drug or other penicillins.

BACAMPICILLIN HYDROCHLORIDE 25

DRUG / CLASS / CATEGORY	DOSAGE FORMS	INDICATIONS / DOSAGES	KEY PRECAUTIONS
bacitracin Baciguent, Baci-IM, Bacitin† *Polypeptide antibiotic* *Systemic antibiotic* Preg. Risk Category: C	*inj:* 10,000-, 50,000-unit vials	*Pneumonia or empyema caused by susceptible staphylococci* — **Infants > 2.5 kg:** 1,000 units/kg IM daily, divided q 8 to 12 hr. **Infants < 2.5 kg:** 900 units/kg IM daily, divided q 8 to 12 hr.	▪ Contraindicated in hypersensitivity or impaired renal function. ▪ Limit IM use to infants with staphylococcal pneumonia.
bacitracin AK-Tracin *Polypeptide antibiotic* *Ophthalmic antibiotic* Preg. Risk Category: NR	*ophth oint:* 500 units/g	*Surface bacterial infections involving conjunctiva and cornea* — **Adults and children:** small amount of oint applied into conjunctival sac ≥ qd or prn until favorable response seen.	▪ Use cautiously in myasthenia gravis and other neuromuscular diseases. ▪ Contraindicated in hypersensitive or atopic patients.
bacitracin Baciguent, Bacitin† *Polypeptide antibiotic* *Topical antibiotic* Preg. Risk Category: C	*oint:* 500 units/g	*Topical infections, abrasions, cuts, and minor burns or wounds* — **Adults and children:** apply thin film qd to tid, depending on severity of condition. Don't use for > 1 wk.	▪ Use cautiously in myasthenia gravis and other neuromuscular diseases. ▪ Contraindicated in hypersensitive or atopic patients.
baclofen Clofen‡, Lioresal, Lioresal Intrathecal *Chlorphenyl derivative* *Skeletal muscle relaxant* Preg. Risk Category: C	*tab:* 10, 20, 25 mg‡; *intrathecal inj:* 500, 2,000 mcg/ml	*Spasticity in multiple sclerosis, spinal cord injury* — **Adults:** 5 mg PO tid for 3 days, then 10 mg tid for 3 days, 15 mg tid for 3 days, 20 mg tid for 3 days. Increase prn to max 80 mg daily. *Management of severe spasticity in patients who can't tolerate or don't respond to oral therapy* — **Adults:** Test dose: 1 ml of 50-mcg/ml dil into intrathecal space by barbotage over ≥ 1 min. Markedly decreased spasms or reduced muscle tone should appear within 4 to 8 hr. If poor response, give 2nd test dose (75 mcg/1.5 ml) 24 hr after 1st. If poor response, give test dose (100 mcg/2 ml) 24 hr later. Patients unresponsive to final test dose shouldn't have implantable pump. Initial maintenance dose titrated per screening	▪ Use cautiously in impaired renal function or seizure disorder or when spasticity used to maintain motor function. ▪ Contraindicated in hypersensitivity to drug. ▪ Don't give orally to treat muscle spasms caused by rheumatic disorders, cerebral palsy, Parkinson's disease, or CVA; efficacy not established.

dose response. Effective dose doubled and given over 24 hr. If screening-dose efficacy maintained for ≥ 12 hr, don't double dose. After 1st 24 hr, may increase dose slowly by 10% to 30% daily.

BCG vaccine
TICE BCG
Bacterial agent
Antineoplastic
Preg. Risk Category: C

percutaneous vaccine: 1 to 0.3 ml
8×10^8

TB exposure — **Adults and children ≥ 1 mo:** 0.2 to 0.3 ml (percutaneous vaccine) applied to cleaned skin, followed by application of multiple-puncture disk. **Infants < 1 mo:** reduce dosage by half by using 2 ml sterile water without preservatives when reconstituting.

- Contraindicated in burns, hypogammaglobulinemia, positive tuberculin reaction (when meant for use as immunoprophylactic after TB exposure) in immunosuppressed patients with fresh smallpox vaccinations; and in patients receiving corticosteroid therapy.
- Avoid giving to pregnant patients.

beclomethasone dipropionate
Becloforte Inhaler‡, Beclovent, Vanceril
Glucocorticoid
Anti-inflammatory/antiasthmatic
Preg. Risk Category: C

oral inhal aerosol: 42, 50‡ mcg/metered spray

Steroid-dependent asthma — **Adults and children ≥ 12 yr:** 2 inhalations tid or qid or 4 inhalations bid; max 20 inhalations daily (840 mcg). **Children 6 to 12 yr:** 1 to 2 inhalations tid or qid or 2 to 4 inhalations bid. Max 10 inhalations daily (420 mcg).

- Use with extreme caution, if at all, in TB, fungal or bacterial infections, ocular herpes simplex, or systemic viral infections. Not for use in asthma controlled by bronchodilators or other noncorticosteroids alone or in nonasthmatic bronchial diseases. Use with caution in patients receiving systemic corticosteroids.
- Contraindicated in hypersensitivity to any component of formulation (fluorocarbons, oleic acid) and in status asthmaticus or other acute asthma episodes.

beclomethasone dipropionate
Beconase AQ Nasal Spray, Beconase Nasal Inhaler, Vancenase AQ Nasal Spray, Vancenase Nasal Inhaler
Glucocorticoid
Anti-inflammatory
Preg. Risk Category: C

nasal aerosol: 42, 50 mcg/ metered spray‡; *nasal spray:* 42, 50 mcg/metered spray‡

Relief of symptoms of seasonal or perennial rhinitis; prevention of recurrence of nasal polyps after surgical removal — **Adults and children > 12 yr:** usual dosage 1 or 2 sprays in each nostril bid, tid, or qid.

- Use cautiously, if at all, in active or quiescent respiratory tract tubercular infections or untreated fungal, bacterial, or systemic viral or ocular herpes simplex infections. Also use cautiously after recent nasal septal ulcers, nasal surgery, or trauma.
- Contraindicated in hypersensitivity to drug.

BECLOMETHASONE DIPROPIONATE 27

†Canadian ‡Australian

DRUG/CLASS/ CATEGORY	DOSAGE FORMS	INDICATIONS/ DOSAGES	KEY PRECAUTIONS
benazepril hydrochloride Lotensin *ACE Inhibitor* *Antihypertensive* Preg. Risk Category: C (D in 2nd and 3rd trimesters)	*tab:* 5, 10, 20, 40 mg	*Hypertension* — **Adults:** in patients not receiving diuretics, 10 mg PO daily initially. Most patients receive 20 to 40 mg daily in 1 or 2 doses; patient receiving diuretic, 5 mg PO daily.	▪ Use cautiously in impaired hepatic or renal function. ▪ Contraindicated in hypersensitivity to ACE inhibitors.
benzonatate Tessalon *Local anesthetic (esther)* *Nonnarcotic antitussive* Preg. Risk Category: C	*cap:* 100 mg	*Symptomatic relief of cough* — **Adults and children > 10 yr:** 100 PO tid; up to 600 mg daily may be needed.	▪ Contraindicated in hypersensitivity to drug or related compounds. ▪ Use cautiously in hypersensitivity to paraminobenzoic acid anesthetics (procaine, tetracaine); cross-sensitivity reactions may occur.
benztropine mesylate Apo-Benztropine†, Bensylate†, Cogentin, PMS Benztropine† *Anticholinergic* *Antiparkinsonian agent* Preg. Risk Category: NR	*tab:* 0.5, 1, 2 mg; *inj:* 1 mg/ml in 2-ml ampules	*Drug-induced extrapyramidal disorders (except tardive dyskinesia)* — **Adults:** 1 to 4 mg PO or IM qd or bid. *Acute dystonic reaction* — **Adults:** 1 to 2 mg IV or IM, followed by 1 to 2 mg PO bid. *Parkinsonism* — **Adults:** 0.5 to 6 mg PO or IM daily. Initial dose 0.5 mg to 1 mg, increased by 0.5 mg q 5 to 6 days. Adjust dosage to meet patient needs.	▪ Use cautiously in hot weather, in mental disorders, and in children ≥ 3 yr. ▪ Contraindicated in hypersensitivity to drug or drug components, in narrow-angle glaucoma, and in children < 3 yr.
bepridil hydrochloride Bepadin†, Vascor *Calcium channel blocker* *Antianginal* Preg. Risk Category: C	*tab:* 200, 300, 400 mg	*Chronic stable angina in patients who can't tolerate or don't respond to other agents* — **Adults:** initially, 200 mg PO daily. After 10 days, increase dosage based on response. Maintenance dosage in most patients 300 mg/day. Max 400 mg daily. Not recommended for use within 3 mo of MI.	▪ Use cautiously in left bundle-branch block, sinus bradycardia, impaired renal or hepatic function, and heart failure. ▪ Contraindicated in hypersensitivity; uncompensated cardiac insufficiency, sick sinus syndrome, or second- or third-degree AV block without pacemaker; hypotension; congenital QT-interval prolongation; history of serious ventricular arrhythmias; treatment with other drugs that prolong QT interval.

beractant (natural lung surfactant)
Survanta
Bovine lung extract
Lung surfactant
Preg. Risk Category: NR

susp for intra-tracheal instillation: 25 mg/ml

Prevention of respiratory distress syndrome (RDS) in premature neonates weighing 1,250 g or less at birth or having symptoms of surfactant deficiency —
Neonates: 4 ml/kg intratracheally; give each dose in 4 quarter-doses; in between, use hand-held resuscitation bag at 60 breaths/min and sufficient O_2 to prevent cyanosis. Give within 15 min of birth, if possible. May repeat in 6 hr. Max 4 doses/48 hr.
Rescue treatment of RDS in premature infants —
Neonates: 4 ml/kg intratracheally; before giving, increase ventilator rate to 60 with inspiratory time of 0.5 sec and FiO_2 of 1. Give each dose in 4 quarter-doses; in between, continue ventilation for ≥ 30 sec or until stable. Give dose as soon as RDS confirmed by X-ray. May repeat in 6 hr. Max 4 doses/48 hr.

- None known.

betamethasone
Betnesol†, Celestone
betamethasone acetate and betamethasone sodium phosphate
Celestone Soluspan
Glucocorticoid
betamethasone sodium phosphate
Celestone Phosate
Anti-inflammatory
Preg. Risk Category: C

tab: 600 mcg; *tab (effery):* 500 mcg†; *syrup:* 600 mcg/5 ml; *acetate and sodium phosphate — inj (susp):* acetate 3 mg and sodium phosphate) per ml; *sodium phosphate: inj:* 4 mg ml in 5-ml vials

Conditions with severe inflammation; conditions requiring immunosuppression — **Adults:** 0.6 to 7.2 mg PO daily; or 0.5 to 9 mg IM, IV, or into joint or soft tissue daily. Betamethasone sodium phosphate-acetate susp 6 to 12 mg injected into large joints or 1.5 to 6 mg injected into smaller joints. May give both injections q 1 to 2 weeks, prn.
Note: Betamethasone sodium phosphate and betamethasone acetate susp combination product should *not* be given IV.

- Use with extreme caution in recent MI or peptic ulcer (only in life-threatening situations).
- Use cautiously in renal disease, hypertension, osteoporosis, diabetes mellitus, hypothyroidism, cirrhosis, diverticulitis, nonspecific ulcerative colitis, recent intestinal anastomoses, thromboembolic disorders, seizures, myasthenia gravis, heart failure, TB, ocular herpes simplex, emotional instability, and psychotic tendencies. Also use cautiously in patients with hypersensitivity to sulfites; formulations contain sulfite preservatives.
- Contraindicated in hypersensitivity to drug and in viral or bacterial infections (except in life-threatening situations) or systemic fungal infections.

DRUG/CLASS/CATEGORY	DOSAGE FORMS	INDICATIONS/DOSAGES	KEY PRECAUTIONS
betamethasone dipropionate Alphatrex, Diprolene, Diprolene AF, Diprosone, Maxivate **betamethasone valerate** Betatrex, Beta-Val, Betnovate‡, Valisone *Topical glucocorticoid Anti-inflammatory* Preg. Risk Category: C	dipropionate — *lotion, oint, cream:* 0.05%; *aerosol:* 0.1%. valerate — *lotion, oint:* 0.1%; *cream:* 0.01%, 0.1%; *aerosol sol:* 0.1%	*Inflammation associated with corticosteroid-responsive dermatoses —* **Adults and children:** clean area; apply cream, oint, lotion, or aerosol spray sparingly. Give dipropionate qd or bid; valerate qd to qid. Max dosage 45 g/wk for Diprolene cream, 50 ml/wk for Diprolene lotion.	▪ Contraindicated in hypersensitivity to corticosteroids.
betaxolol hydrochloride Kerlone *Beta-adrenergic blocker Antihypertensive* Preg. Risk Category: C	*tab:* 10, 20 mg	*Hypertension (used alone or with other antihypertensives) —* **Adults:** initially, 10 mg PO qd; if necessary, 20 mg PO qd if desired response not achieved in 7 to 14 days.	▪ Use cautiously in heart failure controlled by cardiac glycosides and diuretics. ▪ Contraindicated in hypersensitivity to drug, severe bradycardia, > first-degree heart block, cardiogenic shock, or uncontrolled heart failure.
betaxolol hydrochloride Betoptic, Betoptic S, Kerlone *Beta-adrenergic blocker Antiglaucoma agent* Preg. Risk Category: C	*ophth sol:* 0.5%; *ophth susp:* 0.25%	*Chronic open-angle glaucoma and ocular hypertension —* **Adults:** 1 or 2 drops of 0.5% sol or 0.25% susp bid.	▪ Contraindicated in hypersensitivity to drug, sinus bradycardia, > first-degree AV block, cardiogenic shock, or overt heart failure. ▪ Use cautiously in restricted pulmonary function, diabetes mellitus, hyperthyroidism, or history of heart failure.
bethanechol chloride Duvoid, Myotonachol, Urabeth, Urecholine, Urocarb Tablets‡ *Cholinergic agonist Urinary tract and GI tract stimulant* Preg. Risk Category: C	*tab:* 5, 10, 25, 50 mg; *inj:* 5 mg/ml	*Acute postop and postpartum nonobstructive (functional) urine retention, neurogenic atony of urinary bladder with urine retention —* **Adults:** 10 to 50 mg PO tid to qid. Or 2.5 to 5 mg SC. Never give IM or IV. When used for urine retention, some patients may require 50 to 100 mg PO per dose. Use such doses with extreme caution.	▪ Use cautiously in pregnancy. ▪ Contraindicated for IM or IV use and in hypersensitivity to drug; in uncertain strength or integrity of bladder wall; when increased muscular activity of GI or urinary tract is harmful; and in mechanical obstruction of GI or urinary tract, hyperthyroidism, peptic

		ulcers, bronchial asthma, bradycardia or hypotension, vasomotor instability, CAD, seizures, Parkinson's disease, spastic GI disturbances, lesions of GI tract, peritonitis, and marked vagotonia.
bicalutamide Casodex *Nonsteroidal anti-androgen* *Antineoplastic* Preg. Risk Category: X	*tab:* 50 mg	*Test dose:* 2.5 mg SC, repeated at 15- to 30-min in-tervals to total of 4 doses to determine minimal effec-tive dose; then use minimal effective dose q 6 to 8 hr. All doses adjusted individually. *Adjunct therapy in combination with LHRH analogue for treatment of advanced prostate cancer* — **Adults:** 50 mg PO qd in morning or evening.
biperiden hydrochloride Akineton **biperiden lactate** Akineton Lactate *Anticholinergic* *Antiparkinsonian agent* Preg. Risk Category: C	biperiden hy-drochloride: *tab:* 2 mg; biperiden lac-tate: *inj:* 5 mg/ml in 1-ml ampules	*Drug-induced extrapyramidal disorders* — **Adults:** 2 mg PO qd, bid, or tid, depending on severity. Usual dosage 2 mg daily, or 2 mg IM or IV q ½ hr, not to ex-ceed 4 doses or 8 mg daily. *Parkinsonism* — **Adults:** 2 mg PO tid or qid. Dosage individualized and titrated to max 16 mg/24 hr.	• Use cautiously in prostatic hyperplasia, ar-rhythmias, manifest glaucoma, and seizure disorder. • Contraindicated in hypersensitivity to drug, narrow-angle glaucoma, bowel obstruction, and megacolon.
bisacodyl Bisac-Evac, Carter's Little Pills, Da-codyl, Deficol, Dulcagen, Dulcolax, Durolax, Fleet Bisacodyl, Fleet Bisacodyl Prep, Fleet Laxative, Theralax *Diphenylmethane derivative* *Stimulant laxative* Preg. Risk Category: B	*tab: (ent-coat-ed):* 5 mg; *enema:* 0.33 mg/ml, 10 mg/5 ml (mi-croenema)‡; *supp:* 5, 10 mg	*Chronic constipation; preparation for delivery, surgery, or rectal or bowel examination* **Adults and children > 12 yr:** 10 to 15 mg PO in evening or before breakfast. May give up to 30 mg PO or 10 mg PR for evacuation before examination or surgery. **Children 6 to 12 yr:** 5 mg PO or PR hs or before breakfast. Oral form not recommended if unable to swallow tablet whole.	• Contraindicated in hypersensitivity, rectal bleeding, gastroenteritis, intestinal obstruc-tion, or abdominal pain, nausea, vomiting, or other symptoms of appendicitis or acute surgical abdomen.
bismuth subsalicylate Bismatrol, Pepto-Bismol, Pink Bis-muth *Adsorbent* *Antidiarrheal* Preg. Risk Category: NR	*tab (chew):* 262 mg; *cap:* 262 mg; *oral susp:*262, 524 mg/15 ml	*Mild, nonspecific diarrhea* — **Adults:** 30 ml or 2 tabs PO q ½ to 1 hr, to max of 8 doses and for no longer than 2 days. **Children 3 to 6 yr:** 5 ml or ⅓ tab PO. **Children 6 to 9 yr:** 10 ml or ⅔tab PO. **Children 9 to 12 yr:** 15 ml or 1 tab PO.	• Contraindicated in hypersensitivity to salicy-lates. • Use cautiously in patients taking aspirin. Discontinue if tinnitus occurs.

BISMUTH SUBSALICYLATE 31

†Canadian ‡Australian

DRUG/CLASS/CATEGORY	DOSAGE FORMS	INDICATIONS/DOSAGES	KEY PRECAUTIONS
bleomycin sulfate Blenoxane *Antibiotic/antineoplastic (cell cycle—phase specific, G_2 and M phase)* *Antineoplastic* Preg. Risk Category: D	*Inj:* 15-unit vials	Dosage and indications may vary. *Squamous cell carcinoma, lymphosarcoma, reticulum cell carcinoma, testicular carcinoma —* **Adults:** 10 to 20 units/m² IV, IM, or SC once or twice weekly to total of 300 to 400 units. *Hodgkin's disease —* **Adults:** 10 to 20 units/m² IV, IM, or SC once or twice/wk. After 50% response, maintenance dosage 1 unit IM or IV daily or 5 units IM or IV/wk. *Treatment of malignant pleural effusion; prevention of recurrent pleural effusions —* **Adults:** 60 units given as single-dose bolus intrapleural injection.	• Use cautiously in renal or pulmonary impairment. • Contraindicated in hypersensitivity to drug.
botulinum toxin type A Botox, Oculinum *Neurotoxin* *Muscle relaxant* Preg. Risk Category: C	*powder for inj:* 100 units/vial	*Strabismus —* **Adults and children ≥ 12 yr:** inj should be made only by doctors familiar with technique, which involves surg exposure of region and EMG needle guidance. Dosage varies with degree of deviation. For vertical muscles and for horizontal strabismus of < 20 prism D, usual dosage 1.25 to 2.5 units inj into any 1 muscle. For horizontal strabismus of 20 to 50 prism D, 2.5 to 5 units inj into any 1 muscle. For persistent (> 1 mo duration) palsy of 6th cranial nerve, 1.25 to 2.5 units into medial rectus muscle. Don't make subsequent inj for recurrent or residual strabismus until 7 to 14 days after initial dose and unless substantial function has returned to injected and adjacent muscles. May increase dosage up to twice initial dose for patient experiencing incomplete paralysis; don't increase subsequent doses in patient with adequate response. Max single dose for any 1 muscle 25 units. *Blepharospasm —* **Adults:** initially, 1.25 to 2.5 units	• Contraindicated in hypersensitivity to drug or its components.

injected into medial and lateral pretarsal orbicularis oculi of upper lid and lateral pretarsal orbicularis oculi of lower lid. Effects should appear < 3 days and peak < 1 to 2 wk. May double dosage if inadequate paralysis achieved (> 5 units/site produces no apparent benefit). Each treatment lasts about 3 mo and can be repeated indefinitely. Max cumulative dosage: 200 units/mo.

---

bretylium tosylate
Bretylate‡, Bretylol, Critifib‡
Adrenergic blocker
Ventricular antiarrhythmic
Preg. Risk Category: C

inj: 50 mg/ml in 10-ml ampules, vials, and syringes and in 20-ml vials

Ventricular fibrillation or hemodynamically unstable ventricular tachycardia unresponsive to other antiarrhythmics — **Adults:** 5 mg/kg IV push over 1 min. If necessary, increase dose to 10 mg/kg and repeat q 15 to 30 min until 30 to 35 mg/kg given. For continuous suppression, diluted solution given at 1 to 2 mg/min continuously or 5 to 10 mg/kg diluted over more than 8 min q 6 hr.

- Use with extreme caution in fixed cardiac output (aortic stenosis and pulmonary hypertension).
- Contraindicated in digitalized patients unless arrhythmia life-threatening, not caused by cardiac glycoside, and unresponsive to other antiarrhythmics.

---

brompheniramine maleate
Bromphen, Chlorphed, Codimal-A, Dimetane, Veltane
Alkylamine antihistamine
Antihistamine (H₁-receptor antagonist)
Preg. Risk Category: C

tab: 4, 8, 12 mg; **tab (ext-release):** 8, 12 mg; **elixir:** 2 mg/5 ml; **inj:** 10 mg/ml

Rhinitis, allergy symptoms — **Adults:** 4 to 8 mg PO tid or qid; or 8 to 12 mg ext-release PO bid or tid. Max oral dosage 24 mg daily. Or, 5 to 20 mg q 6 to 12 hr IM, IV, or SC. Max parenteral dosage 40 mg daily. **Children 6 to 12 yr:** 2 to 4 mg PO tid or qid; or 8 to 12 mg ext-release PO q 12 hr; or 0.5 mg/kg IM, IV, or SC daily in divided doses tid or qid. **Children < 6 yr:** 0.5 mg/kg PO, IM, IV, or SC daily in divided doses tid or qid.

- Use cautiously in elderly patients and in increased intraocular pressure, diabetes, ischemic heart disease, hyperthyroidism, hypertension, bronchial asthma, and prostatic hyperplasia.
- Contraindicated in hypersensitivity to drug; in acute asthma, hypertension or CAD, angle-closure glaucoma, urine retention, or peptic ulcer; and within 14 days of MAO inhibitor use.

---

budesonide
Rhinocort
Glucocorticoid
Anti-inflammatory
Preg. Risk Category: C

nasal spray: 32 mcg/metered spray (7-g canister)

Symptoms of seasonal or perennial allergic rhinitis — **Adults and children ≥ 6 yr:** 2 sprays in each nostril in morning and evening, or 4 sprays in each nostril in morning. Maintenance dosage should be fewest number of sprays needed to control symptoms.

- Use cautiously in TB; untreated fungal, bacterial, or systemic viral infections; or ocular herpes simplex.
- Contraindicated in hypersensitivity to drug or any component and after recent septal ulcers, nasal surgery, or nasal trauma until total healing has occurred.

DRUG / CLASS / CATEGORY	DOSAGE FORMS	INDICATIONS / DOSAGES	KEY PRECAUTIONS
bumetanide Bumex, Burinex‡ *Loop diuretic* *Diuretic* Preg. Risk Category: C	**tab:** 0.5, 1, 2 mg; **inj:** 0.25 mg/ml	*Edema in heart failure, or hepatic or renal disease —* **Adults:** 0.5 to 2 mg PO qd. If diuretic response inadequate, may give 2nd or 3rd dose at 4- to 5-hr intervals. Max 10 mg/day. May be given IV if PO not feasible. Usual initial dose 0.5 to 1 mg, given IV or IM. If response inadequate, may give 2nd or 3rd dose at 2- to 3-hr intervals. Max 10 mg/day.	▪ Use cautiously in hepatic cirrhosis and ascites and in depressed renal function. ▪ Contraindicated in hypersensitivity to drug or to sulfonamides, in anuria or hepatic coma, and in severe electrolyte depletion.
buprenorphine hydrochloride Buprenex, Temgesic Injection‡ *Narcotic agonist-antagonist* *Opioid partial agonist/analgesic* Preg. Risk Category: C Controlled Sub. Sched.: V	**inj:** 0.324 mg (equiv to 0.3 mg base/ml)	*Moderate to severe pain —* **Adults and children ≥ 13 yr:** 0.3 mg IM or slow IV q 6 hr prn or around the clock; repeat dosage (up to 0.3 mg) if required, 30 to 60 min after initial dose. **Children 2 to 12 yr:** 2 to 6 mcg/kg IM or IV q 4 to 6 hr.	▪ Use cautiously in elderly or debilitated patients; in head injury, intracranial lesions, and increased ICP; severe respiratory, liver, or kidney impairment; CNS depression or coma; thyroid irregularities; adrenal insufficiency; and prostatic hyperplasia, urethral stricture, acute alcoholism, delirium tremens, or kyphoscoliosis. ▪ Contraindicated in hypersensitivity to drug.
bupropion hydrochloride Wellbutrin *Aminoketone* *Antidepressant* Preg. Risk Category: B	**tab:** 75, 100 mg	*Depression —* **Adults:** initially, 100 mg PO bid. increased after 3 days to 100 mg PO tid if needed. If no response after several weeks of therapy, increase to 150 mg tid. No single dose should exceed 150 mg.	▪ Use cautiously in recent history of MI or unstable heart disease and in renal or hepatic impairment. ▪ Contraindicated in hypersensitivity to drug, seizure disorders, within 14 days of MAO inhibitor therapy, and with history of bulimia or anorexia nervosa.
buspirone hydrochloride BuSpar *Azaspirodecanedione derivative* *Antianxiety agent* Preg. Risk Category: B	**tab:** 5, 10 mg	*Anxiety disorders; short-term relief of anxiety —* **Adults:** initially, 5 mg PO tid, increased at 3-day intervals in 5-mg increments. Usual maintenance dosage 20 to 30 mg daily in divided doses. Don't exceed 60 mg daily.	▪ Use cautiously in hepatic or renal failure. ▪ Contraindicated in hypersensitivity to drug or within 14 days of MAO inhibitor therapy.

busulfan
Myleran
Alkylating agent (cell cycle–phase nonspecific)
Antineoplastic
Preg. Risk Category: D

tab: 2 mg

Chronic myelocytic (granulocytic) leukemia — **Adults:** 4 to 8 mg PO qd, up to 12 mg PO qd until WBC count falls to 15,000/mm³; drug stopped until WBC count rises to 50,000/mm³, and then resumed as before; or 4 to 8 mg PO qd until WBC count falls to 10,000 to 20,000/mm³; then daily dosage reduced prn to maintain WBC count at th s level (usually 1 to 3 mg qd). **Children:** 0.06 to 0.12 mg/kg/day or 1.8 to 4.6 mg/m²/day PO; dosage adjusted to maintain WBC count at 20,000/mm³, but never < 10,000/mm³.

- Use cautiously in recent use of other myelo-suppressants or radiation; in low neutrophil or platelet counts, head trauma, or seizures; or in patients taking drugs that reduce seizure threshold.
- Contraindicated in chronic myelogenous leukemia demonstrating prior drug resistance. Not useful with chronic lymphocytic leukemia or acute leukemia or in blastic crisis of chronic myelogenous leukemia.

butoconazole nitrate
Femstat
Synthetic imidazole derivative
Topical fungistat
Preg. Risk Category: C

vag cream: 2% with applicators supplied

Vulvovaginal mycotic infections caused by Candida species — **Adults:** for nonpregnant patient, 1 applicatorful intravaginally hs for 3 days. Treat for another 3 days, prn. For pregnant patient curing 2nd or 3rd trimester, 1 applicatorful intravaginally hs for 6 days.

- Use in 2nd and 3rd trimesters of pregnancy only when potential benefits outweigh possible risks to fetus.
- Contraindicated in hypersensitivity to drug.

butorphanol tartrate
Stadol, Stadol NS
Narcotic agonist-antagonist, opioid partial agonist
Analgesic/adjunct to anesthesia
Preg. Risk Category: C

inj: 1, 2 mg/ml; **nasal spray:** 10 mg/ml

Moderate to severe pain — **Adults:** 1 to 4 mg IM q 3 to 4 hr, prn or around the clock; or 0.5 to 2 mg IV q 3 to 4 hr, prn or around the clock. Not to exceed 4 mg per dose. Alternatively, 1 mg by nasal spray q 3 to 4 hr (1 spray in one nostril); repeated in 60 to 90 min if pain relief inadequate.
Preoperative anesthesia or preanesthesia — **Adults:** 2 mg IM 60 to 90 min before surgery.

- Use cautiously in emotional instability, head injury, increased ICP, acute MI, ventricular dysfunction, coronary insufficiency, respiratory disease or depression, in renal or hepatic dysfunction and with recent use of repeated doses of narcotic analgesics.
- Contraindicated in patients taking repeated doses of narcotics or with narcotic addiction, and in hypersensitivity to drug or preservative (benzethonium chloride).

DRUG/CLASS/ CATEGORY	DOSAGE FORMS	INDICATIONS/ DOSAGES	KEY PRECAUTIONS
caffeine Caffedrine Caplets, Dexitac, NoDoz, Quick Pep, Vivarin *Methylxanthine* *CNS stimulant/analeptic/respiratory stimulant* Preg. Risk Category: C	**tab:** 100, 150, 200 mg; **tab (timed-release):** 200 mg; **cap (timed-release):** 200 mg; **inj:** (250 mg/ml) with sodium benzoate (250 mg/ml)	*CNS stimulant* — **Adults:** 100 to 200 mg anhydrous caffeine PO q 3 to 4 hr, prn. Alternatively, 500 mg to 1 g IM (or slowly IV). Total daily dosage should seldom exceed 2.5 g	▪ Use cautiously in history of peptic ulcer, symptomatic arrhythmias, or palpitations and during first several days to weeks after acute MI. ▪ Contraindicated in hypersensitivity to drug.
calcifediol Calderol *Vitamin D analogue* *Antihypocalcemic* Preg. Risk Category: C	**cap:** 20, 50 mcg	*Metabolic bone disease and hypocalcemia associated with chronic renal failure* — **Adults:** 300 to 350 mcg PO weekly. May be increased at 4-wk intervals.	▪ Contraindicated in hypersensitivity or vitamin D toxicity.
calcipotriene Dovonex *Synthetic vitamin D3 analogue* *Topical antipsoriatic* Preg. Risk Category: C	**oint:** 0.005% in 30, 60, and 100 g aluminum tubes	*Moderate plaque psoriasis* — **Adults:** apply a thin layer to the affected area bid. Rub in gently and completely. Drug should not be used on the face.	▪ Contraindicated in hypersensitivity to drug and in hypercalcemia or vitamin D toxicity. ▪ Use cautiously in breast-feeding or elderly patients.
calcitonin Calcimar (salmon), Cibacalcin (human), Miacalcin (salmon) *Thyroid hormone* *Hypocalcemic* Preg. Risk Category: C	**inj:** 200 IU/ml, 2-ml vials (salmon); 0.5 mg/vial (human); **nasal spray:** 200 IU/activation	*Paget's disease of bone* — **Adults:** 100 IU calcitonin (salmon) SC or IM qd or 0.5 mg calcitonin (human) SC. Maint: 50 to 100 IU calcitonin (salmon) qd or qod or 0.5 mg calcitonin (human) 2 or 3 times/wk or 0.25 mg calcitonin (human) qd. *Hypercalcemia* — **Adults:** 4 IU/kg calcitonin (salmon) IM in 2 ml q 12 hr; increase by 8 IU/kg q 12 hr. *Postmenopausal osteoporosis* — **Adults:** 100 IU calcitonin (salmon) SC or IM qd, or 200 IU (1 spray) qd in alternating nostril.	▪ Contraindicated in hypersensitivity to salmon calcitonin. No contraindications for human calcitonin.

calcitriol Calcijex, Rocaltrol *Vitamin D analogue* *Antihypocalcemic* *Preg. Risk Category: C*	***cap:*** 0.25, 0.5 mcg; ***inj:*** 1, 2 mcg/ml	*Hypocalcemia in patients undergoing chronic dialysis* — **Adults:** 0.25 mcg PO qd. May be increased by 0.25 mcg qd at 4- to 8-wk intervals. Maint.: 0.25 mcg qod up to 0.5 to 1 mcg qd. Or, 0.5 mcg IV 3 times/wk, approx. qod. May be increased by 0.25 to 0.5 mcg at 2- to 4-wk intervals. Maint.: 0.5 to 3 mcg IV 3 times/wk. *Hypoparathyroidism and pseudohypoparathyroidism* — **Adults and children ≥ 6 yr:** 0.25 mcg PO qd in am. May be increased at 2- to 4-wk intervals. Maint.: 0.5 to 2 mcg qd. **Children 1 to 5 yr:** (hypoparathyroidism only) 0.25 to 0.75 mcg qd. *Psoriasis vulgaris* — **Adults:** 0.5 mcg/day PO for 6 months and (0.5 mcg/g petroleum) qd for 8 wks.	▪ Contraindicated in hypercalcemia or vitamin D toxicity.
calcium acetate Phos-Ex, PhosLo **calcium carbonate** Calcarb 600, Cal Carb-HD, Calci-Chew, Os-Cal 500, Rolaids Calcium Rich, Tums **calcium chloride** **calcium citrate** Citracal† Citrical **calcium glubionate** Neo-Calglucon **calcium gluceptate** **calcium gluconate** **calcium lactate**	***inj:*** 0.5 mEq/ml (acetate); 10% sol in 10-ml amp, vials, and syr (chloride); 1.1 g/5-ml amp or 10-ml vials (gluceptate); 10% sol in 10-ml amp and vials or 50-ml vials (gluconate); ***tab/tab (chew);*** strengths vary with product;	*Hypocalcemic emergency* — **Adults:** 7 to 14 mEq calcium IV (as 10% gluconate sol, 2% to 10% chloride sol, or 22% gluceptate sol). **Children:** 1 to 7 mEq calcium IV. **Infants:** up to 1 mEq calcium IV. *Hypocalcemic tetany* — **Adults:** 4.5 to 16 mEq calcium IV. Repeat until controlled. **Children:** 0.5 to 0.7 mEq/kg calcium IV 3 to 4 times/day until controlled. **Neonates:** 2.4 mEq/kg IV qd in divided doses. *Adjunctive treatment of cardiac arrest* — **Adults:** 0.027 to 0.054 mEq/kg calcium chloride IV, 4.5 to 6.3 mEq calcium gluceptate IV, or 2.3 to 3.7 mEq calcium gluconate IV. **Children:** 0.27 mEq/kg calcium chloride IV. May repeat in 10 min; check serum calcium before administering further doses. *Adjunctive treatment of magnesium intoxication* — **Adults:** initially, 7 mEq IV. Subsequent doses based on response.	▪ Use cautiously in sarcoidosis, renal or cardiac disease, cor pulmonale, respiratory acidosis, or respiratory failure and in digitalized patients. ▪ Contraindicated in ventricular fibrillation, hypercalcemia, hypophosphatemia, or renal calculi.

(continued)

†Canadian ‡Australian

DRUG/CLASS/CATEGORY	DOSAGE FORMS	INDICATIONS/DOSAGES	KEY PRECAUTIONS
calcium (continued) **calcium phosphate, dibasic calcium phosphate, tribasic** Posture Calcium supplement Therapeutic agent for electrolyte balance/cardiotonic Preg. Risk Category: C	**tab (effer):** 2,376 mg (cit.); **cap:** 500 mg (acetate); 1.25, 1.5 g (carb.) **oral susp:** 1.25 g/5 ml (carb.); **powder:** 6.5 g (carb.); **syrup:** 1.8 g/5ml (glubionate)	During exchange transfusions — **Adults:** 1.35 mEq IV concurrently with each 100 ml citrated blood. **Neonates:** 0.45 mEq IV after each 100 ml citrated blood. Hyperphosphatemia — **Adults:** 1,334 to 2,000 mg PO acetate tid with meals. Dialysis patients need 3 to 4 tabs with meals. Dietary supplement — **Adults:** 500 mg to 2 g PO daily	▪ Contraindicated in signs of GI obstruction.
calcium polycarbophil Fiberall, FiberCon, FiberLax Hydrophilic agent Bulk laxative/antidiarrheal Preg. Risk Category: NR	**tab:** 500, 625; **tab (chew):** 500, 1,250 mg	Constipation; diarrhea associated with irritable bowel syndrome, as well as acute nonspecific diarrhea — **Adults:** 1 g PO qid prn. Max 6 g in 24-hr period. **2 to 6 yr:** as directed by doctor. 500 mg PO bid prn. Max 1.5 g in 24-hr period. **6 to 12 yr:** 500 mg PO qd to tid prn. Max 3 g in 24-hr period.	
capreomycin sulfate Capastat Sulfate Polypeptide antibiotic Antitubercular agent Preg. Risk Category: C	**inj:** 1 g/vial	Adjunctive treatment of TB — **Adults:** 15 mg/kg/day up to 1 g IM daily injected deep into large muscle mass for 60 to 120 days; then 1 g 2 to 3 times weekly for 18 to 24 mo. Max dosage 20 mg/kg/day. Must give in conjunction with another antitubercular.	▪ Use with extreme caution in patients receiving other ototoxic or nephrotoxic drugs. ▪ Use cautiously in impaired renal function, history of allergies, or hearing impairment. ▪ Contraindicated in hypersensitivity to drug.
captopril Apo-Capto†, Capoten, Novo-Captopril†, Syn-Captopril† ACE inhibitor Antihypertensive/adjunctive treatment of heart failure	**tab:** 12.5, 25, 50, 100 mg	Hypertension — **Adults:** 25 mg PO bid or tid. If BP not controlled in 1 to 2 wk, increase to 50 mg bid or tid. If BP not controlled after another 1 to 2 wk, add diuretic. If further BP reduction needed, may increase dosage to 150 mg tid with diuretic. Max 450 mg daily. Heart failure; to reduce risk of death and to slow development of heart failure after MI — **Adults:** 6.25 to	▪ Use cautiously in impaired renal function, renal artery stenosis, or serious autoimmune disease (especially systemic lupus erythematosus) or in exposure to other drugs known to affect WBC counts or immune response.

Preg. Risk Category: C (D in 2nd and 3rd trimesters)		12.5 mg PO tid initially. Gradually increase to 50 mg tid prn. Max 450 mg daily.
		▪ Contraindicated in hypersensitivity to drug or any other ACE inhibitor.
carbachol (intraocular) Miostat **carbachol (topical)** Isopto Carbachol *Cholinergic agonist* *Miotic* Preg. Risk Category: C	*intraocular inj* 0.01%; *top.* *ophth. sol:* 0.75%, 1.5%, 2.25%, 3%	*To produce pupillary miosis in ocular surgery* — **Adults:** before or after securing sutures, the doctor gently instills 0.5 ml (intraocular form) into anterior chamber. *Open-angle glaucoma* — **Adults:** 1 to 2 drops instilled (topical form) q 4 to 8 hours.	▪ Use cautiously in acute heart failure, bronchial asthma, peptic ulcer, hyperthyroidism, GI spasm, Parkinson's disease, and urinary tract obstruction. ▪ Contraindicated in hypersensitivity to drug or in patients in whom cholinergic effects are undesirable.
carbamazepine Apo-Carbamazepine†, Epitol, Mazepine†, Novocarbamazt†, Tegretol *Iminostilbene derivative; chemically related to TCAs* *Anticonvulsant/analgesic* Preg. Risk Category: C	*tab:* 200 mg; *tab (chew):* 100 mg; *tab* *(ext-re-* *lease)†:* 200, 400 mg; *oral* *susp:* 100 mg/5 ml	*Generalized tonic-clonic and complex partial seizures,* *mixed seizure patterns* — **Adults and children > 12** **yr:** 200 mg PO bid for tab or 1 tsp susp PO qid. Increase at weekly intervals by 200 mg PO qd. in divided doses at 6- to 8-hr intervals. Adjust to min. effective level. Max 1 g/day in ages 12 to 15 or 1.2 g/day in patients > age 15. **Children 6 to 12 yr:** 100 mg PO bid or ½ tsp of susp PO qid. Increase weekly by 100 mg PO qd. Max 1 g/day.	▪ Use cautiously in mixed seizure disorders. ▪ Contraindicated in history of previous bone marrow suppression or hypersensitivity to carbamazepine or TCAs and within 14 days of MAO inhibitor therapy.
carbamide peroxide Debrox *Urea hydrogen peroxide* *Ceruminolytic/topical antiseptic* Preg. Risk Category: NR	*otic sol:* 6.5% in glycerin or glycerin/propy- lene glycol; *oral sol:* 10% with glycerin and propylene glycol; 15% with anhy- drous glycerin, methylparaber, and propylene glycol	*Impacted cerumen* — **Adults and children:** 5 to 10 drops into ear canal bid for up to 4 days. Allow solution to remain in ear canal for 15 to 30 minutes; remove with warm water.	▪ Contraindicated in patients with perforated eardrum.

DRUG / CLASS / CATEGORY	DOSAGE FORMS	INDICATIONS / DOSAGES	KEY PRECAUTIONS
carbidopa-levodopa Sinemet, Sinemet CR *Decarboxylase inhibitor-dopamine precursor* *Antiparkinsonian agent* Preg. Risk Category: NR	**tab:** carb. 10 mg with lev. 100 mg (Sinemet 10-100), carb. 25 mg with lev. 100 mg (Sinemet 25-100), carb. 25 mg with lev. 250 mg (Sinemet 25-250); **tab (ext-release):** carb. 50 mg with lev. 200 mg (Sinemet CR)	*Idiopathic Parkinson's disease, postencephalitic parkinsonism, and symptomatic parkinsonism resulting from carbon monoxide or manganese intoxication* — **Adults:** 1 tab 25 mg carbidopa/100 mg levodopa PO tid, then increase by 1 tab qd or qod pm to max 8 tab daily. 25 mg carbidopa/250 mg levodopa or 10 mg carbidopa/100 mg levodopa tab substituted as required to obtain max response. Optimum dosage determined by individual titration. Patients treated with conventional tab may receive ext-release tab; dosage calculated on current levodopa intake. Initially, ext-release tab dosage should amount to 10% more levodopa per day, increased as needed and tolerated to 30% more per day. Give in divided doses at intervals of 4 to 8 hr.	■ Use cautiously in severe CV, renal, hepatic, endocrine, or pulmonary disorders; history of peptic ulcer; psychiatric illness; MI with residual arrhythmias; bronchial asthma; emphysema; and well-controlled, chronic open-angle glaucoma. ■ Contraindicated in hypersensitivity to drug, narrow-angle glaucoma, melanoma, or undiagnosed skin lesions and within 14 days of MAO inhibitor therapy.
carboplatin Paraplatin, Paraplatin-AQ† *Alkylating agent* *Antineoplastic* Preg. Risk Category: D	**inj:** 50-mg, 150-mg, and 450-mg vials	*Palliative treatment of ovarian cancer* — **Adults:** 360 mg/m² IV on day 1 q 4 weeks; doses not repeated until platelet count > 100,000/mm³ and neutrophil count > 2,000/mm³. Subsequent dosages based on blood counts. Adjust in renal failure.	■ Contraindicated in patients with history of hypersensitivity to cisplatin, platinum-containing compounds, or mannitol or with severe bone marrow suppression or bleeding.
carboprost tromethamine Hemabate *Prostaglandin* *Oxytocic* Preg. Risk Category: C	**inj:** 250 mcg/ml in comb. with 83 mcg tromethamine	*To abort pregnancy between 13th and 20th wk of gestation* — **Adults:** Initially, 250 mcg deep IM. Subsequent doses of 250 mcg administered at intervals of 1½ to 3½ hours, depending on uterine response. Dosage may be increased in increments to 500 mcg if contractility is inadequate after several 250-mcg doses. Total dosage should not exceed 12 mg. *Postpartum hemorrhage caused by uterine atony not managed by conventional methods* — **Adults:** 250	■ Contraindicated in hypersensitivity, acute pelvic inflammatory disease, or active cardiac, pulmonary, renal, or hepatic disease. ■ Use cautiously in history of asthma; hypotension or hypertension; CV, renal, or hepatic disease; anemia; jaundice; diabetes; epilepsy; a compromised uterus; or chorioamnionitis.

		mcg by deep IM injection. Repeat doses administered at 15- to 90-minute intervals, prn. Max total dosage is 2 mg.	
carisoprodol Rela, Sodol, Soma, Soprodol *Carbamate derivative* *Skeletal muscle relaxant* Preg. Risk Category: NR	***tab:*** 350 mg	*As adjunct in acute, painful musculoskeletal conditions* — **Adults:** 350 mg PO tid and hs.	▪ Use cautiously in impaired hepatic or renal function. ▪ Contraindicated in hypersensitivity to related compounds (e.g., meprobamate or tybamate) or in intermittent porphyria.
carmustine (BCNU) BiCNU *Alkylating agent* *Antineoplastic* Preg. Risk Category: D	***inj:*** 100-mg vial (lyophilized) with 3-ml vial of absolute alcohol as diluent	*Brain tumors, Hodgkin's disease, malignant lymphoma, and multiple myeloma* — **Adults:** 75 to 100 mg/m^2 IV by slow inf daily for 2 days; repeated q 6 wk if platelet count > $100,000/mm^3$ and WBC count > $4,000/mm^3$. Dosage reduced by 30% when WBC count is $2,000\text{-}3,000/mm^3$ and platelet count falls.	▪ Contraindicated in patients with hypersensitivity to drug.
carteolol Cartrol *Beta-adrenergic blocker* *Antihypertensive* Preg. Risk Category: C	***tab:*** 2.5, 5 mg	*Hypertension* — **Adults:** initially, 2.5 mg PO as single daily dose; increase gradually to 5 or 10 mg as single daily dose as needed. Dosages > 10 mg daily don't produce greater response (may actually decrease response).	▪ Use cautiously in nonallergic bronchospastic disease, diabetes mellitus, hyperthyroidism, heart failure controlled by cardiac glycosides and diuretics, or decreased pulmonary function and in breast-feeding patients. ▪ Contraindicated in hypersensitivity to any drug component and in bronchial asthma, severe COPD, severe bradycardia, > first-degree heart block, cardiogenic shock, or uncontrolled heart failure.
carteolol hydrochloride Ocupress Ophthalmic Solution, 1% *Beta-adrenergic blocker* *Antihypertensive* Preg. Risk Category: C	***ophth sol:*** 1%	*Chronic open-angle glaucoma, intraocular hypertension* — **Adults:** 1 drop in the conjunctival sac of the affected eye bid	▪ Use cautiously in nonallergic bronchospastic disease, diabetes mellitus, hyperthyroidism, or decreased pulmonary function and in breast-feeding women. ▪ Contraindicated in hypersensitivity, bronchial asthma, severe COPD, sinus bradycardia, second- or third-degree AV block, overt cardiac failure, or cardiogenic shock.

†Canadian ‡Australian

DRUG / CLASS / CATEGORY	DOSAGE FORMS	INDICATIONS / DOSAGES	KEY PRECAUTIONS
cefaclor Ceclor *Second-generation cephalosporin* Antibiotic Preg. Risk Category: B	**cap:** 250, 500 mg; **oral susp:** 125, 250, 187, 375 mg/5 ml	*Respiratory, urinary tract, skin, or soft-tissue infections and otitis media caused by susceptible organisms* — **Adults:** 250 to 500 mg PO q 8 hr. For pharyngitis or otitis media, may give daily dosage in 2 divided doses q 12 hr. **Children:** 20 mg/kg daily PO in divided doses q 8 hr. For pharyngitis or otitis media, may give daily dosage in 2 divided doses q 12 hr. More serious infections, 40 mg/kg daily, max 1 g qd.	▪ Use cautiously in impaired renal function or history of sensitivity to penicillin and in breast-feeding patients. ▪ Contraindicated in hypersensitivity to other cephalosporins.
cefazolin sodium Ancef, Kefzol, Zolicef *First-generation cephalosporin* Antibiotic Preg. Risk Category: B	**inj (parenteral):** 500 mg, 1 g; **infusion:** 500 mg/50-ml vial, 500 mg/100-ml vial; **pharm bulk pkg:** 5, 10, 20 g	*Prophylaxis in contaminated surgery* — **Adults:** 1 g IM or IV 30 to 60 min before surgery; then 0.5 to 1 g IM or IV q 6 to 8 hr for 24 hr. In operations > 2 hr, may give another 0.5 to 1 g IM intraoperatively. Where infection would be devastating, prophylaxis may continue 3 to 5 days. *Respiratory, biliary, GU, skin, soft-tissue, bone and joint infections; septicemia; endocarditis caused by susceptible organisms* — **Adults:** 250 mg IM or IV q 8 hr to 1.5 g PO q 6 hr. Max 12 g/day in life-threatening situations. **Children > 1 mo:** 25 to 50 mg/kg or 1.25 g/m² daily IM or IV in 3 or 4 divided doses. May increase to 100 mg/kg/day.	▪ Use cautiously in impaired renal function or history of sensitivity to penicillin and in breast-feeding patients. ▪ Contraindicated in hypersensitivity to other cephalosporins.
cefixime Suprax *Third-generation cephalosporin* Antibiotic Preg. Risk Category: B	**tab:** 200, 400 mg; **oral susp:** 100 mg/5 ml (after reconstitution)	*Uncomplicated UTI caused by E. coli and P. mirabilis; otitis media caused by H. influenzae, M. (Branhamella) catarrhalis, and S. pyogenes; pharyngitis and tonsillitis caused by S. pyogenes; acute bronchitis and exacerbations of chronic bronchitis caused by S. pneumoniae and H. influenzae* — **Adults and children > 12 yr or weighing > 50 kg:** 400 mg/day PO as 1 400-mg tablet or 200 mg q 12 hr. **Children ≤ 12 yr or weigh-**	▪ Use cautiously and with reduced dosage in renal dysfunction, history of sensitivity to penicillin, and breast-feeding patients. ▪ Contraindicated in hypersensitivity to drug or other cephalosporins.

cefonicid sodium
Monocid
Second-generation cephalosporin
Antibiotic
Preg. Risk Category: B

inj: 500 mg, 1 g; *infusion:* 1 g/100 ml; *pharm bulk pkg:* 10 g

ing ≤ **50 kg:** 8 mg/kg/day susp PO as 1 qd dose or 4 mg/kg q 12 hr. *Uncomplicated gonorrhea caused by N. gonorrhoeae* — **Adults:** 400 mg PO as single dose.

Periop prophylaxis in contaminated surgery — **Adults:** 1 g IM or IV 30 to 60 min before surgery; then 1 g IM or IV daily for 2 days after surgery. For prophylaxis in cesarean section, 1 g IM or IV after umbilical cord is clamped.
Serious infections of lower respiratory and urinary tracts, skin and skin-structure infections, septicemia, bone and joint infections, and preop prophylaxis — **Adults:** usual dosage 1 g IV or IM q 24 hr; in life-threatening infections, 2 g q 24 hr.

- Use cautiously in impaired renal failure or sensitivity to penicillin and in breast-feeding patients.
- Contraindicated in hypersensitivity to drug or other cephalosporins.

---

cefoperazone sodium
Cefobid
Third-generation cephalosporin
Antibiotic
Preg. Risk Category: B

infusion: 1, 2 g piggyback; *parenteral:* 1, 2 g; *pharm bulk pkg:* 10-g vial

Serious respiratory tract infections; intra-abdominal, gyn, and skin infections; bacteremia; and septicemia caused by susceptible organisms — **Adults:** 1 to 2 g q 12 hr IM or IV. In severe infections or those caused by less sensitive organisms, total daily dosage or frequency may increase to 16 g/day in certain situations.

- Use cautiously in impaired renal function or history of sensitivity to penicillin and in breast-feeding patients.
- Contraindicated in hypersensitivity to drug or other cephalosporins.

---

cefotaxime sodium
Claforan
Third-generation cephalosporin
Antibiotic
Preg. Risk Category: B

inj: 500 mg, 1, 2 g; *infusion:* 1, 2 g; *pharm bulk pkg:* 10-g vial

Periop prophylaxis in contaminated surgery — **Adults:** 1 g IM or IV 30 to 60 min before surgery. For cesarean section, 1 g IM or IV as soon as umbilical cord clamped, then 1 g IM or IV 6 and 12 hr later.
Serious infections of lower respiratory and urinary tracts, CNS, skin, bone, and joints; gyn and intra-abdominal infections; bacteremia; and septicemia caused by susceptible organisms — **Adults:** 1 g IV or IM q 6 to 8 hr. Up to 12 g daily can be given in life-threatening infections. **Children ≥ 50 kg:** usual adult dose, but don't exceed 12 g daily. **Children 1 mo to 12 yr weighing < 50 kg:** 50 to 180 mg/kg/day IM or IV in 4 to 6 divided doses. **Neonates to 1 wk:** 50 mg/kg IV q 12 hr. **Neonates 1 to 4 wk:** 50 mg/kg IV q 8 hr.

- Use cautiously in impaired renal function or sensitivity to penicillin and in breast-feeding patients.
- Contraindicated in hypersensitivity to drug or other cephalosporins.

†Canadian ‡Australian

DRUG/CLASS/CATEGORY	DOSAGE FORMS	INDICATIONS/DOSAGES	KEY PRECAUTIONS
cefotetan disodium Cefotan *Second-generation cephalosporin/cephamycin* *Antibiotic* Preg. Risk Category: B	*inj:* 1, 2 g; *infusion:* 1 g, 2 g piggyback; *pharm bulk pkg:* 10-g vial	*Serious UTI and lower respiratory tract infections and gyn, skin and skin-structure, intra-abdominal, and bone and joint infections caused by susceptible organisms* — **Adults:** 1 to 2 g IV or IM q 12 hr for 5 to 10 days. Up to 6 g daily in life-threatening infections. *Periop prophylaxis* — **Adults:** 1 to 2 g IV given once 30 to 60 min before surgery. In cesarean section, give dose as soon as umbilical cord clamped.	▪ Use cautiously in impaired renal function or history of sensitivity to penicillin and in breast-feeding patients. ▪ Contraindicated in hypersensitivity to drug or other cephalosporins.
cefoxitin sodium Mefoxin *Second-generation cephalosporin/cephamycin* *Antibiotic* Preg. Risk Category: B	*inj:* 1, 2 g; *infusion:* 1, 2 g in 50-ml container; *pharm bulk pkg:* 10 g	*Serious infections of respiratory or GU tracts; skin, soft-tissue, bone, and joint infections; bloodstream and intra-abdominal infections caused by susceptible organisms; periop prophylaxis* — **Adults:** 1 to 2 g q 6 to 8 hr in uncomplicated infections. Up to 12 g qd in life-threatening infections. **Children > 3 mo:** 80 to 160 mg/kg daily in 4 to 6 equally divided doses. Max 12 g daily. *Prophylactic use in surgery* — **Adults:** 2 g IM or IV 30 to 60 min before surgery, then 2 g IM or IV q 6 hr for 24 hr (72 hr after prosthetic arthroplasty). **Children ≥ 3 mo:** 30 to 40 mg/kg IM or IV 30 to 60 min before surgery, then 30 to 40 mg/kg q 6 hr for 24 hr (72 hr after prosthetic arthroplasty).	▪ Use cautiously in impaired renal function or history of sensitivity to penicillin and in breast-feeding patients. ▪ Contraindicated in hypersensitivity to drug or other cephalosporins.
ceftazidime Ceptaz, Fortaz, Tazicef, Tazidime *Third-generation cephalosporin* *Antibiotic* Preg. Risk Category: B	*inj (with sodium carbonate):* 500 mg, 1, 2 g; 6 g (pharm bulk); *inj (with arginine):* 1, 2 g; 6, 10 g (pharm	*Serious infections of lower respiratory or urinary tracts; gyn, intra-abdominal, CNS, and skin infections; bacteremia; and septicemia* — **Adults and children ≥ 12 yr:** 1 g IV or IM q 8 to 12 hr; up to 6 g daily in life-threatening infections. **Children 1 mo to 12 yr:** 25 to 50 mg/kg IV q 8 hr (sodium carbonate formulation). **Neonates 0 to 4 wk:** 30 mg/kg IV q 12 hr (sodium carbonate formulation).	▪ Use cautiously in impaired renal failure or history of sensitivity to penicillin and in breast-feeding patients. ▪ Contraindicated in hypersensitivity to drug or other cephalosporins. ▪ Commercially available preparations contain sodium carbonate (Fortaz, Magnacef, Tazicef, Tazidime) or arginine (Ceptaz, Tazidime).

	bulk); **inf:** 1, 2 g in 50-ml, 100-ml vials (premixed)	Pentacef). Safety and efficacy of arginine-containing solutions in children ≤ 12 years is not established.
ceftibuten Cedax *Second-generation cephalosporin* Antibiotic Preg. Risk Category: B	**cap:** 400 mg; **oral susp:** 90, 180 mg/5 ml	*Acute bacterial exacerbation of chronic bronchitis due to susceptible organisms —* **Adults and children ≥ age 12:** 400 mg PO daily for 10 days. *Pharyngitis and tonsillitis due to* S. pyogenes; *acute bacterial otitis media due to* H. influenzae, M. catarrhalis, *or* S. pyogenes *—* **Adults and children ≥ age 12:** 400 mg PO daily for 10 days. **Children < age 12:** 9 mg/kg PO daily for 10 days. **Children > 45 kg:** max dose 400 mg PO daily for 10 days.	▪ Use cautiously in history of hypersensitivity to penicillin or impaired renal function or GI disease (especially colitis) and in elderly or breast-feeding patients. Use in pregnant patients only if clearly needed. ▪ Contraindicated in hypersensitivity to cephalosporins. ▪ Safety and effectiveness in infants < age 6 mo not established.
ceftizoxime sodium Cefizox *Third-generation cephalosporin* Antibiotic Preg. Risk Category: B	**inj:** 500 mg, 1, 2 g; **infusion:** 1, 2 g in 100-mg vials or in 50 ml D₅W; **pharm bulk pkg:** 10 g	*Infections of lower respiratory and urinary tracts; gyn, intra-abdominal, bone, joint, and skin infections; bacteremia; septicemia; and meningitis caused by susceptible microorganisms —* **Adults:** 1 to 2 g IV or IM q 8 to 12 hr up to 2 g q 4 hr. **Children > 6 mo:** 33 to 50 mg/kg IV q 6 to 8 hr. Serious infections: up to 200 mg/kg/day in divided doses. Don't exceed 12 g/day.	▪ Use cautiously in impaired renal function, GI disease (especially colitis), history of sensitivity to penicillin, and breast-feeding patients. ▪ Contraindicated in hypersensitivity to drug or other cephalosporins.
ceftriaxone sodium Rocephin *Third-generation cephalosporin* Antibiotic Preg. Risk Category: B	**inj:** 250, 500 mg, 1, 2 g; **infusion:** 1, 2 g; **pharm bulk pkg:** 10 g	*Most infections caused by susceptible organisms —* **Adults:** 1 to 2 g IM or IV daily or bid. *Serious infections of lower respiratory and urinary tracts; gyn, bone, joint, intra-abdominal, and skin infections; bacteremia; septicemia; and Lyme disease caused by susceptible organisms —* **Adults and children > 12 yr:** 1 to 2 g IM or IV daily or in equally divided doses bid. Max 4 g/day. **Children ≤ 12 yr:** 50 to 75 mg/kg IM or IV, not to exceed 2 g/day, in divided doses q 12 hr. *Meningitis —* **Adults and children:** 100 mg/kg IM or IV (max 4 g); then 100 mg/kg IM or IV once daily or in divided doses q 12 hr, max 4 g, for 7 to 14 days.	▪ Use cautiously in history of sensitivity to penicillin and in breast-feeding patients. ▪ Contraindicated in hypersensitivity to drug or other cephalosporins.

CEFTRIAXONE SODIUM 45

†Canadian ‡Australian

DRUG/CLASS/ CATEGORY	DOSAGE FORMS	INDICATIONS/ DOSAGES	KEY PRECAUTIONS
cefuroxime axetil Ceftin **cefuroxime sodium** Kefurox, Zinacef *Second-generation cephalosporin* *Antibiotic* Preg. Risk Category: B	**cefuroxime axetil — tab:** 125, 250, 500 mg; **susp:** 125 mg/5 ml. **cefuroxime sodium — inj:** 750 mg, 1.5 g; **infusion:** 750 mg, 1.5 g premixed, frozen sol; **pharm bulk pkg:** 7.5 g	*Injectable form used for serious infections and for periop prophylaxis. Oral form used for otitis media, pharyngitis, tonsillitis, infections of urinary and lower respiratory tracts, and skin and skin-structure infections due to susceptible organisms —* **Adults and children ≥ 12 yr:** usual dosage of cefuroxime sodium: 750 mg to 1.5 g IM or IV q 8 hr for 5 to 10 days. For life-threatening infections and less susceptible organisms, 1.5 g IM or IV q 6 hr; for bacterial meningitis, up to 3 g IV q 8 hr. Or, 250 to 500 mg of cefuroxime axetil PO q 12 hr. **Children and infants > 3 mo:** 50 to 100 mg/kg/day of cefuroxime sodium IM or IV in divided doses q 6 to 8 hr. for bacterial meningitis, 200 to 240 mg/kg IV in divided doses q 6 to 8 hr. *Otitis media —* **Children < 2 yr:** 125 mg PO q 12 hr. **Children ≥ 2 yr:** 250 mg PO q 12 hr. *Early Lyme disease caused by B. burgdorferi —* **Adults and children ≥ 13 yr:** 500 mg PO bid for 20 days.	▪ Use cautiously in impaired renal function, history of sensitivity to penicillin, and breast-feeding patients. ▪ Contraindicated in hypersensitivity to drug or other cephalosporins.
cephalexin hydrochloride Keftab **cephalexin monohydrate** Apo-Cephalex†, Bio-cef, Cefanex, C-Lexin, Keflex *First-generation cephalosporin* *Antibiotic* Preg. Risk Category: B	**hydrochloride — tab:** 250, 500 mg. **monohydrate — tab:** 250, 500 mg, 1 g; **cap:** 250, 500 mg; **oral susp:** 100, 125, 250 mg/5 ml	*Respiratory tract, GI tract, skin, soft-tissue, bone, and joint infections and otitis media caused by E. coli and other coliform bacteria, group A beta-hemolytic streptococci, Klebsiella, P. mirabilis, S. pneumoniae, and staphylococci —* **Adults:** 250 mg to 1 g PO q 6 hr. **Children:** 6 to 12 mg/kg PO q 6 hr (monohydrate only). Max 25 mg/kg q 6 hr.	▪ Use cautiously in history of sensitivity to penicillin or renal impairment and in breast-feeding patients. ▪ Contraindicated in hypersensitivity to cephalosporins.

cephapirin sodium
Cefadyl
First-generation cephalosporin
Antibiotic
Preg. Risk Category: B

inj: 500-mg, 1-, 2-g vials; 1-, 2-, 4-g piggyback vials; **pharm bulk pkg:** 20 g

Periop prophylaxis in contaminated or potentially contaminated surgery — **Adults:** 1 to 2 g IM or IV 30 to 60 min before surgery; then 1 to 2 g IM or IV q 6 hr for 24 hr. May give additional doses during procedures > 2 hours. In cases where infection would be devastating, prophylaxis may continue for 3 to 5 days. *Serious infections of respiratory, GU, or GI tract; skin and soft-tissue infections; bone and joint infections (including osteomyelitis); septicemia; and endocarditiscaused by susceptible organisms —* **Adults:** 500 mg to 1 g IM or IV q 4 to 6 hr. In life-threatening infections, up to 12 g/day. **Children > 3 mo:** 10 to 20 mg/kg IM or IV q 6 hr; dose depends on age, weight, and severity of infection.

- Use cautiously in history of sensitivity to penicillin and in breast-feeding patients.
- Contraindicated with hypersensitivity to drug or other cephalosporins.

cephradine
Velosef
First-generation cephalosporin
Antibiotic
Preg. Risk Category: B

cap: 250, 500 mg; **oral susp:** 125, 250 mg/5 ml

Serious infections caused by susceptible organisms; periop prophylaxis — **Adults:** 250 to 500 mg PO q 6 hr. **Children > 9 mo:** 25 to 50 mg/kg PO daily in divided doses.
Otitis media — **Children:** 75 to 100 mg/kg PO daily. Don't exceed 4 g daily. Any patient, regardless of age and weight, may receive doses up to 1 g qid for severe or chronic infections.

- Use cautiously in impaired renal function or history of sensitivity to penicillin and in breast-feeding patients..
- Contraindicated in hypersensitivity to drug or other cephalosporins

cetirizine hydrochloride
Zyrtec
Selective H$_1$-receptor antagonist
Antihistamine agent
Preg. Risk Category: B

tab: 5, 10 mg

Seasonal allergic rhinitis, perennial allergic rhinitis, chronic urticaria — **Adults and children ≥ 12 yr:** 5 or 10 mg PO daily depending on symptom severity; 5 mg PO daily in renal or hepatic impairment.
Seasonal allergic rhinitis, perennial allergic rhinitis, chronic urticaria — **Children 6 to 11 yr:** 5 or 10 mg (1 or 2 tsp) PO qd depending on symptom severity.

- Use cautiously in renal impairment.
- Contraindicated in hypersensitivity to drug or to hydroxyzine.
- Not recommended for breast-feeding patients.
- Safety in children < age 12 not established.

DRUG/CLASS/CATEGORY	DOSAGE FORMS	INDICATIONS/DOSAGES	KEY PRECAUTIONS
chloral hydrate Aquachloral Supprettes, Dormel‡, Noctec, Novo-Chlorhydrate† *General CNS depressant* *Sedative-hypnotic* Preg. Risk Category: C Controlled Sub. Sched.: IV	*cap:* 250, 500 mg; *syrup:* 250, 500 mg/5 ml; *supp:* 324 mg, 500 mg, 648 mg	*Sedation —* **Adults:** 250 mg PO or PR tid after meals. **Children:** 8.3 mg/kg or 250 mg/m² PO or PR tid. Max daily dosage 500 mg tid. *Insomnia —* **Adults:** 500 mg to 1 g PO or PR 15 to 30 min before bedtime. **Children:** 50 mg/kg or 1.5 g/m² PO or PR 15 to 30 min before bedtime. Max single dose 1 g. *Prep —* **Adults:** 500 mg to 1 g PO or PR 30 min before surgery. *Premedication for EEG —* **Children:** 20 to 25 mg/kg PO or PR.	■ Use with extreme caution in mental depression, suicidal tendencies, or history of drug abuse. ■ Contraindicated in hepatic or renal impairment, severe cardiac disease, or hypersensitivity to drug. Oral administration contraindicated in gastric disorders.
chlorambucil Leukeran *Alkylating agent* *Antineoplastic* Preg. Risk Category: D	*tab (sugar-coated):* 2 mg	*Chronic lymphocytic leukemia; malignant lymphomas including lymphosarcoma, giant follicular lymphoma, and Hodgkin's disease —* **Adults:** 0.1 to 0.2 mg/kg PO daily for 3 to 6 weeks; then adjusted for maintenance (usually 4 to 10 mg daily).	■ Contraindicated in hypersensitivity to drug (or other alkylating agents) or resistance to previous therapy. ■ Use cautiously in history of head trauma or seizures and in patients on drugs that lower seizure threshold.
chloramphenicol AK-Chlor, Chloromycetin Ophthalmic, Chloroptic, Chloroptic S.O.P., Chlorsig†, Fenicol†, Isopto Fenicol‡, Ophthoclor Ophthalmic, Pentamycetin†, Sopamycetin† *Dichloroacetic acid derivative* *Antibiotic* Preg. Risk Category: NR	*powder for ophth. sol:* 25 mg/vial; *ophth. oint:* 1%; *ophth. sol:* 0.5%	*Surface bacterial infection involving conjunctiva or cornea —* **Adults and children:** 1 or 2 drops of solution instilled in eye q 3 to 6 hours or more frequently, if necessary. Or, a small amount of ointment applied to lower conjunctival sac q 3 to 6 hours or more frequently, if necessary. Continued for at least 48 hours after eye appears normal.	■ Use cautiously in impaired renal or hepatic function, acute intermittent porphyria, or G6PD deficiency and in patients taking drugs that suppress bone marrow function. ■ Contraindicated in patients with hypersensitivity to chloramphenicol.
chlordiazepoxide Libritabs **chlordiazepoxide hydrochloride**	*tab:* 5, 10, 25 mg. **hydrochloride —** *cap:* 5,	*Mild to moderate anxiety —* **Adults:** 5 to 10 mg PO tid or qid. **Children > 6 yr:** 5 mg PO bid to qid. Max 10 mg PO bid or tid.	■ Use cautiously in mental depression, porphyria, or hepatic or renal disease.

hydrochloride
Librium, Novopoxide†
Benzodiazepine
Antianxiety agent/anticonvulsant/sedative-hypnotic
Preg. Risk Category: NR
Controlled Sub. Sched.: IV

10, 25 mg; **powder for inj**: 100-mg ampule

Severe anxiety — **Adults:** 20 to 25 mg PO tid or qid.
In geri patients, 5 mg bid to qid.
Withdrawal symptoms of acute alcoholism — **Adults:** 50 to 100 mg PO, IM, or IV; repeat in 2 to 4 hr prn. Max 300 mg daily.
Note: Parenteral form not recommended in children < 12 yr.

- Contraindicated in hypersensitivity to drug.
- Avoid giving to pregnant patients, especially in first trimester.

---

chloroquine hydrochloride
Aralen HCl, Chlorquin‡
chloroquine phosphate
Aralen Phosphate, Chlorquin‡
chloroquine sulfate
Nivaquine‡
4-aminoquinoline
Antimalarial/amebicide/antiinflammatory
Preg. Risk Category: C

hydrochloride — **inj**: 50 mg/ml. **phosphate** — **tab**: 250 mg, 500 mg. **sulfate** — **tab**: 200 mg; **syrup**: 68 mg/5 ml

Acute malarial attacks — **Adults:** 600 mg (base) PO, then 300 mg at 6, 24, and 48 hr. Or 160 to 200 mg (base) IM initially; repeat in 6 hr prn. Switch to PO as soon as possible. **Children:** 10 mg (base)/kg PO, then 5 mg (base)/kg at 6, 24, and 48 hr (max < adult dose). Or 5 mg (base)/kg IM initially; repeated in 6 hr prn. Max 10 mg (base)/kg/24 hr. Switch to PO as soon as possible.
Malaria prophylaxis — **Adults and children:** 5 mg (base)/kg PO (max 300 mg) weekly (begun 2 wk before exposure and continued for 4 to 6 wk after.) If treatment begins after exposure, initial dose doubled in 2 divided doses PO q 6 hr.

- Use with extreme caution in severe GI, neurologic, or blood disorders.
- Use cautiously in hepatic disease, alcoholism, G6PD deficiency, or psoriasis.
- Contraindicated in hypersensitivity to drug, in retinal or visual field changes, or in porphyria.

---

chlorothiazide
Chlotride‡, Diurigen, Diuril
chlorothiazide sodium
Diuril Sodium
Thiazide diuretic
Diuretic/antihypertensive
Preg. Risk Category: C

chlorothiazide — **tab**: 250, 500 mg; **oral susp**: 250 mg/5 ml. **sodium** — **inj**: 500-mg vial

Edema, hypertension — **Adults:** 500 mg to 1 g PO or IV daily or bid.
Diuresis, hypertension — **Children 6 mo to 12 yr:** 10 to 20 mg/kg PO daily or in 2 divided doses; max 1,000 mg/day in children > 2 yr; in children < 2 yr, max dose is 375 mg/day. **Children < 6 mo:** up to 30 mg/kg PO daily in 2 divided doses.

- Contraindicated in anuria or hypersensitivity to other thiazides or sulfonamide-derived drugs.

DRUG / CLASS / CATEGORY	DOSAGE FORMS	INDICATIONS / DOSAGES	KEY PRECAUTIONS
chlorpheniramine maleate Aller-Chlor L, Chlor-Trimeton, Novopheniram‡, Teldrin *Propylamine-derivative antihistamine* *Antihistamine (H₁-receptor antagonist)* Preg. Risk Category: B	**tab:** 4, 8, 12 mg; **tab (chew):** 2 mg; **tab (timed-release):** 8, 12 mg; **cap (timed-release):** 6, 8, 12 mg; **syrup:** 2 mg/5 ml; **inj:** 10, 100 mg/ml	*Rhinitis, allergy symptoms —* **Adults:** 4 mg PO q 4 to 6 hr, not to exceed 24 mg/day; or 8 to 12 mg timed-release PO q 8 to 12 hr, not to exceed 24 mg daily. Or, 5 to 20 mg IM, IV, or SC as single dose. Max 40 mg/24 hr. **Children 6 to 12 yr:** 2 mg PO q 4 to 6 hr, not to exceed 12 mg/day. Alternatively, may give 8 mg timed-release PO hs. **Children 2 to 6 yr:** 1 mg PO q 4 to 6 hr, not to exceed 4 mg daily.	■ Use cautiously in elderly patients and in increased intraocular pressure, hyperthyroidism, CV or renal disease, hypertension, bronchial asthma, urine retention, prostatic hyperplasia, bladder-neck obstruction, and stenosing peptic ulcerations. ■ Contraindicated during acute asthmatic attacks and breast-feeding.
chlorpromazine hydrochloride Chlorpromanyl-5†, Chlorpromanyl-20†, Chlorpromanyl-40†, Ormazine, Thorazine *Aliphatic phenothiazine* *Antipsychotic/antiemetic* Preg. Risk Category: NR	**tab:** 10, 25, 50, 100, 200 mg; **cap (contr-release):** 30, 75, 150, 200, 300 mg; **oral conc:** 30, 100 mg/ml; **syrup:** 10 mg/5 ml; **inj:** 25 mg/ml; **supp:** 25, 100 mg	*Psychosis —* **Adults:** 25 to 75 mg PO qd in 2 to 4 divided doses. Increase by 20 to 50 mg twice weekly until symptoms controlled. May need 800 mg daily. Or, 25 to 50 mg IM q 1 to 4 hr, prn. IM doses gradually increased to max 400 mg q 4 to 6 hr. Switch to PO as soon as possible. **Children ≥ 6 mo:** 0.55 mg/kg PO q 4 to 6 hr or IM q 6 to 8 hr; or 1.1 mg/kg PR q 6 to 8 hr. Max IM in < 5 yr or < 22.7 kg: 40 mg. Max IM in 5 to 12 yr or 22.7 to 45.5 kg: 75 mg. *Nausea and vomiting —* **Adults:** 10 to 25 mg PO q 4 to 6 hr, prn; or 50 to 100 mg PR q 6 to 8 hr, prn; or 25 to 50 mg IM q 3 to 4 hr prn. **Children ≥ 6 mo:** 0.55 mg/kg q 4 to 6 hr or IM q 6 to 8 hr; or 1.1 mg/g PR q 6 to 8 hr. Max IM in < 5 yr or < 22.7 kg: 40 mg. Max IM in 5 to 12 yr or 22.7 to 45.5 kg: 75 mg.	■ Use cautiously in acutely ill or dehydrated children; elderly or debilitated patients; or in hepatic or renal disease, severe CV disease, glaucoma, prostatic hyperplasia, respiratory or seizure disorders, hypocalcemia, reaction to insulin or electroconvulsive therapy, or exposure to extreme heat or cold (including antipyretic therapy) or to organophosphate insecticides. ■ Contraindicated in hypersensitivity to drug or in CNS depression, bone marrow suppression, subcortical damage, and coma.
chlorthalidone Apo-Chlorthalidone†, Hygroton, Novo-Thalidone†, Thalitone, Uridon†	**tab:** 15, 25, 50, 100 mg	*Edema, hypertension —* **Adults:** 25 to 100 mg PO qd, or up to 200 mg PO on alternate days. **Children:** 2 mg/kg or 60 mg/m² PO 3 times/wk.	■ Use cautiously in severe renal disease and impaired hepatic function.

Thiazide-like diuretic *Diuretic/antihypertensive* Preg. Risk Category: B			▪ Contraindicated in anuria or hypersensitivity to thiazides or other sulfonamide-derived drugs.
cholestyramine Cholybar, Prevalite, Questran, Questran Light *Anion exchange resin* *Antilipemic/bile acid sequestrant* Preg. Risk Category: NR	**powder:** 378-g cans, 9-g single-dose pkt.; **tab:** 1 g	*Primary hyperlipidemia or pruritus caused by partial bile obstruction; adjunct for reduction of elevated serum cholesterol in primary hypercholesterolemia* — **Adults:** 4 g qd or bid. Maintenance: 8 to 16 g daily divided into 2 doses. Max 24 g daily.	▪ Use cautiously in predisposition to constipation and in conditions aggravated by constipation, such as severe, symptomatic CAD. ▪ Contraindicated in hypersensitivity to bile-acid sequestering resins and in complete biliary obstruction.
choline magnesium trisalicylate (choline salicylate and magnesium salicylate) Tricosal, Trilisate *Salicylate* *Nonnarcotic analgesic/antipyretic/ anti-inflammatory* Preg. Risk Category: C	**tab:** 500, 750, 1,000 mg salicylate; **sol:** 500 mg salicylate/5 ml	*Rheumatoid arthritis (RA) and other inflammatory conditions* — **Adults:** initially, 1.5 to 2.5 g PO daily as single dose or in 2 or 3 divided doses. Adjust dosage according to response. Maintenance: 1 to 4.5 g daily. *Juvenile RA* — **Children:** 60 to 110 mg/kg/day PO in divided doses (q 6 to 8 hr). *Mild to moderate pain and fever* — **Adults:** 2 to 3 g PO daily in divided doses q 4 to 6 hr. **Children ≤ 37 kg:** 25 mg/kg PO bid. **Children > 37 kg:** 2,250 mg/day.	▪ Use cautiously in renal insufficiency, hepatic impairment, peptic ulcer disease, or gastritis. ▪ Contraindicated in hypersensitivity to drug, hemophilia, bleeding ulcers, and hemorrhagic states. ▪ Don't give to children or teenagers with chickenpox or flulike illness. Febrile, dehydrated children can develop toxicity rapidly.
choline salicylate Arthropan, Teejel† *Salicylate* *Nonnarcotic analgesic/antipyretic/ anti-inflammatory* Preg. Risk Category: NR	**liq:** 870 mg/5 ml; **gel:** 87 mg/g†	*Rheumatoid arthritis, osteoarthritis, mild to moderate pain or fever* — **Adults and children > 12 yr:** ½ to 1 tsp (435 to 870 mg) PO q 4 hr, prn. If tolerated and needed, increase to 8 tsp daily. Not to exceed 8 tsp daily. *Relief of pain from inflamed gums* — **Adults and children > 2 yr:** apply 1 cm of gel to affected area q 3 to 4 hr and hs, prn.	▪ Use cautiously in renal insufficiency, hepatic impairment, peptic ulcer disease, and gastritis. ▪ Contraindicated in hypersensitivity to drug, hemophilia, bleeding ulcers, and hemorrhagic states. ▪ Epidemiologic association with Reye's syndrome; don't give to children or teenagers with chickenpox or flulike illness.

CHOLINE SALICYLATE   51

†Canadian   †Australian

DRUG/CLASS/ CATEGORY	DOSAGE FORMS	INDICATIONS/ DOSAGES	KEY PRECAUTIONS
cidofovir Vistide *Nucleotide analogue* *Antiviral* Preg. Risk Category: C	*inj*: 75 mg/ml in 5-ml vial	*CMV retinitis in patients with AIDS* — **Adults**: initially, 5 mg/kg IV infused over 1 hr once weekly for 2 consecutive wk, then maintenance dosage of 5 mg/kg IV infused over 1 hr once q 2 wk. Must give probenecid and prehydration with 0.9% NaCl solution IV concomitantly (may reduce potential for nephrotoxicity).	▪ Use cautiously in impaired renal function. ▪ Contraindicated in hypersensitivity to drug or history of clinically severe hypersensitivity to probenecid or other sulfur-containing drug. ▪ Don't give as direct intraocular injection. ▪ Don't administer to breast-feeding patients.
cimetidine Tagamet, Tagamet HB, Tagamet HCl, Tagamet Tiltab *Histamine₂-receptor antagonist* *Antiulcer agent* Preg. Risk Category: B	*tab*: 100, 200, 300, 400, 800 mg; *oral liq*: 300 mg/5 ml; *efferv tab*: 800 mg‡; *inj*: 100 mg/ml‡; 300 mg/2 ml; 300 mg in 50 ml 0.9% NaCl solution	*Duodenal ulcer (short-term treatment and maintenance)* — **Adults and children ≥ 16 yr**: 800 mg PO hs. Alternatively, 400 mg PO bid or 300 mg qid with meals and hs. Maintenance therapy: 400 mg hs. Parenteral therapy: 300 mg diluted to 20 ml by IV push over at least 5 min q 6 hr; or 300 mg diluted in 50 ml D₅W or other compatible IV solution by IV infusion over 15 to 20 min q 6 hr; or 300 mg IM q 6 hr (no dilution necessary). Max 2,400 mg daily prn. Alternatively, 900 mg/day (37.5 mg/hr) IV diluted in 100 to 1,000 ml by continuous IV infusion. *Active benign gastric ulceration* — **Adults**: 800 mg PO hs, or 300 mg PO qid (with meals and hs) for up to 6 wk. *Gastroesophageal reflux disease* — **Adults**: 800 mg PO bid or 400 mg qid before meals and hs for up to 12 wk.	▪ Use cautiously in elderly or debilitated patients. ▪ Contraindicated in hypersensitivity to drug.
ciprofloxacin Cipro, Cipro IV, Ciproxin‡ *Fluroquinolone antibiotic* *Antibiotic* Preg. Risk Category: C	*tab (film-coated)*: 250, 500, 750 mg; *infusion (premixed)*: 200 mg in 100 ml	*Mild to moderate UTI caused by susceptible organisms* — **Adults**: 250 mg PO or 200 mg IV q 12 hr. *Severe or complicated UTI or mild to moderate bone, joint, skin, or skin structure infections caused by susceptible organisms* — **Adults**: 500 mg PO or 400 mg IV q 12 hr.	▪ Use cautiously in CNS disorders, such as severe cerebral arteriosclerosis or seizure disorders, and in patients at increased risk for seizures.

	Chronic bacterial prostatitis caused by E. coli *or* P. mirabilis — **Adults:** 500 mg PO q 12 hr for 28 days.	▪ Contraindicated in sensitivity to fluoro-quinolones.
ciprofloxacin hydrochloride Ciloxan *Fluoroquinolone* *Antibacterial agent* Preg. Risk Category: C	**ophth. sol:** 0.3% (base) in 2.5- and 5-ml containers	*Corneal ulcers caused by susceptible organisms* — **Adults and children over 12 years:** 2 drops in the affected eye q 15 minutes for the first 6 hours; then 2 drops q 30 minutes for the remainder of the first day. On days 2, 2 drops hourly. On days 3 to 14, 2 drops q 4 hours. *Bacterial conjunctivitis caused by susceptible organisms* — **Adults and children over 12 years:** 1 or 2 drops into the conjunctival sac of the affected eye q 2 hours while awake for the first 2 days. Then 1 or 2 drops q 4 hours while awake for the next 5 days.	▪ Use cautiously in CNS disorders or patients at risk for seizures. ▪ Contraindicated in sensitivity to fluoro-quinolone antibiotics.
cisapride Propulsid *Serotonin-4 receptor agonist* *GI prokinetic agent* Preg. Risk Category: C	**tab:** 10 mg, 20 mg; **susp:** 1 mg/ml	*Symptoms of nocturnal heartburn caused by gastro-esophageal reflux disease* — **Adults:** initially, 10 mg PO qid 15 minutes before meals and hs. If response is inadequate, increased to 20 mg qid.	
cisplatin (cis-platinum, CDDP) Platamine‡, Platinol, Platinol AQ *Alkylating agent* *Antineoplastic* Preg. Risk Category: D	**inj:** 10-mg and 50-mg vials (lyophilized); 50-mg and 100-mg vials (aqueous)	*Adjunctive therapy in metastatic testicular cancer* — **Adults:** 20 mg/m² IV qd for 5 days. Repeated q 3 wk for 3 cycles or longer. *Adjunctive therapy in metastatic ovarian cancer* — **Adults:** 100 mg/m² IV: repeated q 4 weeks. Or 75 to 100 mg/m² IV once q 4 wk in combination with cy-clophosphamide. *Advanced bladder cancer* — **Adults:** 50 to 70 mg/m² IV q 3 to 4 weeks. Patients who have received other antineoplastic agents or radiation therapy should receive 50 mg/m² q 4 weeks.	▪ Contraindicated in hypersensitivity to drug or to other platinum-containing compounds and in severe renal disease, hearing impair-ment, or myelosuppression.

D₅W, 400 mg in 200 ml D₅W; **inj:** 200, 400 mg	

CISPLATIN 53

DRUG / CLASS / CATEGORY	DOSAGE FORMS	INDICATIONS / DOSAGES	KEY PRECAUTIONS
cladribine (2-chlorodeoxyadeno-sine, CdA) Leustatin *Purine nucleoside analogue Antineoplastic* Preg. Risk Category: D	*inj:* 1 mg/ml, 10-mg vial	*Active hairy cell leukemia* — **Adults:** 0.09 mg/kg daily by continuous IV infusion for 7 days.	▪ Use cautiously in patients with renal or hepatic impairment. ▪ Contraindicated in hypersensitivity to drug.
clarithromycin Biaxin *Macrolide Antibiotic* Preg. Risk Category: C	*tab (film-coat-ed):* 250, 500 mg; *susp:* 125, 250 mg/5 ml	*Pharyngitis or tonsillitis caused by* S. pyogenes — **Adults:** 250 mg PO q 12 hr for 10 days. **Children:** 15 mg/kg/day PO in divided doses q 12 hr for 10 days. *Acute maxillary sinusitis caused by* S. pneumoniae, H. influenzae, *or* M. (Branhamella) catarrhalis — **Adults:** 500 mg PO q 12 hr for 14 days. **Children:** 15 mg/kg/day PO in divided doses q 12 hr for 10 days. M. avium *complex disease in HIV infection* — **Adults:** 500 mg PO q 12 hr, with other antimycobacterial drugs, for life. **Children:** 7.5 mg/kg PO (max 500 mg) q 12 hr, with other antimycobacterial drugs, for life. H. pylori *infection* — **Adults:** 500 mg PO q 8 hr for 14 days with omeprazole 40 mg PO q am. Continue omeprazole (20 mg PO q am) for 28 days.	▪ Use cautiously in hepatic or renal impairment. ▪ Contraindicated in hypersensitivity to erythromycin or other macrolides and in patients receiving astemizole who have preexisting cardiac abnormalities or electrolyte disturbances.
clemastine fumarate Tavist, Tavist-1 *Ethanolamine-derivative antihistamine Antihistamine (H₁-receptor antagonist)* Preg. Risk Category: C	*tab:* 1.34, 2.68 mg; *syrup:* 0.67 mg per 5 ml	*Rhinitis, allergy symptoms* — **Adults and children ≥ 12 yr:** 1.34 mg PO q 12 hr, or 2.68 mg PO qd to tid prn. Don't exceed 8.04 mg/day. **Children 6 to 12 yr:** 0.67 to 1.34 mg PO bid. Don't exceed 4.02 mg/day. Children < 12 years should use only as directed by doctor.	▪ Use cautiously in elderly patients, angle-closure glaucoma, increased IOP, hyperthyroidism, CV or renal disease, hypertension, asthma, prostatic hyperplasia, bladder-neck or pyloroduodenal obstruction, or stenosing peptic ulcerations. ▪ Contraindicated in hypersensitivity, acute asthma, in neonates or premature infants, and in breast-feeding patients.

clindamycin hydrochloride
Cleocin HCl, Dalacin C†‡
clindamycin palmitate hydrochloride
Cleocin Pediatric, Dalacin C Palmitate ‡
clindamycin phosphate
Cleocin Phosphate, Cleocin T, Dalacin C†‡
Lincomycin derivative
Antibiotic
Preg. Risk Category: B

clindamycin hydrochloride — *cap:* 75, 150, 300 mg. clindamycin palmitate hydrochloride — *granules for oral sol:* 75 mg/5 ml. clindamycin phosphate — *inj:* 150 mg base/ml, 300 mg base/2 ml, 600 mg base/4 ml, 900 mg base/6 ml, 9,000 mg base/60 ml; *inj. infusion (in 5% dextrose):* 300, 600, 900 mg (50 ml)

Infections caused by sensitive aerobic and anaerobic organisms — **Adults:** 150 to 450 mg PO q 6 hr; or 300 to 600 mg IM or IV q 6, 8, or 12 hr. **Children >1 mo:** 8 to 20 mg/kg PO daily in divided doses q 6 to 8 hr; or 20 to 40 mg/kg IM or IV daily in divided doses q 6 or 8 hr.

Endocarditis prophylaxis for dental procedures in patients allergic to penicillin — **Adults:** initially, 300 mg PO 1 hr before procedure; then 150 mg 6 hr later. **Children:** initially, 10 mg/kg PO 1 hr before procedure; then half of initial dose 6 hr later.

Pelvic inflammatory disease — **Adults:** 900 mg IV q 8 hr in conjunction with gentamicin. Continue at least 48 hr after symptoms improve; then switch to oral clindamycin 450 mg 5 times daily for total course of 10 to 14 days.

- Use cautiously in neonates and in renal or hepatic disease, asthma, history of GI disease, or significant allergies.
- Contraindicated in hypersensitivity to this drug or lincomycin and in history of ulcerative colitis, regional enteritis, antibiotic-associated colitis, or atopic reactions.
- Doesn't penetrate blood-brain barrier.

---

clobetasol propionate
Dermovate†, Temovate
Topical adrenocorticoid
Anti-inflammatory
Preg. Risk Category: C

cream: 0.05%; *lotion:* 0.05%; *oint:* 0.05%

Inflammation associated with corticosteroid-responsive dermatoses — **Adults:** apply a thin layer to affected skin areas bid, in the morning and evening for a maximum of 14 days. Total dosage should not exceed 50 g weekly.

- Contraindicated in hypersensitivity to corticosteroids.

CLOBETASOL PROPIONATE 55

DRUG/CLASS/CATEGORY	DOSAGE FORMS	INDICATIONS/DOSAGES	KEY PRECAUTIONS
clofazimine Lamprene *Substituted iminophenazine dye Leprostatic* Preg. Risk Category: C	*cap:* 50, 100 mg	*Dapsone-resistant leprosy (Hansen's disease)* — **Adults:** 100 mg PO daily in combination with other antileprotics for 3 yr. Then, clofazimine alone, 100 mg daily. *Erythema nodosum leprosum* — **Adults:** 100 to 200 mg PO daily for up to 3 mo.	▪ Use cautiously in GI dysfunction, such as abdominal pain and diarrhea.
clomiphene citrate Clomid, Milophene, Serophene *Chlorotrianisene derivative Ovulation stimulant* Preg. Risk Category: NR	*tab:* 50 mg	*To induce ovulation* — **Adults:** 50 mg PO daily for 5 days starting on day 5 of the menstrual cycle (first day of menstrual flow is day 1) if bleeding occurs or at any time if patient has not had recent uterine bleeding. If ovulation does not occur, may increase dose to 100 mg PO daily for 5 days as soon as 30 days after previous course. Repeated until conception occurs or until three courses of therapy are completed.	▪ Contraindicated during pregnancy and with undiagnosed abnormal genital bleeding, ovarian cyst not due to polycystic ovarian syndrome, hepatic disease or dysfunction, uncontrolled thyroid or adrenal dysfunction, or presence of organic intracranial lesion.
clomipramine hydrochloride Anafranil *Tricyclic antidepressant Antiobsessional agent* Preg. Risk Category: C	*cap:* 25, 50, 75 mg	*Obsessive-compulsive disorder* — **Adults:** initially, 25 mg PO daily with meals, gradually increased to 100 mg daily in divided doses during first 2 wk. Thereafter, increase to max 250 mg daily in divided doses with meals, prn. After titration, total daily dosage may be given hs. **Children and adolescents:** initially, 25 mg PO daily with meals, gradually increased over first 2 wk to daily max 3 mg/kg or 100 mg in divided doses, whichever is smaller. Max daily dosage 3 mg/kg or 200 mg, whichever is smaller; may be given hs after titration. Periodic reassessment and adjustment necessary.	▪ Use cautiously in history of seizure disorders; in brain damage of varying etiology; in patients receiving other drugs that lower seizure threshold; in patients at risk for suicide; in history of urine retention or angle-closure glaucoma, increased intraocular pressure, CV disease, impaired hepatic or renal function, or hyperthyroidism; in adrenal medulla tumors; in patients receiving thyroid medication or electroconvulsive therapy; and in patients undergoing elective surgery. ▪ Contraindicated in hypersensitivity to drug or other TCAs, within 14 days of MAO inhibitor use, and during acute recovery period after MI.

clonazepam
Klonopin
Benzodiazepine
Anticonvulsant
Preg. Risk Category: NR
Controlled Sub. Sched.: IV

tab: 0.5, 1, 2 mg

Lennox-Gastaut syndrome; atypical absence seizures; akinetic and myoclonic seizures — **Adults:** initially, not to exceed 1.5 mg PO daily in 3 divided doses. May increase by 0.5 to 1 mg q 3 days until seizures controlled. If given in unequal doses, give largest dose hs. Max recommended daily dosage 20 mg. **Children ≤ 10 yr or 30 kg:** initially, 0.01 to 0.03 mg/kg PO daily (not to exceed 0.05 mg/kg daily), in 2 or 3 divided doses. Increase by 0.25 to 0.5 mg PO q third day to max maintenance dosage: 0.1 to 0.2 mg/ kg daily as needed.

- Use cautiously in mixed seizure type; may trigger generalized tonic-clonic seizures. Also use cautiously in children and in chronic respiratory disease or open-angle glaucoma.
- Contraindicated in significant hepatic disease, sensitivity to benzodiazepines, or acute angle-closure glaucoma.

clonidine
Catapres-TTS
clonidine hydrochloride
Catapres, Dixarit‡
Centrally acting adrenergic agent
Antihypertensive
Preg. Risk Category: C

clonidine — *transderm:* TTS-1 (releases 0.1 mg/24 hr), TTS-2 (releases 0.2 mg/24 hr), TTS-3 (releases 0.3 mg/24 hr); **clonidine hydrochloride** —*tab:* 0.025 mg ‡, 0.1 mg, 0.2 mg, 0.3 mg

Essential and renal hypertension — **Adults:** initially, 0.1 mg PO bid; then increase by 0.1 to 0.2 mg daily on weekly basis. Usual range 0.2 to 0.8 mg daily in divided doses. Infrequently, dosages up to 2.4 mg daily used. Or, as transdermal patch applied to non-hairy area of intact skin on upper arm or torso q 7 days, starting with 0.1-mg system and titrated with another 0.1-mg or larger system.

- Use cautiously in severe coronary insufficiency, recent MI, cerebrovascular disease, chronic renal failure, or impaired liver function.
- Contraindicated in hypersensitivity to drug. Transdermal form contraindicated in hypersensitivity to any component of adhesive layer.

clorazepate dipotassium
Apo-Clorazepate†, Gen-XENE, Novoclopate†, Tranxene, Tranxene-SD, Tranxene-T-Tab

tab: 3.75, 7.5, 11.25, 15, 22.5 mg; *cap:* 3.75, 7.5, 15 mg

Acute alcohol withdrawal — **Adults:** day 1: 30 mg PO initially, then 30 to 60 mg PO in divided doses; day 2: 45 to 90 mg PO in divided doses; day 3: 22.5 to 45 mg PO in divided doses; day 4: 15 to 30 mg PO in di-vided doses; then gradually reduce dosage to 7.5 to

- Contraindicated in hypersensitivity to drug or other benzodiazepines and acute angle-closure glaucoma.
- Avoid giving during pregnancy, especially first trimester.

(continued)

†Canadian ‡Australian

DRUG/CLASS/CATEGORY	DOSAGE FORMS	INDICATIONS/DOSAGES	KEY PRECAUTIONS
clorazepate dipotassium *(continued)* *Benzodiazepine* *Antianxiety agent/anticonvulsant/sedative-hypnotic* Preg. Risk Category: D Controlled Sub. Sched.: IV		15 mg daily. Max recommended daily dosage 90 mg. *Adjunct in partial seizure disorder* — **Adults and children > 12 yr:** Max recommended initial dosage 7.5 mg PO tid. Increase no more than 7.5 mg/wk to max 90 mg daily. **Children 9 to 12 yr:** max recommended initial dosage 7.5 mg PO bid. Increase no more than 7.5 mg/wk, to max 60 mg daily.	▪ Use cautiously in suicidal tendencies, renal or hepatic impairment, or history of drug abuse.
clotrimazole Canestent, Gyne-Lotrimin, Lotrimin, Mycelex, Mycelex-7, Mycelex-G, Mycelex-OTC *Synthetic imidazole derivative* *Antifungal* Preg. Risk Category: B	**vag tab:** 500 mg; **top cream:** 1%; **top lotion:** 1%; **top sol:** 1%; **loz:** 10 mg	*Superficial fungal infections (tinea pedis, tinea cruris, tinea corporis, or tinea versicolor; candidiasis)* — **Adults and children:** apply thinly and massage into affected and surrounding area, morning and evening, for 2 to 4 weeks. If no improvement occurs after 4 weeks, patient should be reevaluated. *Vulvovaginal candidiasis* — **Adults:** two 100-mg vaginal tablets inserted daily hs for 7 consecutive days, or one 500-mg vaginal tablet daily hs for 1 day; or 1 applicatorful vaginal cream daily hs for 7 days. *Oropharyngeal candidiasis treatment* — **Adults and children 3 years and older:** dissolve lozenge over 15 to 30 minutes in mouth five times daily for 14 consecutive days. *Prevention of oropharyngeal candidiasis in patients immunocompromised by such conditions as chemotherapy, radiotherapy, or steroid therapy in the treatment of leukemia, solid tumors, or renal transplantation* — **Adults and children:** dissolve lozenge over 15 to 30 minutes in mouth three times daily for duration of chemotherapy or until steroid is reduced to maintenance levels.	▪ Contraindicated in hypersensitivity or ophthalmic use.

cloxacillin sodium Alcox‡, Apo-Cloxi†, Cloxapen, Novo-Cloxin†, Tegopen *Penicillinase-resistant penicillin* *Antibiotic* Preg. Risk Category: B	**cap:** 250, 500 mg; **oral sol:** 125 mg/5 ml (after reconstitution)	*Systemic infections caused by penicillinase-producing staphylococci* — **Adults and children > 20 kg:** 250 to 500 mg PO q 6 hr. **Children ≤ 20 kg:** 50 to 100 mg/kg PO daily in divided doses q 6 hr.	▪ Use cautiously in other drug allergies or in mononucleosis. ▪ Contraindicated in hypersensitivity to drug or other penicillins.
clozapine Clozaril *Tricyclic dibenzodiazepine derivative* *Antipsychotic* Preg. Risk Category: B	**tab:** 25, 100 mg	*Schizophrenia in severely ill patients unresponsive to other therapies* — **Adults:** initially, 12.5 mg PO qd or bid, titrated upward at 25 to 50 mg daily (if tolerated) to 300 to 450 mg daily by end of 2 wk. Individual dosage based on clinical response, patient tolerance, and adverse reactions. Don't increase subsequent dosage more than once or twice weekly, and don't exceed 100 mg. Many patients respond to dosage of 300 to 600 mg daily, but some may need up to 900 mg. Don't exceed 900 mg daily.	▪ Use cautiously in prostatic hyperplasia or angle-closure glaucoma, hepatic or renal impairment, or cardiac disease or in patients receiving general anesthesia. ▪ Contraindicated in uncontrolled epilepsy; myelosuppressive disorders; history of clozapine-induced agranulocytosis; WBC count < 3,500/mm³; severe CNS depression or coma; and in patients taking other drugs that suppress bone marrow function.
codeine phosphate Paveral **codeine sulfate** *Opioid* *Analgesic/antitussive* Preg. Risk Category: C Controlled Sub. Sched.: II	**codeine phosphate — oral sol:** 15 mg/5 ml, 10 mg/ml; **inj:** 30 mg/ml; **sol tablets:** 30, 60 mg. **codeine sulfate — tab:** 15, 30, 60 mg	*Mild to moderate pain* — **Adults:** 15 to 60 mg PO or 15 to 60 mg (phosphate) SC, IM, or IV q 4 to 6 hr, prn. **Children > 1 yr:** 0.5 mg/kg PO, SC, or IM q 4 hr, prn. *Nonproductive cough* — **Adults:** 10 to 20 mg PO q 4 to 6 hr. Max 120 mg/day. **Children 6 to 12 yr:** 5 to 10 mg PO q 4 to 6 hr. Max 60 mg/day. **Children 2 to 6 yr:** 2.5 to 5 mg PO q 4 to 6 hr. Don't exceed 30 mg/day.	▪ Use cautiously in head injury, increased ICP, increased CSF pressure, hepatic or renal disease, hypothyroidism, Addison's disease, acute alcoholism, seizures, severe CNS depression, bronchial asthma, COPD, respiratory depression, and shock. Use with extreme caution in elderly or debilitated patients. ▪ Contraindicated in hypersensitivity to drug.
colchicine Colchicine MR‡, Colgout‡, Colsalide, Novocolchicine† *Colchicum autumnale alkaloid*	**inj:** 1 mg (1/60 grain)/2 ml ampule; **tab:**	*Prevention of acute gout attacks as prophylactic or maintenance therapy* — **Adults:** 0.5 or 0.6 mg PO daily. Dosage and its frequency may vary with severity and frequency of attacks.	▪ Contraindicated in hypersensitivity, blood dyscrasias, or serious CV, renal, or GI disease.

(continued)

DRUG/CLASS/ CATEGORY	DOSAGE FORMS	INDICATIONS/ DOSAGES	KEY PRECAUTIONS
colchicine *(continued)* *Antigout agent* Preg. Risk Category: C (oral), D (IV)	0.6 mg (1/100 grain), 0.5 mg (1/120 grain) as sugar-coat-ed granules	*Prevention of gout attacks in patients undergoing surgery —* **Adults:** 0.5 to 0.6 mg PO tid 3 days before and 3 days after surgery. *Acute gout, acute gouty arthritis —* **Adults:** 0.5 to 1.3 mg PO, then 0.5 or 0.6 mg q 1 to 2 hours until pain is relieved; nausea, vomiting, or diarrhea ensues; or max 8 mg is reached. Or, 2 mg IV, then 0.5 mg IV q 6 hours if necessary. Total IV dosage over 24 hours (one course of treatment) should not exceed 4 mg.	▪ Use cautiously in elderly or debilitated pa-tients and in those with early signs of CV, renal, or GI disease.
colestipol hydrochloride Colestid *Anion exchange resin* *Antilipemic* Preg. Risk Category: NR	**granules:** 300- and 500-g bot-tles, 5-g pkt; **tab:** 1 g	*Primary hypercholesterolemia —* **Adults:** granules: 5 to 30 g PO qd or in divided doses; tab: 2 to 16 g/day given once or in divided doses.	▪ Use cautiously in predisposition to constipa-tion and in conditions aggravated by consti-pation, such as severe, symptomatic CAD. ▪ Contraindicated in hypersensitivity reactions to bile-acid sequestering resins.
corticotropin (adreno-corticotropic hormone, ACTH) ACTH, Acthar **repository corticotropin** Acthar Gel (H.P.)†, ACTH Gel, H.P. Acthar Gel *Anterior pituitary hormone* *Diagnostic aid/replacement hor-mone/multiple sclerosis and non-suppurative thyroiditis treatment* Preg. Risk Category: C	**aqueous inj:** 25, 40 unit/vial; **repository inj:** 40, 80 units/ml	*Diagnostic test of adrenocortical function —* **Adults:** 40 units IV infusion q 12 hr for 48 hr; or IM q 12 hr for 1 to 2 days; or 10 to 25 units aqueous form in 500 ml of D_5W IV over 8 hr, between blood samplings. Individual dosages vary with adrenal glands' sensitivi-ty to stimulation and with specific disease. Infants and younger children require larger doses per kg. *For therapeutic use —* **Adults:** 40 units aqueous form SC or IM in 4 divided doses; or 40 to 80 units q 24 to 72 hr (repository form).	▪ Use cautiously in pregnant patients, women of childbearing age, patients being immu-nized, and in latent TB or tuberculin reactivity, hypothyroidism, cirrhosis, renal insufficiency, acute gouty arthri-tis, psychotic tendencies, ocular herpes simplex, nonspecific ulcerative colitis, diverticulitis, thromboembolic disorders, seizures, uncon-trolled hypertension, or myasthenia gravis. ▪ Contraindicated in peptic ulcer, scleroder-ma, osteoporosis, systemic fungal infec-tions, ocular herpes simplex, peptic ulcera-tion, heart failure, hypertension, sensitivity to pork and pork products, adrenocortical hyperfunction or primary insufficiency, Cushing's syndrome, or recent surgery.

cortisone acetate
Cortate‡, Cortone Acetate
Glucocorticoid/mineralocorticoid
Anti-inflammatory/replacement
therapy
Preg. Risk Category: C

tab: 5, 10, 25
mg; ***inj (susp):***
50 mg/ml

Adrenal insufficiency, allergy, inflammation — **Adults:**
25 to 300 mg PO or 20 to 300 mg IM daily. Dosages
highly individualized, depending on disease severity.

- Use cautiously in GI ulcer, renal disease, recent MI, hypertension, osteoporosis, diabetes, hypothyroidism, cirrhosis, diverticulitis, nonspecific ulcerative colitis, recent intestinal anastomoses, thromboembolism, seizures, myasthenia gravis, heart failure, TB, ocular herpes simplex, emotional instability, or psychotic tendencies.
- Contraindicated in hypersensitivity and in systemic fungal infections.

cosyntropin
Cortrosyn
Anterior pituitary hormone
Diagnostic agent
Preg. Risk Category: C

inj: 0.25 mg-
vial

Diagnostic test of adrenocortical function — **Adults**
and children ≥ 2 yr: 0.25 IM or IV (unless label prohibits IV route) between blood samplings. **Children <
2 yr:** 0.125 mg IM or IV.

- Use cautiously in hypersensitivity to natural corticotropin.
- Contraindicated in hypersensitivity to drug.

co-trimoxazole
(sulfamethoxazole-
trimethoprim)
Apo-Sulfatrim†, Bactrim, Bactrim
DS, Bactrim IV Infusion, Cotrim,
Novotrimel†, Protrin†, Roubac†,
Septra, Septra DS, Septra IV Infusion, SMZ-TMP, Sulfatrim, UroPlus
DS, UroPlus SS
Sulfonamide and folate antagonist
Antibiotic
Preg. Risk Category: C

tab: trimeth.
80 mg and sul-
fameth. 400
mg; trimeth.
160 mg and
sulfameth. 800
mg; ***susp:***
trimeth. 40 mg
and sulfameth.
200 mg/5 ml;
inj: trimeth. 80
mg and sul-
fameth. 400
mg/5 ml

UTI and shigellosis — **Adults:** 1 DS or 2 reg.-strength
tab PO q 12 hr for 10 to 14 days or 5 days for shigellosis. Or, 8 to 10 mg/kg IV qd in 2 to 4 divided doses ≤
14 days (5 days for shigellosis). Max 960 mg qd. **Children > 2 months:** 8 mg/kg trimeth and 40 mg/kg sulfameth PO qd in 2 divided doses q 12 hr (10 days for
UTI; 5 for shigellosis). *Otitis media* — **Children > 2
months:** 8 mg/kg trimeth and 40 mg/kg sulfameth PO
qd, in 2 divided doses q 12 hr for 10 days. *Pneumocystis carinii pneumonitis* — **Adults and children > 2
months:** 15 to 20 mg/kg trimeth and 75 to 100 mg/kg
sulfameth PO qd in divided doses, q 6 to 8 hr for 14 to
21 days. *Chronic bronchitis* — **Adults:** 1 DS or 2 reg.-
strength tab q 12 hr for 14 days. *Traveler's diarrhea* —
Adults: 1 DS or 2 reg.-strength tab q 12 hr for 5 days.

- Use cautiously in impaired renal or hepatic function, severe allergies, severe bronchial asthma, G6PD deficiency, or blood dyscrasia. Dosages adjusted for impaired renal function.
- Contraindicated in hypersensitivity to trimethoprim or sulfonamides, severe renal impairment, porphyria, megaloblastic anemia caused by folate deficiency, at-term pregnancy, and in breast-feeding women and children under 2 months.

DRUG / CLASS / CATEGORY	DOSAGE FORMS	INDICATIONS / DOSAGES	KEY PRECAUTIONS
cromolyn sodium (sodium cromoglycate) Crolom, Intal, Intal Aerosol Spray, Intal Nebulizer Solution, Nasalcrom *Chromone derivative* *Mast cell stabilizer/antiasthmatic* Preg. Risk Category: B	*cap (for oral sol):* 100 mg; *aerosol:* 800 mcg/metered spray; *nasal sol:* 5.2 mg/metered spray (40 mg/ml); *sol (for nebulization):* 20 mg/2 ml; *ophth sol:* 4%	*Mild to moderate persistent asthma* — **Adults and children ≥ 5 yr:** 2 metered sprays using inhaler qid at regular intervals. Alternatively, 20 mg via nebulization qid at regular intervals. *Prevention and treatment of seasonal and perennial allergic rhinitis* — **Adults and children > 5 yr:** 1 spray in each nostril tid or qid, up to 6 times daily. *Prevention of exercise-induced bronchospasm* — **Adults and children ≥ 5 yr:** 2 metered sprays inhaled no more than 1 hr before anticipated exercise. *Conjunctivitis* — **Adults and children ≥ 4 yr:** 1 to 2 drops in each eye 4 to 6 times daily at regular intervals.	▪ Use inhalation form cautiously in CAD or history of arrhythmias. ▪ Use cautiously in children. Use of oral inhalation solution *not* recommended in children < 2 yr; powder or aerosol for oral inhalation not recommended in children < 5 yr; ophthalmic solution not recommended in children < 4 yr; nasal solution not recommended in children < 6 yr. ▪ Contraindicated in acute asthma attacks, status asthmaticus, and hypersensitivity to drug.
cyanocobalamin (vitamin B₁₂) Anacobin†, Bedoz†, Crystamine, Crysti-12, Cyanoject Crysti-12, Cyanoject **hydroxocobalamin (vitamin B₁₂)** Codroxomin, Hydrobexan, Hydro-Cobex, Hydro-Crysti-12, LA-12 *Water soluble vitamin* *Vitamin/nutritional supplement* Preg. Risk Category: NR	**cyanocobalamin — *inj*:** 30, 100 mcg/ml, 1,000 mcg/ml; **hydroxocobalamin — *inj*:** 100, 1,000 mcg/ml	*Vitamin B₁₂ deficiency* — **Adults:** 30 mcg hydroxocobalamin IM daily for 5 to 10 days, depending on severity. Maint.: 100 to 200 mcg IM q mo. **Children:** 1 to 5 mg hydroxocobalamin spread over ≥ 2 wk in doses of 100 mcg IM, depending on severity. Maint.: 30 to 50 mcg/mo IM. *Pernicious anemia or vitamin B₁₂ malabsorption* — **Adults:** 100 mcg cyanocobalamin IM or SC qd for 6 to 7 days, then 100 mcg IM or SC q mo. **Children:** 30 to 50 mcg IM or SC qd over ≥ 2 wk; then 100 mcg IM or SC q mo for life. *Methylmalonic aciduria* — **Neonates:** 1,000 mcg cyanocobalamin IM daily.	▪ Contraindicated in hypersensitivity to vitamin B₁₂ or cobalt and in early Leber's disease. ▪ Use cautiously in anemic patients with cardiac, pulmonary, or hypertensive disease and those with severe vitamin B₁₂-dependent deficiencies.
cyclobenzaprine hydrochloride Flexeril *Tricyclic antidepressant derivative*	*tab:* 10 mg	*Short-term treatment of muscle spasm* — **Adults:** 10 mg PO tid. Max 60 mg daily; max duration of treatment 2 to 3 wk.	▪ Use cautiously in history of urine retention, acute angle-closure glaucoma, or increased IOP and in elderly or debilitated patients.

Skeletal muscle relaxant
Preg. Risk Category: B

- Contraindicated < 14 days of MAO inhibitor therapy; during acute recovery phase of MI; and in hyperthyroidism, hypersensitivity, heart block, arrhythmias, conduction disturbances, or heart failure.

cyclopentolate hydrochloride
AK-Pentolate, Cyclogyl
Anticholinergic agent
Cycloplegic mydriatic
Preg. Risk Category: NR

ophth sol: 0.5, 1, 2%

Diagnostic procedures requiring mydriasis and cycloplegia — **Adults:** 1 or 2 drops of 0.5%, 1%, or 2% solution instilled into the eyes followed by 1 or 2 drops in 5 to 10 minutes, if needed. **Children:** 1 drop of 0.5%, 1%, or 2% solution instilled into each eye, followed in 5 to 10 minutes with 1 drop 0.5% or 1% solution, if necessary.

- Use cautiously in children, elderly, and patients with increased intraocular pressure.
- Contraindicated in glaucoma, hypersensitivity to drug or belladonna alkaloids, or adhesions between iris and lens.

cyclophosphamide
Cycloblastin‡, Cytoxan, Cytoxan Lyophilized, Endoxan-Asta‡, Neosar‡, Procytox†
Alkylating agent
Antineoplastic
Preg. Risk Category: D

tab: 25 mg, 50 mg; **inj:** 100-mg, 200-mg, 500-mg, 1-g, 2-g vials

Breast and ovarian cancers; Hodgkin's disease; chronic lymphocytic leukemia; chronic myelocytic leukemia; acute lymphoblastic leukemia; acute myelocytic and monocytic leukemia; neuroblastoma; retinoblastoma; malignant lymphoma; multiple myeloma; mycosis fungoides; sarcoma — **Adults and children:** initially, 40 to 50 mg/kg IV in divided doses over 2 to 5 days. Or, 10 to 15 mg/kg IV q 7 to 10 days, 3 to 5 mg/kg IV twice weekly, or 1 to 5 mg/kg PO daily, depending on patient tolerance.
"Minimal change" nephrotic syndrome in children — **Children:** 2.5 to 3 mg/kg PO daily for 60 to 90 days.

- Contraindicated in hypersensitivity or severe bone marrow suppression.
- Use cautiously in impaired renal or hepatic function, leukopenia, thrombocytopenia, or malignant cell infiltration of bone marrow and in patients who have recently undergone radiation therapy or chemotherapy.

cyclosporine (cyclosporin)
Neoral, Sandimmun‡, Sandimmune
Polypeptide antibiotic
Immunosuppressant
Preg. Risk Category: C

cap: 25 mg, 50 mg, 100 mg; **oral sol:** 100 mg/ml; **inj:** 50 mg/ml

Prophylaxis of organ rejection in kidney, liver, or heart transplantation — **Adults and children:** 15 mg/kg PO 4 to 12 hours before transplantation and continued daily postoperatively for 1 to 2 weeks. Then dosage reduced by 5% each wk to maintenance level of 5 to 10 mg/kg/day. Or, 5 to 6 mg/kg IV concentrate 4 to 12 hours before transplantation. Postoperatively, dosage repeated daily until patients can tolerate oral form.

- Contraindicated in hypersensitivity to drug or polyoxyethylated castor oil.

†Canadian ‡Australian

DRUG/CLASS/ CATEGORY	DOSAGE FORMS	INDICATIONS/ DOSAGES	KEY PRECAUTIONS
cysteamine bitartrate Cystagon *Aminothiol* *Cystine depletor* Preg. Risk Category: C	*cap:* 50 mg, 150 mg	*Management of nephropathic cystinosis* — **Adults and children > 12 yr and weighing > 50 kg:** one-fourth to one-sixth of the maintenance dosage, then increased over 4 to 6 wk to achieve maint. dosage. Maint: 2 g (free base) PO in 4 divided doses. **Children ≤ 12 yr:** one-fourth to one-sixth of maint. dosage, then increased over 4 to 6 wk to achieve maint. dosage. Maint: 1.3 g/m² (free base) PO qd in 4 divided doses.	▪ Contraindicated in hypersensitivity to cysteamine or penicillamine.
cytarabine (ara-C, cytosine arabinoside) Alexant, Cytosart, Cytosar-U *Antimetabolite* *Antineoplastic* Preg. Risk Category: D	*inj:* 100-mg, 500-mg, 1-g, 2-g vials	*Acute nonlymphocytic leukemia, acute lymphocytic leukemia, blast phase of chronic myelocytic leukemia* — **Adults and children:** 100 mg/m² daily by continuous IV infusion or 100 mg/m² IV q 12 hours. Given for 7 days and repeated q 2 weeks. For maintenance, 1 mg/kg SC once or twice a week. *Meningeal leukemia* — **Adults and children:** from 5 mg/m² to 75 mg/m² intrathecally. Frequency varies from once a day for 4 days to once q 4 days.	▪ Contraindicated in hypersensitivity to drug. ▪ Use cautiously in impaired hepatic function, hepatic or renal compromise, gout, or myelosuppression.
cytomegalovirus immune globulin (human), intravenous (CMV-IGIV) CytoGam *Immune globulin* *Immune serum* Preg. Risk Category: C	*inj:* 2.5 g as lyophilized powder with 50 ml sterile water (supplied)	*To attenuate primary CMV disease in seronegative kidney transplant recipients who receive a kidney from CMV seropositive donor* — **Adults:** admin. IV based on time after transplantation: within 72 hr, 150 mg/kg; 2, 4, 6, and 8 wk after: 100 mg/kg; 12 and 16 wk after: 50 mg/kg. Initial dose: 15 mg/kg/hour. Increased to 30 mg/kg/hour after 30 min if no untoward reactions, then to 60 mg/kg/hour after another 30 min if no reactions. Volume max 75 ml/hour. Add. doses may be given at 15 mg/kg/hour for 15 minutes, increasing q 15 min in steps to 60 mg/kg/hour.	▪ Contraindicated in sensitivity to other human immunoglobulin preparations or with selective immunoglobulin A (IgA) deficiency.

d

dactinomycin (actinomycin D) Cosmegen *Antibiotic antineoplastic (cell cycle-phase nonspecific) Antineoplastic* Preg. Risk Category: C	***inj:*** 500-mcg vial	Dosage and indications vary. *Sarcoma, trophoblastic tumors in women, testicular cancer* — **Adults:** 500 mcg IV qd for 5 days. Max 15 mcg/kg/day, or 400 to 600 mcg/m²/day for 5 days. *Wilms' tumor, rhabdomyosarcoma, Ewing's sarcoma* — **Children:** 10 to 15 mcg/kg or 450 mcg/m²/day IV for 5 days. Max 500 mcg/day. Or 2.5 mg/m² IV in divided daily doses over 7 days. May repeat in adults or children after bone marrow recovery.	• Contraindicated in chickenpox or herpes zoster.

dalteparin sodium Fragmin *Low-molecular-weight heparin Anticoagulant* Preg. Risk Category: B	***syringe:*** 2,500 anti-factor Xa IU/0.2 ml	*Prophylaxis against DVT in patients undergoing abdominal surgery who are at risk for thromboembolic complications* — **Adults:** 2,500 IU SC daily, starting 1 to 2 hr before surgery and repeated qd for 5 to 10 days postop.	• Use cautiously in history of heparin-induced thrombocytopenia or in severe uncontrolled hypertension, bacterial endocarditis, congenital or acquired bleeding disorders, active ulceration and angiodysplastic GI disease, hemorrhagic CVA, or shortly after brain, spinal, or ophth surg; in bleeding diathesis, thrombocytopenia, or platelet defects; severe liver or kidney insufficiency; hypertensive or diabetic retinopathy; or recent GI bleeding. • Contraindicated in hypersensitivity to drug, heparin, or pork products; in active major bleeding; and in thrombocytopenia associated with positive in vitro tests for antiplatelet antibody in presence of drug.

danaparoid sodium Orgaran *Glycosaminoglycan Anticoagulant/antithrombotic* Preg. Risk Category: B	***amp:*** 750 anti-Xa units/0.6 ml; ***syringe:*** 750 anti-Xa units/0.6 ml	*Prophylaxis against postop DVT in patients undergoing elective hip replacement surgery* — **Adults:** 750 anti-Xa units SC bid starting 1 to 4 hr preop, and then not sooner than 2 hr after surgery. Treatment continued for 7 to 10 days postop or until risk of DVT diminished.	• Contraindicated in hypersensitivity to drug or pork products, severe hemorrhagic diathesis, major bleeding, or thrombocytopenia with positive in vitro tests for antiplatelet antibody in presence of drug. • Contains sodium sulfite (can cause allergic reactions, particularly in asthmatics).

DANAPAROID SODIUM 65

†Canadian ‡Australian

DRUG / CLASS / CATEGORY	DOSAGE FORMS	INDICATIONS / DOSAGES	KEY PRECAUTIONS
danazol Cyclomen†, Danocrine Androgen Antiestrogen/androgen Preg. Risk Category: X	**cap:** 50, 100, 200 mg	*Mild endometriosis* — **Women:** initially, 100 to 200 mg PO bid uninterrupted for 3 to 6 mo; may continue for 9 mo. Subsequent dosage based on patient response. *Moderate to severe endometriosis* — **Women:** 400 mg PO bid uninterrupted for 3 to 6 mo; may continue for 9 mo. *Fibrocystic breast disease* — **Women:** 100 to 400 mg PO daily in 2 divided doses uninterrupted for 2 to 6 mo.	▪ Use cautiously in seizure disorders or migraine headache. ▪ Contraindicated in undiagnosed abnormal genital bleeding, porphyria, or impaired renal, cardiac, or hepatic function; during pregnancy; and in breast-feeding patients. ▪ Avoid use in women of childbearing age until pregnancy ruled out.
dantrolene sodium Dantrium *Hydantoin derivative* Skeletal muscle relaxant Preg. Risk Category: NR	**cap:** 25, 50, 100 mg; **inj:** 20 mg/vial	*Spasticity and sequelae secondary to severe chronic disorders (such as multiple sclerosis, cerebral palsy, spinal cord injury, CVA)* — **Adults:** 25 mg PO qd. Increase gradually in 25-mg increments, up to 100 mg bid to qid, to max 400 mg qd. **Children:** initially, 0.5 mg/kg PO bid; increase to tid, then qid. Increase prn by 0.5 mg/kg qd to 3 mg/kg bid to qid, to max 100 mg qid.	▪ Use cautiously in severely impaired cardiac or pulmonary function or preexisting hepatic disease, in women (especially those taking estrogen), and in patients > 35 yr. ▪ Contraindicated in patients who use spasticity to maintain motor function, in upper motor neuron disorders, for spasms in rheumatic disorders, in active hepatic disease, and in breast-feeding patients. ▪ Contraindicated in combination with verapamil in management of malignant hyperthermia.
dapsone Avlosulfon†, Dapsone 100‡ *Synthetic sulfone* Antileprotic/antimalarial Preg. Risk Category: C	**tab:** 25, 100 mg	*All forms of leprosy (Hansen's disease)* — **Adults:** 100 mg PO daily, indefinitely; give with rifampin 600 mg PO daily for 6 mo. **Children:** 1.4 mg/kg PO daily for min 3 yr. *Dermatitis herpetiformis* — **Adults:** 50 mg PO daily; increase to 300 mg daily prn.	▪ Use cautiously in chronic renal, hepatic, or CV disease; refractory anemia; and G6PD deficiency. ▪ Contraindicated in hypersensitivity to drug.

daunorubicin hydrochloride Cerubidin†, Cerubidine *Antibiotic antineoplastic (cell cycle–phase nonspecific) Antineoplastic* Preg. Risk Category: D	*inj:* 20-mg vial	Dosage and indications vary. *Remission induction in acute nonlymphocytic (myelogenous, monocytic, erythroid) leukemia —* **Adults:** in combination, 30 to 45 mg/m²/day IV on days 1, 2, and 3 of 1st course and on days 1 and 2 of subsequent courses with cytarabine infusions. *Remission induction in acute lymphocytic leukemia —* **Adults:** in combination, 45 mg/m²/day IV on days 1, 2, and 3 of 1st course. **Children ≥ 2 yr:** 25 mg/m² IV on day 1 q 1 wk, for up to 6 wk, if needed. **Children < 2 yr or BSA < 0.5 m²:** dose calculated based on body weight (1 mg/kg).	▪ Use cautiously in myelosuppression or impaired cardiac, renal, or hepatic function.
deferoxamine mesylate Desferal, Desferal Mesylate *Chelating agent Heavy metal antagonist* Preg. Risk Category: C	*powder for inj:* 500 mg	*Adjunctive treatment of acute iron intoxication —* **Adults and children:** 1 g IM, then 500 mg IM for 2 doses q 4 hr; then 500 mg IM q 4 to 12 hr. Max 6 g/24 hr. Give IV by slow inf (15 mg/kg/hr or less) only in CV collapse. *Chronic iron overload from multiple transfusions —* **Adults and children:** 500 mg to 1 g IM qd and 2 g by slow IV infusion in separate solution along with each unit of blood transfused. Max 6 g qd. Or, 20 to 40 mg/kg/day via SC infusion pump.	▪ Use cautiously in impaired renal function. ▪ Contraindicated in severe renal disease or anuria.
demecarium bromide Humorsol *Cholinesterase inhibitor Antiglaucoma agent* Preg. Risk Category: X	*ophth sol:* 0.125%, 0.25%	*Acute angle-closure glaucoma after iridectomy; primary open-angle glaucoma —* **Adults:** 1 drop instilled qd or bid. *Treatment of convergent strabismus (uncomplicated) —* **Adults:** 1 drop qd for 2 to 3 wk, then 1 drop q 2 days for 3 to 4 wk. After reevaluation, 1 drop once or twice weekly to once q 2 days per condition. Reevaluate q 4 to 12 wk; adjust dosage prn. Discontinue after 4 mo if dosage of 1 drop q 2 days required. *Diagnosis of convergent strabismus —* **Adults:** 1 drop instilled daily for 2 wk, then 1 drop q 2 days for 2 to 3 wk.	▪ Use cautiously in history or risk of retinal detachment, marked vagotonia, bronchial asthma, spastic GI conditions, urinary tract obstruction, peptic ulcer, severe bradycardia, hypotension, hypertension, hyperthyroidism, acute cardiac failure, recent MI, epilepsy, marked vasomotor instability, parkinsonism, or with corneal abrasion. ▪ Contraindicated in hypersensitivity to drug, acute angle-closure glaucoma before iridectomy, and other forms of glaucoma (except primary open-angle glaucoma).

DEMECARIUM BROMIDE 67

†Canadian ‡Australian

DRUG/CLASS/ CATEGORY	DOSAGE FORMS	INDICATIONS/ DOSAGES	KEY PRECAUTIONS
demeclocycline hydrochloride Declomycin, Ledermycin‡ *Tetracycline antibiotic* Antibiotic Preg. Risk Category: D	*film-coated* **tab:** 150, 300 mg; **cap:** 150 mg	*Infections caused by susceptible gram-pos and gram-neg organisms, rickettsiae, M. pneumoniae, C. trachomatis; psittacosis; granuloma inguinale* — **Adults:** 150 mg PO q 6 hr or 300 mg PO q 12 hr. **Children > 8 yr:** 6 to 12 mg/kg PO daily in divided doses q 6 to 12 hr. *Gonorrhea* — **Adults:** initially, 600 mg PO; then 300 mg PO q 12 hr for 4 days (total 3 g).	▪ Use cautiously in impaired renal or hepatic function. Use during last half of pregnancy and in children < 8 yr may cause permanent tooth discoloration, enamel defects, and bone growth retardation. ▪ Contraindicated in hypersensitivity to drug or other tetracyclines.
desipramine hydrochloride Norpramin, Pertofran‡, Pertofrane *Dibenzazepine tricyclic antidepressant* Antidepressant Preg. Risk Category: NR	**tab:** 10, 25, 50, 75, 100, 150 mg; **cap:** 25, 50 mg	*Depression* — **Adults:** 100 to 200 mg PO daily in divided doses, increased to max 300 mg daily. Or give entire dosage hs. **Elderly and adolescents:** 25 to 100 mg PO daily in divided doses, increased gradually to max 150 mg daily if needed.	▪ Use with extreme caution in CV disease, glaucoma, thyroid disease, history of urine retention or seizure disorders, and in patients on thyroid medication. ▪ Contraindicated in hypersensitivity to drug, within 14 days of MAO inhibitor therapy, and during acute recovery phase of MI.
desmopressin acetate DDAVP, Minirin‡, Stimate *Posterior pituitary hormone* Antidiuretic/hemostatic Preg. Risk Category: B	**nasal sol:** 0.1 mg/ml; **inj:** 4 mcg/ml	*Nonnephrogenic diabetes insipidus, temporary polyuria and polydipsia with pituitary trauma* — **Adults:** 0.1 to 0.4 ml intranasally qd in 1 to 3 doses. Adjust morning and evening doses separately for adequate diurnal rhythm of water turnover. Or, give injectable form 0.5 to 1 ml IV or SC qd, usually in 2 divided doses. **Children 3 mo to 12 yr:** 0.05 to 0.3 ml intranasally qd in 1 or 2 doses.	▪ Use cautiously in coronary artery insufficiency, hypertensive CV disease, or conditions associated with fluid and electrolyte imbalances (such as cystic fibrosis). ▪ Use cautiously in breast-feeding patients. ▪ Contraindicated in hypersensitivity to drug and in type IIB von Willebrand's disease.
desonide DesOwen, Tridesilon *Topical adrenocorticoid* Anti-inflammatory Preg. Risk Category: C	**cream:** 0.05%; **oint:** 0.05%; **lotion:** 0.05%	*Inflammation associated with corticosteroid-responsive dermatoses* — **Adults and children:** clean area; apply sparingly bid to qid.	▪ Contraindicated in hypersensitivity to drug.

desoximetasone Topicort *Topical adrenocorticoid* *Anti-inflammatory* Preg. Risk Category: C	**cream:** 0.05%, 0.25%; **gel:** 0.05%; **oint:** 0.25%	*Inflammation associated with corticosteroid-responsive dermatoses* — **Adults and children:** clean area; apply sparingly bid.	▪ Contraindicated in hypersensitivity to drug.
dexamethasone Decadron, Hexadrol **dexamethasone acetate** Dalalone D.P., Decadron-LA, Dexasone-LA **dexamethasone sodium phosphate** Dalalone, Decadron Phosphate, Dexasone *Glucocorticoid* *Anti-inflammatory/immunosuppressant* Preg. Risk Category: C	**tab:** 0.25, 0.5, 0.75, 1, 1.5, 2, 4, 6 mg; **oral** **sol:** 0.5, 1 mg/ ml; **elixir:** 0.5 mg/5 ml. **acetate** — **inj:** 8, 16 mg/ ml susp. **sodium phosphate** — **inj:** 4, 10, 20, 24 mg/ml	*Cerebral edema* — **Adults:** initially, 10 mg (sodium phosphate) IV; then 4 to 6 mg IM q 6 hr until symptoms subside (usually 2 to 4 days); then taper over 5 to 7 days. *Inflammatory conditions, allergic reactions, neoplasias* — **Adults:** 0.75 to 9 mg/day PO or 0.5 to 9 mg/day (sodium phosphate) IM; or 4 to 16 mg (acetate) IM into joint or soft tissue q 1 to 3 wk; or 0.8 to 1.6 mg (acetate) into lesions q 1 to 3 wk. *Shock* — **Adults:** 1 to 6 mg/kg (sodium phosphate) IV as single dose; or 40 mg IV q 2 to 6 hr, prn; continue only until patient stabilized.	▪ Use cautiously in recent MI, GI ulcer, renal disease, hypertension, osteoporosis, diabetes mellitus, hypothyroidism, cirrhosis, diverticulitis, nonspecific ulcerative colitis, recent intestinal anastomoses, thromboembolic disorders, seizures, myasthenia gravis, heart failure, TB, ocular herpes simplex, emotional instability, and psychotic tendencies. Some formulations contain sulfite preservatives; also use cautiously in sulfite sensitivity. ▪ Contraindicated in hypersensitivity to any component of drug and in systemic fungal infections.
dexamethasone Maxidex Ophthalmic Suspension **dexamethasone sodium phosphate** Decadron Phosphate Ophthalmic, Maxidex Ophthalmic *Glucocorticoid* *Ophthalmic anti-inflammatory* Preg. Risk Category: C	**dexamethasone** — **ophth** **susp:** 0.1%; **sodium phosphate** — **ophth oint:** 0.05% **ophth** **sol:** 0.1%	*Uveitis; iridocyclitis; inflammatory conditions of eyelids, conjunctiva, cornea, anterior segment of globe; corneal injury from chemical or thermal burns, or penetration of foreign bodies; allergic conjunctivitis; suppression of graft rejection after keratoplasty* — **Adults and children:** 1 to 2 drops susp or sol of 1.25 to 2.5 cm oint into conjunctival sac. In severe disease, drops may be used hourly, tapering to discontinuation as condition improves. In mild conditions, drops may be used up to 6 times daily or oint applied tid or qid. As condition improves, dosage tapered to bid, then qd.	▪ Use cautiously in corneal abrasions that may be infected (especially with herpes) and in glaucoma (any form). Glaucoma medications may need to be increased to compensate. ▪ Contraindicated in acute superficial herpes simplex (dendritic keratitis), vaccinia, varicella, or other fungal or viral diseases of cornea and conjunctiva; ocular TB; acute, purulent, untreated eye infections; or hypersensitivity to any component of formulation and after uncomplicated removal of superficial corneal foreign body.

DRUG/CLASS/CATEGORY	DOSAGE FORMS	INDICATIONS/DOSAGES	KEY PRECAUTIONS
dexamethasone Aeroseb-Dex, Decaderm, Decaspray **dexamethasone sodium phosphate** Decadron Cream *Glucocorticoid* *Anti-inflammatory* Preg. Risk Category: C	**dexamethasone —** *aerosol:* 0.01%, 0.04%; *gel:* 0.1%; **sodium phosphate —** *cream:* 0.1%	*Inflammation associated with corticosteroid-responsive dermatoses* — **Adults and children:** clean area; apply sparingly tid to qid. For aerosol use on scalp, shake can gently and apply to dry scalp after shampooing. Slide applicator tube under hair to touch scalp. Spray (about 2 sec) while moving tube to all affected areas, keeping it under hair and in contact with scalp. Spot-spray inadequately covered areas. Don't massage drug into scalp or spray forehead or near eyes.	▪ Contraindicated in hypersensitivity to drug.
dexamethasone sodium phosphate inhalation Decadron Phosphate Respihaler *Glucocorticoid* *Anti-inflammatory/antiasthmatic* Preg. Risk Category: C	**inh aerosol:** 84 mcg dexamethasone/ metered spray	*Persistent asthma* — **Adults:** initially, 3 inhalations tid or qid. Decrease as needed and tolerated; most patients respond to 2 inhalations bid. Max 12 inhalations daily. **Children:** 2 inhalations tid or qid. Decrease as needed and tolerated; most patients respond to 2 inhalations bid. Max 8 inhalations daily.	▪ Use cautiously in ocular herpes simplex, nonspecific ulcerative colitis, diverticulitis, fresh intestinal anastomoses, peptic ulcer, renal insufficiency, hypertension, osteoporosis, and myasthenia gravis. ▪ Contraindicated in hypersensitivity, status asthmaticus, persistent positive sputum cultures for *C. albicans*, or systemic fungal infections. Not for use in asthma controlled by bronchodilators or other noncorticosteroids alone or in nonasthmatic bronchial diseases.
dextran, high-molecular-weight (dextran 70, dextran 75) Dextran 75, Gendex 75, Gentran 70, Gentran 75, Macrodex *Glucose polymer* *Plasma volume expander* Preg. Risk Category: C	**inj:** 6% dextran 70 in 0.9% NaCl sol or D₅W; 6% dextran 75 in 0.9% NaCl sol or D₅W	*Plasma expander* — **Adults:** 30 g (500 ml of 6% sol) IV. In emergencies, may give at 1.2 to 2.4 g (20 to 40 ml)/min. In normovolemic or nearly normovolemic patients, infusion rate shouldn't exceed 240 mg (4 ml)/min. Total dosage during 1st 24 hr not to exceed 1.2 g/kg; actual dosage depends on amount of fluid loss and resultant hemoconcentration and must be determined for each patient.	▪ Use cautiously in hemorrhage, thrombocytopenia, impaired renal clearance, chronic liver disease, and abdominal conditions or in patients undergoing bowel surgery. ▪ Contraindicated in hypersensitivity to dextran and in marked hemostatic defects, marked cardiac decompensation, renal disease with severe oliguria or anuria, hypervolemic conditions, and severe bleeding disorders.

Drug	Forms	Indications & dosages	Precautions
dextran, low-molecular-weight (dextran 40) Dextran 40, Gentran 40, 10% LMD, Rheomacrodex *Glucose polymer* *Plasma volume expander* Preg. Risk Category: C	*inj:* 10% dextran 40 in D$_5$W or 0.9% NaCl sol	*Plasma volume expansion* — **Adults:** dosage by IV infusion depends on amount of fluid loss. Infuse 1st 10 ml/kg rapidly with CVP monitoring; infuse remaining dose slowly. Total dosage not to exceed 20 ml/kg/day. If therapy continues > 24 hr, don't exceed 10 ml/kg/day, continued no longer than 5 days. *Prophylaxis of venous thrombosis* — **Adults:** 10 ml/kg (500 to 1,000 ml) IV on day of procedure; 500 ml on days 2 and 3. *Hemodilution in extracorporeal circulation* — **Adults:** 10 to 20 ml/kg added to perfusion circuit, not to exceed total dosage of 20 ml/kg.	▪ Use cautiously in hemorrhage, thrombocytopenia, or diabetes mellitus. ▪ Contraindicated in hypersensitivity to drug and in marked hemostatic defects, marked cardiac decompensation, and renal disease with severe oliguria or anuria.
dextroamphetamine sulfate Dexedrine, Dexedrine Spansule, Oxydess II, Robese, Spancap #1 *Amphetamine* *CNS stimulant/short-term adjunctive anorexigenic/sympathomimetic amine* Preg. Risk Category: C Controlled Sub. Sched.: II	*tab:* 5, 10 mg; *cap (sust-release):* 5, 10, 15 mg	*Narcolepsy* — **Adults:** 5 to 60 mg PO qd in divided doses. **6 to 12 yr:** 5 mg PO qd, with 5-mg increments/wk, prn. **Children ≥ 12 yr:** 10 mg PO qd, with 10-mg increments/wk, prn. First dose on awakening; add. doses (1 or 2) q 4 to 6 hr. *Short-term adjunct in exogenous obesity* — **Adults and children ≥ 12 yr:** 5 to 30 mg PO qd 30 to 60 min before meals in divided doses of 5 to 10 mg, OR one 10- or 15-mg sust-release cap qd in am. *Attention deficit disorder with hyperactivity* — **Children 3 to 5 yr:** 2.5 mg PO qd, with 2.5-mg increments/wk, prn. **Children ≥ 6 yr:** 5 mg PO qd or bid, with 5-mg increments/wk, prn.	▪ Use cautiously in motor and phonic tics, Tourette syndrome, and agitated states. ▪ Contraindicated in hypersensitivity or idiosyncrasy to sympathomimetic amines, hyperthyroidism, mod. to severe hypertension, symptomatic CV disease, glaucoma, advanced arteriosclerosis, history of drug abuse, and < 14 days of MAO inhibitor use. ▪ Not recommended as first-line treatment of obesity. Use as anorexigenic agent prohibited in some states.
dextromethorphan hydrobromide Benylin DM, Pertussin Cough Suppressant, Robitussin Pediatric, Vicks Formula 44 Pediatric Formula *Levorphanol derivative* *Antitussive (nonnarcotic)* Preg. Risk Category: C	*liq (ext-release):* 30 mg/5 ml; *lozenges:* 5, 7.5 mg; *sol:* 3.5, 5, 7.5, 10, 15 mg/5 ml; 15 mg/15 ml	*Nonproductive cough* — **Adults and children ≥ 12 yr:** 10 to 20 mg PO q 4 hr, or 30 mg q 6 to 8 hr. Or, 60 mg ext-release liq bid. Max 120 mg daily. **Children 6 to 12 yr:** 5 to 10 mg PO q 4 hr, or 15 mg q 6 to 8 hr. Or, 30 mg ext-release liq bid. Max 60 mg daily. **Children 2 to 6 yr:** 2.5 to 5 mg PO q 4 hr, or 7.5 mg q 6 to 8 hr. Or, 15 mg ext-release liq bid. Max 30 mg daily. **Children < 2 yr:** dosages must be individualized.	▪ Use with caution in atopic children, sedated or debilitated patients, and in patients confined to supine position. Also use cautiously in aspirin sensitivity. ▪ Contraindicated in patients currently taking MAO inhibitors or within 2 wk of discontinuing MAO inhibitors.

†Canadian   ‡Australian

DIAZEPAM 72

DRUG/CLASS/CATEGORY	DOSAGE FORMS	INDICATIONS/DOSAGES	KEY PRECAUTIONS
diazepam Apo-Diazepam†, Diazepam Intensol, T-Quil, Valium, Zetran *Benzodiazepine* *Antianxiety agent/skeletal muscle relaxant/amnesic agent/anticonvulsant/sedative-hypnotic* Preg. Risk Category: D Controlled Sub. Sched.: IV	*tab:* 2, 5, 10 mg; *cap (ext-release):* 15 mg; *oral sol:* 5 mg/5 ml, 5 mg/ml; *inj:* 5 mg/ml; *sterile emulsion for inj:* 5 mg/ml	*Anxiety* — **Adults:** 2 to 10 mg PO bid to qid, or 15 to 30 mg ext-release cap PO qd. Or, 2 to 10 mg IM or IV q 3 to 4 hr, prn. **Elderly patients:** 2 to 2.5 mg qd or bid; increased gradually. **Children ≥ 6 mo:** 1 to 2.5 mg PO tid or qid, increased gradually. *Muscle spasm* — **Adults:** 2 to 10 mg PO bid to qid or 15 to 30 mg ext-release cap qd. Or, 5 to 10 mg IM or IV initially, then 5 to 10 mg IM or IV q 3 to 4 hr, prn. **Children > 30 days to 5 yr:** 1 to 2 mg IM or IV slowly, repeated q 3 to 4 hr, prn. **Children ≥ 5 yr:** 5 to 10 mg IM or IV q 3 to 4 hr, prn. *Status epilepticus and severe recurrent seizures* — **Adults:** 5 to 10 mg IV (preferred) or IM. Repeat q 10 to 15 min, prn, to max 30 mg. Repeat q 2 to 4 hr p.r.n. **Children > 30 days to 5 yr:** 0.2 to 0.5 mg IV slowly q 2 to 5 min to max 5 mg. Repeat q 2 to 4 hr, prn. **Children ≥ 5 yr:** 1 mg IV q 2 to 5 min to max 10 mg. Repeat q 2 to 4 hr, prn.	▪ Use cautiously in hepatic or renal impairment, depression, or chronic open-angle glaucoma and in elderly and debilitated patients. ▪ Contraindicated in hypersensitivity or angle-closure glaucoma; in shock, coma, or acute alcohol intoxication (parenteral form); and in children < 6 mo (oral form). ▪ Avoid during pregnancy, especially first trimester.
diclofenac potassium Cataflam **diclofenac sodium** Fenac†, Voltaren, Voltaren SR *Nonsteroidal anti-inflammatory* *Antiarthritic/anti-inflammatory* Preg. Risk Category: B	*tab:* 50 mg; *tab (enteric-coated):* 25, 50, 75 mg; *tab (slow-release):* 100 mg; *supp:* 50†, 100 mg†	*Ankylosing spondylitis* — **Adults:** 25 mg PO qid (and hs, prn). *Osteoarthritis* — **Adults:** 50 mg PO bid or tid, or 75 mg PO bid (sodium form only). *Rheumatoid arthritis* — **Adults:** 50 mg PO tid or qid. Or, 75 mg PO bid (sodium form only) or 50 to 100 mg PR hs as substitute for last PO dose of day. Max 225 mg qd. *Analgesia and primary dysmenorrhea* — **Adults:** 50 mg PO tid (potassium form only).	▪ Use cautiously in history of peptic ulcer disease, hepatic or renal dysfunction, cardiac disease, hypertension, or conditions associated with fluid retention. ▪ Contraindicated in hypersensitivity to drug, in hepatic porphyria, or in history of asthma, urticaria, or other allergic reactions to aspirin or other NSAIDs. Not recommended during late pregnancy or breast-feeding.

diclofenac sodium 0.1%
Voltaren Ophthalmic
Nonsteroidal anti-inflammatory
Anti-inflammatory
Preg. Risk Category: B

ophth sol: 0.1%

Postop inflammation following cataract removal — **Adults:** 1 drop in conjunctival sac qid, beginning 24 hr after surg and continuing throughout 1st 2 wk of postop period.

- Use cautiously in hypersensitivity to aspirin, phenylacetic acid derivatives, and other NSAIDs; in surg patients with known bleeding tendencies; and in patients receiving medications that may prolong bleeding time.
- Contraindicated in hypersensitivity to any component of drug and in patients who wear soft contact lenses.
- Avoid use during late pregnancy.

---

dicloxacillin sodium
Dycill, Dynapen, Pathocil
Penicillinase-resistant penicillin
Antibiotic
Preg. Risk Category: NR

cap: 250, 500 mg; *oral susp:* 62.5 mg/5 ml (after reconstitution)

Systemic infections caused by penicillinase-producing staphylococci — **Adults and children > 40 kg:** 125 to 250 mg PO q 6 hr. **Children ≤ 40 kg:** 12.5 to 25 mg/kg PO daily, in divided doses q 6 hr depending on severity.

- Use cautiously in other drug allergies or in mononucleosis.
- Contraindicated in hypersensitivity to drug or other penicillins.

---

dicyclomine hydrochloride
Antispas, Bemote, Bentyl, Neoquess, Spasmoban†
Anticholinergic
Antimuscarinic/GI antispasmodic
Preg. Risk Category: B

tab: 10, 20 mg; *cap:* 10, 20 mg; *syrup:* 5, 10 mg/5 ml; *inj:* 10 mg/ml

Irritable bowel syndrome and other functional GI disorders — **Adults:** initially, 20 mg PO qid, increased to 40 mg qid, or 20 mg IM q 4 to 6 hr.

- Use cautiously in autonomic neuropathy, hyperthyroidism, CAD, arrhythmias, heart failure, hypertension, hiatal hernia, hepatic or renal disease, prostatic hyperplasia, and ulcerative colitis.
- Contraindicated in obstructive uropathy, obstructive GI tract disease, reflux esophagitis, severe ulcerative colitis, myasthenia gravis, hypersensitivity to anticholinergics, unstable CV status in acute hemorrhage, glaucoma, breast-feeding patients, and children < 6 mo.

---

didanosine (ddI)
Videx
Purine analogue
Antiviral agent
Preg. Risk Category: B

tab (buff, chew): 25, 50, 100, 150 mg; *powder for oral sol (buff):* 100, 167, 250,

Treatment of HIV infection when antiretroviral therapy warranted — **Adults ≥ 60 kg:** 200 mg (tab) PO q 12 hr; or 250 mg buff powder PO q 12 hr. **Adults < 60 kg:** 125 mg (tab) PO q 12 hr; or 167 mg buff powder PO q 12 hr. **Children:** 120 mg/m² PO q 12 hr.

- Use very cautiously in history of pancreatitis. Also use cautiously in peripheral neuropathy, renal or hepatic impairment, or hyperuricemia.

(continued)

DIDANOSINE   **73**

---

†Canadian   †Australian

DRUG/CLASS/CATEGORY	DOSAGE FORMS	INDICATIONS/DOSAGES	KEY PRECAUTIONS
didanosine *(continued)*	375 mg/pkt; *powder for oral sol (ped):* 10 mg/ml in 2- and 4-g bottles		▪ Contraindicated in history of hypersensitivity to any component of formulation.
diethylstilbestrol (stilboestrol) diethylstilbestrol diphosphate DES, Honvol, Stilphostrol *Estrogen* *Estrogen replacement/antineoplastic* Preg. Risk Category: X	**diethylstilbestrol** — *tab:* 1, 5 mg. **diphosphate** — *tab:* 50, 83 mg. *inj:* 50 mg/ml	*Prostate cancer* — **Men:** initially, 1 to 3 mg PO qd; may reduce to 1 mg qd or 50 mg PO diphosphate tid. Then increase to 200 mg or more prn tid or 0.5 g IV, followed by 1 g qd for 5 or more days prn. Maint: 0.25 to 0.5 g IV once or twice per wk. *Metastatic, advanced breast cancer* — **Men and post-menopausal women:** 15 mg PO qd.	▪ Use cautiously in hypertension, cerebrovascular disease, CAD, mental depression, bone disease, migraine, seizures, diabetes mellitus, or cardiac, hepatic, or renal dysfunction. ▪ Contraindicated in men with known or suspected breast cancer, except in selected patients being treated for metastatic disease; in active thromboembolic disorders, estrogen-dependent neoplasia, and undiagnosed abnormal genital bleeding; during pregnancy; and in history of thrombophlebitis, thrombosis, or thromboembolic disorders associated with estrogen use.
diflorasone diacetate Florone, Flutone, Maxiflor, Psorcon *Topical adrenocorticoid* *Anti-inflammatory* Preg. Risk Category: C	*cream:* 0.05%; *oint:* 0.05%	*Inflammation associated with corticosteroid-responsive dermatoses* — **Adults and children:** clean area; apply sparingly in thin film. Apply cream bid to qid; apply emollient cream and oint qd to tid.	▪ Contraindicated in hypersensitivity to drug.
diflunisal Dolobid *Nonsteroidal anti-inflammatory/salicylic acid derivative*	*tab:* 250, 500 mg	*Mild to moderate pain, osteoarthritis, rheumatoid arthritis* — **Adults:** 500 to 1,000 mg PO daily in 2 divided doses, usually q 12 hr. Max 1,500 mg daily. **Adults > 65 yr:** half of usual adult dose.	▪ Use cautiously in GI bleeding, history of peptic ulcer disease, renal impairment, and compromised cardiac function, hypertension, or other conditions predisposing patient to fluid retention.

*Nonnarcotic analgesic/antipyretic/
anti-inflammatory*
Preg. Risk Category: C

- Contraindicated in hypersensitivity to drug or for patients in whom aspirin or other NSAIDs trigger acute asthma attacks, urticaria, or rhinitis.
- Don't give to children or teenagers with chickenpox or flulike illness due to risk of Reye's syndrome.

---

digoxin
Digoxin, Lanoxicaps, Lanoxin, Novodigoxin†
Cardiac glycoside
Antiarrhythmic/inotropic
Preg. Risk Category: C

tab: 0.125, 0.25, 0.5 mg; *cap*: 0.05, 0.1, 0.2 mg; *elixir*: 0.05 mg/ml; *inj*: 0.05 mg/ml†, 0.1 mg/ml (ped), 0.25 mg/ml

Heart failure, PSVT, atrial fibrillation and flutter —
Adults: loading dose 0.5 to 1 mg IV or PO in divided doses over 24 hr; maint.: 0.125 to 0.5 mg IV or PO qd (average: 0.25 mg). **Adults > 65 yr:** 0.125 mg PO qd as maint dose. **Premature neonates:** loading dose 0.015 to 0.025 mg/kg IV in 3 divided doses over 24 hr; maint: 0.01 mg/kg qd, divided q 12 hr. **Neonates:** loading dose 0.025 to 0.035 mg/kg PO, divided q 8 hr over 24 hr; IV loading dose 0.02 to 0.03 mg/kg; maint: 0.01 mg/kg PO qd, divided q 12 hr. **Children 1 mo to 2 yr:** loading dose 0.035 to 0.06 mg/kg PO in 3 divided doses over 24 hr; IV loading dose 0.03 to 0.05 mg/kg; maint: 0.01 to 0.02 mg/kg PO qd, divided q 12 hr. **Children > 2 yr:** loading dose 0.02 to 0.04 mg/kg PO qd, divided q 8 hr over 24 hr; IV loading dose 0.015 to 0.035 mg/kg; maint: 0.012 mg/kg PO qd, divided q 12 hr.

- Use with extreme caution in elderly patients and in acute MI, incomplete AV block, sinus bradycardia, PVCs, chronic constrictive pericarditis, hypertrophic cardiomyopathy, renal insufficiency, severe pulmonary disease, or hypothyroidism. Reduce dosage in renal impairment.
- Contraindicated in hypersensitivity to drug, digitalis-induced toxicity, ventricular fibrillation, or ventricular tachycardia unless caused by heart failure.
- Hypothyroid patients are extremely sensitive to cardiac glycosides; hyperthyroid patients may need larger doses.

---

digoxin immune FAB (ovine)
Digibind
Antibody fragment
Cardiac glycoside antidote
Preg. Risk Category: C

inj: 38-mg vial

Potentially life-threatening digoxin or digitoxin intoxication — **Adults and children:** IV dosage varies according to amount of digoxin or digitoxin to be neutralized. Each vial binds about 0.5 mg of digoxin or digitoxin. Avg dosage 6 vials (228 mg). However, if toxicity resulted from acute digoxin ingestion and neither serum digoxin level nor estimated ingestion amount known, 20 vials (760 mg) may be needed. See pkg insert for complete, specific dosage instructions.

- Use cautiously in known allergy to ovine proteins or in patients who have previously received antibodies (in these high-risk patients, skin testing recommended).

DIGOXIN IMMUNE FAB 75

†Canadian †Australian

DRUG / CLASS / CATEGORY	DOSAGE FORMS	INDICATIONS / DOSAGES	KEY PRECAUTIONS
dihydroergotamine mesylate D.H.E. 45, Dihydergot‡ *Ergot alkaloid* *Vasoconstrictor* Preg. Risk Category: X	*inj:* 1 mg/ml	*To prevent or abort vascular or migraine headache* — **Adults:** 1 mg IM or IV. Repeat q 1 to 2 hr, prn, to total of 2 mg IV or 3 mg IM per attack. Max wkly dosage 6 mg.	▪ Contraindicated in hypersensitivity to drug, during pregnancy or breast-feeding, and in peripheral and occlusive vascular disease, CAD, uncontrolled hypertension, severe hepatic or renal dysfunction, and sepsis.
dihydrotachysterol AT-10‡, DHT Intensol, Hytakerol *Vitamin D analogue* *Antihypocalcemic* Preg. Risk Category: C	*tab:* 0.125, 0.2, 0.4 mg; *cap:* 0.125 mg; *oral sol:* 0.2 mg/5 ml, 0.2 mg/ml (DHT Intensol), 0.25 mg/ml (in sesame oil)	*Hypocalcemia associated with hypoparathyroidism and pseudohypoparathyroidism* — **Adults:** initially, 0.75 to 2.5 mg PO daily for 4 days. Maintenance 0.2 to 1.5 mg daily. **Children:** initially, 1 to 5 mg PO for 4 days. Maintenance 0.5 to 1.5 mg daily. *Prophylaxis of hypocalcemic tetany following thyroid surgery* — **Adults:** 0.25 mg PO daily (with calcium supplements). *Note:* 1 mg dihydrotachysterol = 120,000 units ergocalciferol (vitamin D$_2$).	▪ Contraindicated in hypercalcemia or vitamin D toxicity.
diltiazem hydrochloride Apo-Diltiaz†, Cardizem, Cardizem CD, Cardizem SR, Vasocardol SR‡ *Calcium channel blocker* *Antianginal* Preg. Risk Category: C	*tab:* 30, 60, 90, 120 mg; *cap (ext-release; Cardizem CD):* 120, 180, 240, 300 mg; *cap (sust-release; Cardizem SR; Vasocardol SR‡):* 60, 90, 120, 180, 240 mg; *inj:* 5 mg/ml	*Vasospastic angina (Prinzmetal's [variant] angina) and classic chronic stable angina pectoris* — **Adults:** 30 mg PO tid or qid before meals and hs. Increase gradually to max 360 mg/day in divided doses. Or, 120 or 180 mg (ext-release cap). Titrate prn to max 480 mg daily. *Hypertension* — **Adults:** 60 to 120 mg PO bid (sust-release). Titrate to effect. Max dosage 360 mg/day. Or, 180 to 240 mg daily (ext-release). Adjust prn. *Atrial fibrillation or flutter; PSVT* — **Adults:** 0.25 mg/kg as IV bolus injection over 2 min. If response inadequate, 0.35 mg/kg IV after 15 min followed with continuous infusion of 10 mg/hr; max dose 15 mg/hr. Some respond well to rates of 5 mg/hr.	▪ Use cautiously in elderly patients, in heart disease, or in impaired hepatic or renal function. ▪ Contraindicated in sick sinus syndrome or second- or third-degree AV block in absence of artificial pacemaker, systolic BP < 90, hypersensitivity to drug, acute MI, and pulmonary congestion (documented by X-ray).

dimenhydrinate

Dimetabs, Dinate, Dommanate, Dramamine, Nauseatol†

Ethanolamine-derivative antihistamine

Antihistamine (H₁-receptor antagonist)/antiemetic/antivertigo agent

Preg. Risk Category: B

tab: 50 mg; **tab (chew):** 50 mg; **cap:** 50 mg; **elixir:** 15 mg/5 ml†; **syrup:** 12.5 mg/4 ml, 15.62 mg/5 ml; **inj:** 50 mg/ml

Prevention and treatment of motion sickness — **Adults and children ≥ 12 yr:** 50 to 100 mg PO q 4 to 6 hr; 50 mg IM, prn; or 50 mg IV diluted in 10 ml NaCl for injection, injected over 2 min. Max 400 mg daily. **Children 6 to 12 yr:** 25 to 50 mg PO q 6 to 8 hr, not to exceed 150 mg in 24 hr. **Children 2 to 6 yr:** 12.5 to 25 mg PO q 6 to 8 hr, not to exceed 75 mg in 24 hr. **Children > 2 yr:** 1.25 mg/kg or 37.5 mg/m² IM qid. Max 300 mg daily.

- Use cautiously in seizures, acute angle-closure glaucoma, or enlarged prostate gland and in patients receiving ototoxic drugs.
- Contraindicated in hypersensitivity to drug or its components. IV product contains benzyl alcohol, associated with fatal "gasping syndrome" in premature and low-birth-weight infants.

dimercaprol

BAL in Oil

Chelating agent

Heavy metal antagonist

Preg. Risk Category: NR

inj: 100 mg/ml

Severe arsenic or gold poisoning — **Adults and children:** 3 mg/kg deep IM q 4 hr for 2 days, then qid on 3rd day, then bid for 10 days.

Mild arsenic or gold poisoning — **Adults and children:** 2.5 mg/kg deep IM qid for 2 days, then bid on 3rd day, then qd for 10 days.

Mercury poisoning — **Adults and children:** 5 mg/kg deep IM, then 2.5 mg/kg daily or bid for 10 days.

Acute lead encephalopathy or lead level > 100 mcg/ml — **Adults and children:** 4 mg/kg deep IM, then q 4 hr with edetate calcium disodium for 2 to 7 days. Use separate sites.

- Use cautiously in hypertension, G6PD deficiency, or oliguria.
- Avoid in pregnant patients, unless required to treat life-threatening acute poisoning.
- Contraindicated in hepatic dysfunction (except postarsenical jaundice); iron, cadmium, or selenium poisoning; and in peanut allergy.

dinoprostone

Prepidil, Prostin E₂

Prostaglandin

Oxytocic

Preg. Risk Category: C

vag supp: 20 mg; **endocerv gel:** 0.5 mg/ application (2.5-ml syringe)

To abort 2nd-trimester pregnancy; to evacuate uterus in missed abortion, intrauterine fetal deaths up to 28 wk of gestation, or benign hydatidiform mole — **Adults:** 20-mg supp inserted high into posterior vag fornix. Repeat q 3 to 5 hr until abortion complete.

Ripening of unfavorable cervix in pregnant patients at or near term — **Adults:** gel contents of 1 syringe given intravaginally; if cervix unfavorable after 6 hr, repeat. Don't give > 1.5 mg within 24-hr period.

- Use supp cautiously in asthma; seizure disorders; anemia; diabetes; hypertension or hypotension; jaundice; CV, renal, or hepatic disease; scarred uterus; cervicitis; or acute vaginitis. Use gel cautiously in asthma or history of asthma, glaucoma or increased IOP, renal or hepatic dysfunction, or ruptured membranes.
- Gel contraindicated where prolonged uterine contractions inappropriate, in hypersensitivity to prostaglandins or gel constituents,

(continued)

DINOPROSTONE 77

DRUG/CLASS/CATEGORY	DOSAGE FORMS	INDICATIONS/DOSAGES	KEY PRECAUTIONS
dinoprostone *(continued)*			and in patients with placenta previa or unexplained vag bleeding during this pregnancy and in whom vag delivery not indicated. ■ Supp contraindicated in hypersensitivity, acute pelvic inflammatory disease, and active cardiac, pulmonary, renal, or hepatic disease. ■ Vag insert contraindicated in known hypersensitivity to prostaglandins, with suspicion or definite evidence of marked cephalopelvic disproportion or fetal distress where delivery imminent, in unexplained vag bleeding in pregnancy, in multiparity with 6 or more previous term pregnancies, and in patients already receiving oxytocic drugs.
diphenhydramine hydrochloride Allerdryl, Benadryl, Hydramine, Nytol Maximum Strength, Sominex Formula 2 *Ethanolamine-derivative antihistamine* Antihistamine/antiemetic/antivertigo agent/antitussive/sedative-hypnotic/antidyskinetic Preg. Risk Category: B	**tab:** 25, 50 mg; **cap:** 25, 50 mg; **elixir:** 12.5 mg/5 ml (14% alcohol); **syrup:** 12.5 mg/5 ml; **inj:** 10, 50 mg/ml	*Rhinitis, allergy symptoms, motion sickness, Parkinson's disease* — **Adults and children ≥ 12 yr:** 25 to 50 mg PO tid or qid; or 10 to 50 mg deep IM or IV. Max IM or IV dosage 400 mg daily. **Children < 12 yr:** 5 mg/kg qd PO, deep IM, or IV in divided doses qid. Max 300 mg daily. *Sedation* — **Adults:** 25 to 50 mg PO, or deep IM, prn. *Nonproductive cough* — **Adults:** 25 mg PO q 4 to 6 hr (max 150 mg daily). **Children 6 to 12 yr:** 12.5 mg PO q 4 to 6 hr (max 75 mg daily). **Children 2 to 6 yr:** 6.25 mg PO q 4 to 6 hr (max 25 mg/day).	■ Use with extreme caution in angle-closure glaucoma, prostatic hyperplasia, pyloroduodenal and bladder-neck obstruction, asthma, COPD, increased IOP, hyperthyroidism, CV disease, hypertension, and stenosing peptic ulcer. ■ Contraindicated in hypersensitivity to drug, during acute asthmatic attacks, in newborns or premature neonates, and in breast-feeding patients.

dipivefrin Propine *Sympathomimetic Antiglaucoma agent* Preg. Risk Category: B	**ophth sol:** 0.1%	*IOP reduction in chronic open-angle glaucoma —* **Adults:** for initial glaucoma therapy, 1 drop of 0.1% sol q 12 hr. Adjust dosage based on patient response as determined by tonometric readings.	▪ Use cautiously in aphakia or CV disease, history of hypersensitivity to epinephrine, and asthma. ▪ Contraindicated in angle-closure glaucoma or hypersensitivity to drug.
dipyridamole IV Persantine, Persantin‡, Persantine *Pyrimidine analogue Coronary vasodilator/platelet aggregation inhibitor* Preg. Risk Category: B	**tab:** 25, 50, 75 mg; **inj:** 10 mg/2 ml	*Inhibition of platelet adhesion in prosthetic heart valves —* **Adults:** 75 to 100 mg PO qid. *Alternative to exercise in CAD evaluation during thallium (2017) myocardia perfusion scintigraphy —* **Adults:** 0.57 mg/kg as IV infusion at constant rate over 4 min (0.142 mg/kg/min). *Acute coronary insufficiency —* **Adults:** 10 mg IV or IM.	▪ Use cautiously in hypotension. ▪ Contraindicated in hypersensitivity to drug.
dirithromycin Dynabac *Macrolide Antibiotic* Preg. Risk Category: C	**tab (enteric-coated):** 250 mg	*Acute bacterial exacerbations of chronic bronchitis or secondary bacterial infection of acute bronchitis due to M. catarrhalis or S. pneumoniae; uncomplicated skin-structure infections due to S. aureus (methicillin-susceptible strains) —* **Adults and children ≥ 12 yr:** 500 mg PO qd for 7 days. *Community-acquired pneumonia due to L. pneumophila, M. pneumoniae, or S. pneumoniae —* **Adults and children ≥ 12 yr:** 500 mg PO qd for 14 days.	▪ Use cautiously in hepatic insufficiency and in breast-feeding women. ▪ Contraindicated in hypersensitivity to drug, erythromycin, or any other macrolide antibiotic. ▪ Safety in children < 12 yr not established.
disopyramide Rythmodan† **disopyramide phosphate** Norpace, Norpace CR, Rythmodan LA‡ *Pyridine derivative antiarrhythmic Antiarrhythmic* Preg. Risk Category: C	**disopyramide — cap:** 100, 150 mg†. **phosphate — tab (sust-release):** 250 mg‡; **cap:** 100, 150 mg; **cap (contr-release):** 100, 150 mg	*Ventricular tachycardia and ventricular arrhythmias thought to be life-threatening —* **Adults > 50 kg:** 150 mg q 6 hr with conventional capsules or 300 mg q 12 hr with ext-release prep. **Adults ≤ 50 kg:** highly individualized. **Children < 1 yr:** 10 to 30 mg/kg PO qd. **Children 1 to 4 yr:** 10 to 20 mg/kg PO qd. **Children 4 to 12 yr:** 10 to 15 mg/kg PO qd. **Children 12 to 18 yr:** 6 to 15 mg/kg PO qd. For pediatric dosages, divide into equal amounts and give q 6 hr.	▪ Use with extreme caution in heart failure. ▪ Use cautiously in underlying conduction abnormalities, urinary tract diseases, hepatic or renal impairment, myasthenia gravis, or acute angle-closure glaucoma. ▪ Contraindicated in hypersensitivity, sick sinus syndrome, cardiogenic shock, or second- or third-degree heart block in absence of artificial pacemaker.

(continued)

†Canadian ‡Australian

DRUG / CLASS / CATEGORY	DOSAGE FORMS	INDICATIONS / DOSAGES	KEY PRECAUTIONS
disopyramide *(continued)*			- Sust- or contr-release forms not for use to achieve rapid control of ventricular arrhythmias, when therapeutic blood levels must be rapidly attained, in cardiomyopathy or possible cardiac decompensation, or in severe renal impairment.
disulfiram Antabuse *Aldehyde dehydrogenase inhibitor* *Alcoholic deterrent* Preg. Risk Category: NR	***tab:*** 250, 500 mg	*Adjunct in management of chronic alcoholism* — **Adults:** 250 to 500 mg PO as single dose in morning for 1 to 2 wk or in evening if drowsiness occurs. Maintenance dosage 125 to 500 mg PO daily (avg dosage 250 mg) until permanent self-control established. Treatment may continue for months or years.	- Use with extreme caution in diabetes, hypothyroidism, seizure disorder, cerebral damage, nephritis or hepatic cirrhosis or insufficiency, and concurrent phenytoin therapy. - Contraindicated during alcohol intoxication and within 12 hr of alcohol ingestion; in hypersensitivity to drug or other thiuram derivatives used in pesticides and rubber vulcanization; psychoses, myocardial disease, or coronary occlusion; pregnancy; and patients receiving metronidazole, paraldehyde, alcohol, or alcohol-containing forms.
dobutamine hydrochloride Dobutrex *Adrenergic, beta₁ agonist* *Inotropic* Preg. Risk Category: B	***inj:*** 12.5 mg/ml in 20-ml vials (parenteral)	*To increase cardiac output in short-term treatment of cardiac decompensation caused by depressed contractility, such as during refractory heart failure, and as adjunct in cardiac surgery* — **Adults:** 2.5 to 10 mcg/kg/min IV infusion. Rates up to 40 mcg/kg/min may be needed (rare).	- Use cautiously in history of hypertension. May trigger exaggerated pressor response. - Contraindicated in hypersensitivity to drug or any drug component and in idiopathic hypertrophic subaortic stenosis.
docetaxel Taxotere *Taxoid* *Antineoplastic* Preg. Risk Category: D	***inj:*** 20, 80 mg in single-dose vials	*Treatment of patients with locally advanced or metastatic breast cancer who have progressed during anthracycline-based therapy or have relapsed during anthracycline-based adjuvant therapy* — **Adults:** 60 to 100 mg/m² IV over 1 hr q 3 wk.	- Contraindicated in history of severe hypersensitivity to drug or other formulations containing polysorbate 80 or when neutrophil count < 1,500 cells/mm³.

docusate calcium
Dioctocal, Surfak

docusate sodium
Colace, Doxinate, Genasoft
Surfactant
Emollient laxative
Preg. Risk Category: C

calcium —
cap: 50, 240
mg. **sodium** —
cap: 50, 60,
100, 240, 250
mg; *oral liq:*
150 mg/15 ml;
oral sol: 50
mg/ml; *syrup:*
50, 60 mg/15
ml

Stool softener — **Adults and children > 12 yr:** 50 to
500 mg PO (calcium or sodium) qd until bowel
movements normal. **Children < 3 yr:** 10 to 40 mg
(sodium) PO qd. **Children 3 to 6 yr:** 20 to 60 mg
(sodium) PO qd. **Children 6 to 12 yr:** 40 to 120 mg
(sodium) PO qd.

- Contraindicated in hypersensitivity, intestinal obstruction, undiagnosed abdominal
pain, vomiting or other signs of appendicitis, fecal impaction, or acute surgical abdomen.
- Laxative of choice for patients who should
not strain during defecation, including those
recovering from MI or rectal surgery; for
those with rectal or anal disease that makes
passage of firm stools difficult; and for
those with postpartum constipation.

donepezil hydrochloride
Aricept
Acetylcholinesterase inhibitor
CNS agent for Alzheimer's disease
Preg. Risk Category: C

tab: 5, 10 mg

Mild to moderate dementia of Alzheimer's type —
Adults: initially, 5 mg PO qd hs. After 4 to 6 wk, may
increase to 10 mg qd.

- Use cautiously in CV disease, asthma,
COPD, urinary outflow impairment, or history of ulcer disease and in patients currently
taking NSAIDs.
- Contraindicated in known hypersensitivity to
drug or piperidine derivatives. Use in pregnancy only if benefit justifies risk to fetus.
Women taking drug shouldn't breast-feed.
Safety and effectiveness in pediatric patients
not established.

dopamine hydrochloride
Intropin, Revimine†‡
Adrenergic
Inotropic, vasopressor
Preg. Risk Category: C

inj: 40, 80, 160
mg/ml conc for
inj for IV inf;
0.8 mg/ml (200
or 400 mg) in
D₅W,1.6 mg/ml
(400 or 800
mg) in D₅W,
3.2 mg/ml (800
mg) in D₅W inj
for IV inf

*To treat shock and correct hemodynamic imbalances;
to improve perfusion to vital organs; to increase cardiac output; to correct hypotension* — **Adults:** initially, 1 to 5 mcg/kg/min by IV infusion. Titrate dosage to
desired hemodynamic or renal response; may increase infusion by 1 to 4 mcg/kg/min at 10- to 30-
min intervals.

- Use cautiously in occlusive vascular disease, cold injuries, diabetic endarteritis, and
arterial embolism; in pregnant patients; and
in patients taking MAO inhibitors.
- Contraindicated in uncorrected tachyarrhythmias, pheochromocytoma, or ventricular
fibrillation.

DOPAMINE HYDROCHLORIDE   81

†Canadian ‡Australian

DRUG / CLASS / CATEGORY	DOSAGE FORMS	INDICATIONS / DOSAGES	KEY PRECAUTIONS
dornase alfa Pulmozyme *Recombinant human deoxyribo- nuclease 1, mucolytic enzyme* *Respiratory inhalant* Preg. Risk Category: B	*inhal sol:* 2.5- mg ampule (1 mg/ml)	*To improve pulmonary function and decrease fre- quency of moderate to severe respiratory infections in cystic fibrosis —* **Adults and children ≥ 5 yr:** 1 am- pule (2.5 mg) inhaled qd. Treatment usually takes 10 to 15 min. Use only with approved nebulizer.	• Contraindicated in hypersensitivity to drug or to Chinese hamster ovary cell–derived products. • Safety and efficacy in children < 5 yr or with forced vital capacity < 40% of normal value not established.
dorzolamide hydrochloride Trusopt *Sulfonamide* *Antiglaucoma agent* Preg. Risk Category: C	*ophth sol:* 2%	*Treatment of increased IOP in patients with ocular hy- pertension or open-angle glaucoma —* **Adults:** 1 drop in conjunctival sac of affected eye tid.	• Use with caution in hepatic or renal impair- ment. • Contraindicated in hypersensitivity to any component of drug.
doxazosin mesylate Cardura *Alpha-adrenergic blocker* *Antihypertensive* Preg. Risk Category: C	*tab:* 1, 2, 4, 8 mg	*Essential hypertension —* **Adults:** 1 mg PO qd, and determine effect on standing and supine BP at 2 to 6 hr and 24 hr after dosing. If necessary, increase to 2 mg daily. Titrate slowly. May increase to 4 mg qd, then 8 mg. Max 16 mg. *Benign prostatic hyperplasia —* **Adults:** initially, 1 mg PO qd in morning or evening; may increase to 2 mg qd and, thereafter, 4 mg and 8 mg qd, as needed. Rec- ommended titration interval 1 to 2 wk.	• Use cautiously in impaired hepatic function. • Contraindicated in hypersensitivity to drug and quinazoline derivatives (including pra- zosin and terazosin).
doxepin hydrochloride Deptran‡, Novo-Doxepin†, Sinequan, Triadapin† *Tricyclic antidepressant* *Antidepressant* Preg. Risk Category: NR	*cap:* 10, 25, 50, 75, 100, 150 mg; *oral conc:* 10 mg/ml	*Depression or anxiety —* **Adults:** initially, 25 to 75 mg PO daily in divided doses to max 300 mg daily. Alter- natively, give entire maintenance dosage qd with max 150 mg PO.	• Contraindicated in hypersensitivity to drug, glaucoma, or tendency to urine retention, within 14 days of MAO inhibitor therapy, or during acute recovery phase of an MI. • Decrease dosage in elderly or debilitated pa- tients, adolescents, and those receiving oth- er medications. Avoid in children < 12 yr.

doxorubicin hydrochloride
Adriamycin‡, Adriamycin PFS, Adriamycin RDF, Rubex
Antineoplastic antibiotic (cell cycle–phase nonspecific)
Antineoplastic
Preg. Risk Category: D

inj (preservtree): 2 mg/ml; *powder for inj:* 10-, 20-, 50-, 100-, 150-mg vials

Dosage and indications vary. Check treatment protocol.

Bladder, breast, lung, ovarian, stomach, and thyroid cancers; Hodgkin's disease; acute lymphoblastic and myeloblastic leukemia; Wilms' tumor; neuroblastoma; lymphoma; sarcoma — **Adults:** 60 to 75 mg/m² IV as single dose q 3 wk; or 30 mg/m² IV in single qd dose, days 1 to 3 of 4-wk cycle. Or, 20 mg/m² IV once weekly. Max cumulative dosage 550 mg/m².

■ Contraindicated in marked myelosuppression induced by previous treatment with other antitumor agents or by radiotherapy and in patients who have received lifetime cumulative dosage of 550 mg/m² of doxorubicin or daunorubicin.

---

doxycycline calcium
Vibramycin

doxycycline hyclate
Doryx, Doxy-100, Doxy-200, Doxy-Caps, Vibramycin, Vibra-Tabs

doxycycline hydrochloride
Cyclidox‡, Doryx‡, Doxylin‡, Vibramycin‡, Vibra-Tabs 50‡

doxycycline monohydrate
Monodox, Vibramycin
Tetracycline
Antibiotic
Preg. Risk Category: D

calcium—oral susp: 50 mg/5 ml. *hyclate — cap:* 50 mg, 100 mg; *tab:* 100 mg; *inj:* 100 mg, 200 mg. *hydrochloride — tab:* 50 mg‡, 100 mg‡; *cap:* 50 mg‡, 100 mg‡, 250 mg‡; *inj:* 100 mg‡; *monohydrate — cap:* 50 mg, 100 mg; *oral susp:* 25 mg/5 ml

Infections caused by sensitive organisms — **Adults and children > 8 yr and ≥ 45 kg:** 100 mg PO q 12 hr on day 1, then 100 mg PO qd; or 200 mg IV on day 1 in one or two infusions, then 100 to 200 mg IV qd. **Children > 8 yr and < 45 kg:** 4.4 mg/kg PO or IV qd, divided q 12 hr day 1, then 2.2 to 4.4 mg/kg qd. Give IV infusion slowly (min 1 hr). Complete infusion by 12 hr by 6 hr in lactated Ringer's solution or dextrose 5% in lactated Ringer's solution).
Gonorrhea in patients allergic to penicillin — **Adults:** 100 mg PO bid for 7 days.
C. trachomatis, nongonococcal urethritis, and uncomplicated urethral, endocervical, or rectal infections — **Adults:** 100 mg PO bid for at least 7 days.
Acute epididymo-orchitis caused by C. trachomatis or N. gonorrhoeae — **Adults:** 100 mg PO bid for at least 10 days.
Prophylaxis for malaria — **Adults:** 100 mg PO once daily. Begin 1 to 2 days before travel to malarious areas; qd while in affected area, and for 4 wk after return. **Children > 8 yr:** 2 mg/kg PO qd as one dose; max 100 mg qd. Use adult dosage schedule.

■ Use cautiously in impaired renal or hepatic function.
■ Use during last half of pregnancy and in children < 8 yr may cause permanent discoloration of teeth, enamel defects, and bone growth retardation.
■ Contraindicated in hypersensitivity to drug or other tetracyclines.

†Canadian ‡Australian

DRUG/CLASS/ CATEGORY	DOSAGE FORMS	INDICATIONS/ DOSAGES	KEY PRECAUTIONS
d-penicillamine Cuprimine, Depen, D-Penamine‡ *Chelating agent* *Anti-inflammatory* Preg. Risk Category: NR	*tab:* 125 mg‡; 250 mg; *cap:* 125, 250 mg	*Wilson's disease* — **Adults and children:** 250 mg PO qid 30 to 60 min before meals. Adjust dosage to achieve urinary copper excretion of 0.5 to 1 mg daily. *Cystinuria* — **Adults:** 250 mg to 1 g PO qid before meals. Adjust dosage to urinary cystine excretion < 100 mg daily with calculi present or 100 to 200 mg daily when no calculi present. Max 4 g daily. **Children:** 30 mg/kg PO daily, divided qid before meals. Dosage adjusted to achieve urinary cystine excretion < 100 mg daily when renal calculi present, or 100 to 200 mg qd with no calculi. *Rheumatoid arthritis* — **Adults:** initially, 125 to 250 mg PO daily, with increases of 125 to 250 mg q 1 to 3 months, if necessary. Max 1.5 g daily.	• Use with extreme caution, if at all, in hypersensitivity to penicillin. • Contraindicated in pregnant patients with cystinuria, in penicillamine-related aplastic anemia or granulocytosis, and in rheumatoid arthritis accompanied by renal insufficiency.
dronabinol (delta-g-tetrahydrocannabinol) Marinol *Cannabinoid* *Antiemetic/appetite stimulant* Preg. Risk Category: C Controlled Sub. Sched.: II	*cap:* 2.5, 5, 10 mg	*Nausea and vomiting associated with cancer chemotherapy* — **Adults:** 5 mg/m² PO 1 to 3 hr before chemotherapy. Then same dose q 2 to 4 hr after chemotherapy for total of 4 to 6 doses per day. If needed, increase in 2.5-mg/m² increments to max 15 mg/m² per dose. *Anorexia and weight loss in patients with AIDS* — **Adults:** 2.5 mg PO bid before lunch and dinner. If unable to tolerate, decrease dose to 2.5 mg PO, given as single dose daily in evening or hs. May gradually increase to max 20 mg/day.	• Use cautiously in elderly, pregnant, or breast-feeding patients and in heart disease, psychiatric illness, and history of drug abuse. • Contraindicated in hypersensitivity to sesame oil or cannabinoids.

e

echothiophate iodide (ecothiopate iodide) Phospholine Iodide *Cholinesterase inhibitor* *Miotic* Preg. Risk Category: C	**ophth powder for sol:** for reconstitution to make 0.03%, 0.06%, 0.125%, 0.25% sol	*Primary open-angle glaucoma, conditions obstructing aqueous outflow* — **Adults and children:** 1 drop 0.03% to 0.125% sol instilled into conjunctival sac daily. Max 1 drop bid. Lowest possible dosage used for continuous IOP control. *Diagnosis of convergent strabismus* — **Adults:** 1 drop 0.125% sol instilled daily at hs for 2 to 3 wk. *Treatment of convergent strabismus* — **Adults:** initially, 1 drop 0.125% sol instilled into each eye daily at hs for 2 to 3 wk. Decrease dosage to 1 drop 0.125% sol qod or 1 drop 0.06% sol daily. For some patients, 0.03% sol may be used instead.	■ Use with extreme caution in seizure disorders, vasomotor instability, parkinsonism, asthma, spastic GI conditions, urinary tract obstruction, peptic ulcer, severe bradycardia or hypotension, vascular hypertension, MI, or history or risk of retinal detachment. Use cautiously in corneal abrasion. ■ Contraindicated in hypersensitivity to drug or iodine, uveal inflammation, acute angle-closure glaucoma before iridectomy, and other forms of glaucoma (except primary open-angle).
econazole nitrate Ecostatin†, Spectazole *Synthetic imidazole derivative* *Antifungal* Preg. Risk Category: C	**cream:** 1%	*Tinea pedis, tinea cruris, tinea corporis, and tinea versicolor; cutaneous candidiasis* — **Adults and children:** rub into affected areas qd for ≥ 2 wk. *Cutaneous candidiasis* — **Adults and children:** rub into affected areas bid.	■ Contraindicated in hypersensitivity to drug.
edetate calcium disodium Calcium Disodium Versenate, Calcium EDTA *Chelating agent* *Heavy metal antagonist* Preg. Risk Category: NR	**inj:** 200 mg/ml	*Acute lead encephalopathy or blood lead levels > 70 mcg/dl* — **Adults and children:** 1 to 1.5 g/m² IV or IM qd in 2 divided doses q 12 hr for 3 to 5 days, with dimercaprol. May give 2nd course after drug-free ≥ 2 days. *Lead poisoning without encephalopathy or asymptomatic with blood levels < 70 mcg/dl* — **Children:** 1 g/m² IV or IM qd in divided doses for 5 days.	■ Use with extreme caution and at reduced dosages in mild renal disease. ■ Contraindicated in anuria, hepatitis, and acute renal disease.
edetate disodium Disodium EDTA, Disotate, Endrate *Chelating agent* *Heavy metal antagonist* Preg. Risk Category: NR	**inj:** 150 mg/ml	*Hypercalcemic crisis* — **Adults:** 50 mg/kg/day by slow IV infusion added to 500 ml D₅W or 0.9% NaCl sol administered over ≥ 3 hr. Max 3 g/day. **Children:** 40 to 70 mg/kg/day by slow IV infusion, diluted to max conc 30 mg/ml in D₅W or 0.9% NaCl sol given over ≥ 3 hr. Max 70 mg/kg/day.	■ Use cautiously in limited cardiac reserve, heart failure, or hypokalemia. ■ Contraindicated in hypersensitivity, anuria, known or suspected hypocalcemia, significant renal disease, active or healed tubercular lesions, or history of seizures or intracranial lesions.

EDETATE DISODIUM **85**

ENALAPRILAT   86

DRUG/CLASS/CATEGORY	DOSAGE FORMS	INDICATIONS/DOSAGES	KEY PRECAUTIONS
enalaprilat Vasotec IV **enalapril maleate** Amprace‡, Renitec‡, Vasotec *ACE inhibitor* *Antihypertensive* Preg. Risk Category: C (D in 2nd and 3rd trimesters)	**enalaprilat** — *inj:* 1.25 mg/ml in 2-ml vials. **enalapril maleate** — *tab:* 2.5, 5, 10, 20 mg	*Hypertension* — **Adults:** if patient not on diuretics, initially 5 mg PO qd, then adjust based on response. Usual dosage range 10 to 40 mg daily as single dose or 2 divided doses. Or, 1.25 mg IV infusion q 6 hr over 5 min. For patient on diuretics, initially 2.5 mg PO qd. Or, 0.625 mg IV over 5 min; repeat in 1 hr if needed, then 1.25 mg IV q 6 hr. *To switch from IV to oral therapy* — **Adults:** initially, 5 mg PO qd; if patient was receiving 0.625 mg IV q 6 hr, then 2.5 mg PO qd. Adjust dosage to response. *To convert from oral to IV therapy* — **Adults:** 1.25 mg IV over 5 min q 6 hr.	▪ Use cautiously in renal impairment. ▪ Contraindicated in hypersensitivity to drug or history of angioedema related to previous ACE inhibitor therapy.
enoxaparin sodium Lovenox *Low-molecular-weight heparin* *Anticoagulant* Preg. Risk Category: B	*inj:* 30 mg/0.3 ml	*To prevent pulmonary embolism and DVT after hip or knee replacement surgery* — **Adults:** 30 mg SC q 12 hr for 7 to 10 days. Give initial dose between 12 and 24 hr postop if hemostasis established.	▪ Use with extreme caution in history of heparin-induced thrombocytopenia and in bacterial endocarditis, congenital or acquired bleeding disorders, ulcer disease, angiodysplastic GI disease, hemorrhagic CVA, or recent spinal, eye, or brain surgery, threatened abortion, aneurysms, or uncontrolled hypertension. ▪ Contraindicated in hypersensitivity to drug, heparin, or pork products; major bleeding or thrombocytopenia; and demonstrated antiplatelet antibodies in presence of drug.
ephedrine sulfate Vicks Vatronol Nose Drops *Adrenergic* *Bronchodilator/nasal decongestant* Preg. Risk Category: NR	*nasal sol:* 0.5%	*Nasal congestion* — **Adults and children:** 2 to 3 drops of 0.5% sol into each nostril. Don't use more frequently than q 4 hr.	▪ Use cautiously in hyperthyroidism, hypertension, diabetes mellitus, prostatic hyperplasia, or nervous or excitable states. ▪ Contraindicated in hypersensitivity to drug or other sympathomimetics; in porphyria,

severe CAD, arrhythmias, angle-closure glaucoma, psychoneurosis, angina pectoris, substantial organic heart disease, CV disease; and in patients taking MAO inhibitors.

- Use with extreme caution in long-standing bronchial asthma and emphysema accompanied by degenerative heart disease. Also use cautiously in elderly patients and in hyperthyroidism, CV disease, hypertension, psychoneurosis, and diabetes.
- Contraindicated in angle-closure glaucoma, shock (other than anaphylactic), organic brain damage, cardiac dilation, arrhythmias, coronary insufficiency, or cerebral arteriosclerosis. Also contraindicated during general anesthesia with halogenated hydrocarbons or cyclopropane and during labor.
- Commercial products containing sulfites contraindicated in sulfite allergies, except when used to treat serious allergic reactions or other emergency situations.

---

epinephrine (adrenaline)
Adrenalin, Bronkaid Mist, Bronkaid Mistometer†, Primatene Mist

epinephrine bitartrate
AsthmaHaler, Bronitin Mist, Bronkaid Mist Suspension, MediHaler-Epi

epinephrine hydrochloride
Adrenalin Chloride, AsthmaNefrin†, Epi-Pen, Epi-Pen Jr., Racepinephrine†, Sus-Phrine, Vaponefrine
Adrenergic
Bronchodilator/vasopressor/ cardiac stimulant
Preg. Risk Category: C

aerosol inhaler: 160, 200, 220, 250 mcg/metered spray; *neb inhaler:* 1% (1:100)†, 1.25%†; *inj:* 2.25%†; *inj:* 0.01 mg/ml (1:100,000), 0.1 mg/ml (1:10,000), 0.5 mg/ml (1:2,000), 1 mg/ml (1:1,000) parenteral; 5 mg/ml (1:200) parenteral susp; *ophth sol:* 0.1, 0.25, 0.5, 1, 2%

Bronchospasm, hypersensitivity reactions, anaphylaxis — **Adults:** 0.1 to 0.5 ml of 1:1,000 SC or IM. Repeat q 10 to 15 min, prn. Or, 0.1 to 0.25 ml of 1:1,000 IV slowly over 5 to 10 min. **Children:** 0.01 ml (10 mcg) of 1:1,000/kg SC; repeat q 20 min to 4 hr, prn. Or, 0.004 to 0.005 ml/kg of 1:200 (Sus-Phrine) SC; repeat q 8 to 12 hr, prn.
Acute asthmatic attacks — **Adults and children ≥ 4 yr:** 160 to 250 mcg (metered aerosol), equiv to 1 inh; repeated once prn after ≥ 1 min; don't give add. doses for ≥ 3 hr. Or, 1% (1:100) sol epinephrine or 2.25% sol racepinephrine by hand-bulb nebulizer as 1 to 3 deep inh, repeated q 3 hr prn.
To restore cardiac rhythm in cardiac arrest — **Adults:** 0.5 to 1 mg IV. May repeat q 3 to 5 min prn. Higher-dose epinephrine may be used: 3 to 5 mg (approx 0.1 mg/kg) repeated q 3 to 5 min. **Children:** usual dose 0.01 mg/kg (0.1 ml/kg 1:10,000 injection) IV Usual dose through ET tube 0.1 mg/kg (0.1 ml/kg 1:1,000 inj) diluted in 1 to 2 ml 0.45% or 0.9% NaCl sol. Add. IV or intratracheal doses 0.1 to 0.2 mg/kg (0.1 to 0.2 ml/kg of 1:1,000 injection). May repeat q 3 to 5 min.

---

epinephrine hydrochloride
Adrenalin Chloride
Adrenergic
Topical antihemorrhagic
Preg. Risk Category: NR

nasal sol: 0.1%

Nasal congestion, local superficial bleeding — **Adults and children ≥ 6 yr:** instill 1 or 2 drops of sol.

- Use cautiously in hyperthyroidism, CAD, hypertension, or diabetes mellitus.
- Contraindicated in hypersensitivity to drug.

†Canadian ‡Australian

DRUG / CLASS / CATEGORY	DOSAGE FORMS	INDICATIONS / DOSAGES	KEY PRECAUTIONS
epinephrine hydrochloride Epifrin, Glaucon *Adrenergic* *Antiglaucoma agent* Preg. Risk Category: C	**ophth sol:** 0.1, 0.25, 0.5, 1, 2%	*Open-angle glaucoma* — **Adults:** 1 or 2 drops 1% or 2% sol qd or bid. Adjust dosage according to tonometric readings.	▪ Use cautiously in elderly patients and in diabetes mellitus, hypertension, Parkinson's disease, hyperthyroidism, aphakia, cardiac disease, cerebral arteriosclerosis, or bronchial asthma. ▪ Contraindicated in angle-closure glaucoma or when glaucoma nature not established. Also contraindicated in hypersensitivity to drug or sulfites, in organic mental syndromes, and in hypertensive CV disease or CAD.
epoetin alfa (erythropoietin) Epogen, Procrit *Glycoprotein* *Anti-anemic agent* Preg. Risk Category: C	**inj:** 2,000, 3,000, 4,000, 10,000 units/ml	*Anemia due to reduced production of endogenous erythropoietin caused by end-stage renal disease* — **Adults:** dosage individualized. 50 to 100 units/kg IV 3 times weekly. (Can use SC or IV in nondialysis patients with chronic renal failure or those on cont. peritoneal dialysis.) Reduce dosage when target Hct reached or if Hct > 4 pts in any 2-wk period. Increase if Hct doesn't increase by 5 to 6 pts after 8 wk of therapy. Maint dosage highly individualized. *Adjunctive treatment of HIV-infected patients with anemia secondary to zidovudine therapy* — **Adults:** 100 units/kg IV or SC 3 times weekly for 8 wk or until target Hgb level reached. If response unsatisfactory after 8 wk, may increase by 50 to 100 units/kg IV or SC 3 times weekly. After 4 to 8 wk, may increase in increments of 50 to 100 units/kg 3 times weekly, to max 300 units/kg IV or SC 3 times weekly. *Anemia secondary to cancer chemotherapy* — **Adults:** 150 units/kg SC 3 times weekly for 8 wk or until target Hgb level reached.	▪ Contraindicated in uncontrolled hypertension or hypersensitivity to mammalian cell-derived products or to albumin (human).

ergotamine tartrate

Ergodryl Mono‡, Ergomar, Ergostat, Gynergen†, Medihaler Ergotamine

Ergot alkaloid
Vasoconstrictor
Preg. Risk Category: X

cap: 1 mg†; **tab:** 1 mg†; **tab (SL):** 2 mg; **aerosol inhaler:** 360 mcg/metered spray

Vascular or migraine headache — **Adults:** initially, 2 mg PO or SL, then 1 to 2 mg PO q hr or SL q ½ hr, to max 6 mg daily and 10 mg weekly. Alternatively, aerosol inhaler: 1 spray (360 mcg) initially, repeated q 5 min prn to max of 6 sprays (2.16 mg) per 24 hr or 15 sprays (5.4 mg) per wk.

- Contraindicated in hypersensitivity to ergot alkaloids, peripheral and occlusive vascular diseases, CAD, hypertension, hepatic or renal dysfunction, severe pruritus, or sepsis and in pregnancy.

erythromycin

Akne-mycin, Erycette, EryDerm, EryGel, Ery-Sol†

Erythromycin
Antibiotic
Preg. Risk Category: C

oint: 2%; **topical gel:** 2%; **topical sol:** 1.5, 2%; **pledgets:** 2%

Inflammatory acne vulgaris — **Adults and children:** apply in thin film to affected areas bid.

- Contraindicated in hypersensitivity to drug or other macrolides.

erythromycin

Ilotycin Ophthalmic Ointment

Erythromycin
Antibiotic
Preg. Risk Category: NR

ophth oint: 0.5%

Acute and chronic conjunctivitis, trachoma, other eye infections — **Adults and children:** 1-cm length applied directly to infected eye up to 6 times daily, depending on severity of infection.
Prophylaxis of ophthalmia neonatorum due to N. gonorrhoeae or C. trachomatis — **Neonates:** ribbon of oint approx 1 cm long applied in lower conjunctival sac of each eye shortly after birth.

- Contraindicated in hypersensitivity to drug or other macrolides.

erythromycin base
E-Mycin, Eramycin, Robimycin
erythromycin estolate
Ilosone, Ilosone pulvules
erythromycin ethylsuccinate
EryPed, EryPed 200
erythromycin lactobionate
Erythrocin

base — tab (ent-coated): 250, 333, 500 mg; **tab (filmtabs):** 250, 500 mg; **pellets:** 250 mg. **estol. — tab:** 500 mg; **cap:** 250 mg; **oral susp:** 125, 250 mg/5 ml.

Acute PID caused by N. gonorrhoeae — **Adults:** 500 mg IV (lacto.) q 6 for 3 days, then 250 mg (base, estolate, stearate) or 400 mg (ethyl.) PO q 6 for 7 days.
Endocarditis prophylaxis for dental procedures in patients allergic to penicillin — **Adults:** 800 mg (ethyl.) or 1 g (stearate) PO 1½ to 2 hr before; then 400 mg (ethyl.) or 500 mg (stearate) PO 6 hr later. **Children:** 20 mg/kg (ethyl., stearate) PO 1½ to 2 hr before procedure; half amount 6 hr later.

- Use erythromycin salts cautiously in impaired hepatic function.
- Erythromycin estolate not recommended during pregnancy.
- Contraindicated in hypersensitivity to drug or other macrolides. Erythromycin estolate contraindicated in hepatic disease.

(continued)

ERYTHROMYCIN LACTOBIONATE

†Canadian ‡Australian

DRUG/CLASS/ CATEGORY	DOSAGE FORMS	INDICATIONS/ DOSAGES	KEY PRECAUTIONS
erythromycin *(continued)* **erythromycin stearate** Erythrocin Stearate *Erythromycin* *Antibiotic* Preg. Risk Category: B	**ethyl. — tab** *(film-coated):* 400 mg; **tab** *(chew):* 200 mg; *oral susp:* 200, 400 mg/5 ml, 100 mg/2.5 ml. **lacto.** — *inj:* 500-mg, 1-g vials. **stearate — tab:** 250, 500 mg	*Mild to mod. severe respiratory tract, skin, and soft-tissue infections —* **Adults:** 250 to 500 mg (base, es-tolate, stearate) PO q 6 hr; or 400 to 800 mg (ethyl.) PO q 6 hr; or 15 to 20 mg/kg IV daily (ethyl.) continu-ous inf or divided doses q 6 hr for 10 days. **Children:** 30 to 50 mg/kg (oral salts) PO qd, divided doses q 6 hr; or 15 to 20 mg/kg IV qd, divided doses q 4 to 6 hr for 10 days.	▪ Use cautiously in impaired renal function, diabetes, or bronchospasm. ▪ Contraindicated in sinus bradycardia, heart block > first degree, cardiogenic shock, or overt heart failure.
esmolol hydrochloride Brevibloc *Beta₁-adrenergic blocker* *Antiarrhythmic* Preg. Risk Category: C	*inj:* 10 mg/ml in 10-ml vials, 250 mg/ml in 10-ml ampules	*SVT; to control ventricular rate in atrial fibrillation or flutter in periop, postop, or other emergent circum-stances; noncompensatory sinus tachycardia when HR requires specific interventions —* **Adults:** loading dose: 500 mcg/kg/min by IV infusion over 1 min, then 4-min maint infusion of 50 mcg/kg/min. If no ade-quate response in 5 min, repeat loading dose and then maint infusion of 100 mcg/kg/min for 4 min. Re-peat loading dose and increase maint infusion by 50-mcg/kg/min increments. Max maint infusion for tachycardia 200 mcg/kg/min. *Periop and postop tachycardia or hypertension —* **Adults:** for periop treatment of tachycardia or hyper-tension, 80 mg (approx 1 mg/kg) IV bolus over 30 sec, followed by 150 mcg/kg/min IV infusion, if need-ed. Adjust rate prn to max 300 mcg/kg/min.	

esterified estrogens
Estratab, Menest, Neo-Estrone†

Estrogen

Estrogen replacement/antineoplastic

Preg. Risk Category: X

tab: 0.3, 0.625, 1.25, 2.5 mg; *tab (film-coated)*: 0.3, 0.625, 1.25, 2.5 mg

Inoperable prostate cancer — **Men:** 1.25 to 2.5 mg PO tid.

Breast cancer — **Men and postmenopausal women:** 10 mg PO tid for ≥3 mo.

Female hypogonadism — **Women:** 2.5 to 7.5 mg qd in divided doses in cycles of 20 days on, 10 days off.

Female castration, primary ovarian failure — **Women:** 1.25 mg qd in cycles of 3 wk on, 1 wk off. Adjust for symptoms.

- Use cautiously in history of hypertension; mental depression; cardiac, hepatic, or renal dysfunction; bone disease; migraine; seizures; or diabetes mellitus.
- Contraindicated in breast cancer (except metastatic disease), estrogen-dependent neoplasia, thrombophlebitis or thromboembolic disorders, undiagnosed abnormal genital bleeding, hypersensitivity, history of thromboembolic disease, or pregnancy.

---

estradiol (oestradiol)
Climara, Estrace, Estraderm
estradiol cypionate
depGynogen, Depo-Estradiol, E-Cypionate, Estrofem
estradiol valerate (oestradiol valerate)
Climara Patch, Delestrogen, Dioval, Estradiol L.A., Estra-L 20, Estra-L 40, Estraval, Femogex, Gynogen LA, LAE, Menaval, Primogyn Depot‡
polyestradiol phosphate
Estradurin

Estrogen

Estrogen replacement/antineoplastic

Preg. Risk Category: X

estradiol — tab (micronized): 0.5, 1, 2 mg; *transderm*: 4 mg/10 cm² (0.05 mg/24 hr); 8 mg/20 cm² (0.1 mg/24 hr); *vag cream*: 0.1 mg/g. *cypionate — inj (in oil)*: 5 mg/ml. *valerate — inj (in oil)*: 10 mg/ml, 20 mg/ml, 40 mg/ml.

polyestradiol phosphate — inj: 40 mg/2 ml

Vasomotor menopausal symptoms, female hypogonadism, female castration, primary ovarian failure — **Adults:** 1 to 2 mg PO (estradiol) daily in cycles of 21 days on and 7 days off, or cycles of 5 days on and 2 days off; or 1 transdermal system (Estraderm) delivering 0.05 mg/24 hr, or as system (Climara) delivering either 0.05 mg/24 hr or 0.1 mg/24 hr and applied q wk in cycles of 3 wk on and 1 wk off. Alternatively, 1 to 5 mg (cypionate) IM q 3 to 4 wk, or 10 to 20 mg (valerate) IM q 4 wk, prn.

Palliative treatment of advanced, inoperable breast cancer — **Men and postmenopausal women:** 10 mg PO (estradiol) tid for 3 mo.

Palliative treatment of advanced inoperable prostate cancer — **Men:** 30 mg (valerate) IM q 1 to 2 wk, or 1 to 2 mg PO (estradiol) tid. Polyestradiol phosphate injection: 40 mg IM q 2 to 4 wk.

- Use cautiously in cerebrovascular disease; CAD; asthma; bone diseases; migraine; seizures; cardiac, hepatic or renal dysfunction; or in women with strong family history of breast cancer or who have breast nodules, fibrocystic disease, or abnormal mammographic findings.
- Contraindicated in thrombophlebitis or thromboembolic disorders, estrogen-dependent neoplasia, breast or reproductive organ cancer (except for palliative treatment), or undiagnosed abnormal genital bleeding and during pregnancy. Also contraindicated in history of thrombophlebitis or thromboembolic disorders associated with previous estrogen use (except for palliative treatment of breast and prostate cancer).

---

†Canadian ‡Australian

ESTRADIOL 91

DRUG/CLASS/ CATEGORY	DOSAGE FORMS	INDICATIONS/ DOSAGES	KEY PRECAUTIONS
estramustine phosphate sodium Emcyt, Estracyt‡ *Estrogen/alkylating agent Antineoplastic* Preg. Risk Category: NR	*cap:* 140 mg	*Palliative treatment of metastatic or progressive prostate cancer —* **Adults:** 10 to 16 mg/kg/day PO in 3 or 4 divided doses. Usual dosage 14 mg/kg daily. Continue therapy for up to 3 mo and, if successful, maintain as long as patient responds.	▪ Use cautiously in history of throm-bophlebitis or thromboembolic disorders and in cerebrovascular disease or CAD. ▪ Contraindicated in hypersensitivity to estra-diol or nitrogen mustard and in active thrombophlebitis or thromboembolic disor-ders (except when tumor mass is cause of thromboembolism).
estrogens, conjugated (estrogenic substances, conjugated; oestrogens, conjugated) C.E.S†, Premarin, Premarin Intravenous *Estrogen Estrogen replacement/ antineoplastic/antiosteoporotic* Preg. Risk Category: X	*tab:* 0.3, 0.625, 0.9, 1.25, 2.5 mg; *inj:* 25 mg/5 ml; *vag cream:* 0.625%	*Abnormal uterine bleeding (hormonal imbalance) —* **Women:** 25 mg IV or IM, repeated in 6 to 12 hr prn. *Female castration, primary ovarian failure —* **Women:** 1.25 mg PO daily in cycles of 3 wk on and 1 wk off. *Osteoporosis —* **Postmenopausal women:** 0.625 mg PO daily in cyclic regimen (3 wk on, 1 wk off).	▪ Use cautiously in cerebrovascular disease; CAD; asthma; bone disease; migraine; seizures; cardiac, hepatic, or renal dysfunc-tion; or in women with family history of breast or genital tract cancer or who have breast nodules, fibrocystic disease, or ab-normal mammographic findings. ▪ Contraindicated in thrombophlebitis or thromboembolic disorders, estrogen-depen-dent neoplasia, breast or reproductive organ cancer (except for palliative treatment), or undiagnosed abnormal genital bleeding and during pregnancy.
estropipate (piperazine estrone sulfate) Ogen, OrthoEST *Estrogen Estrogen replacement* Preg. Risk Category: X	estropipate as estrone sodi-um sulfate — *tab:* 0.625, 1.25, 2.5 mg	*Primary ovarian failure, female castration, female hy-pogonadism —* **Women:** 1.25 to 7.5 mg PO daily for first 3 wk, followed by rest period of 8 to 10 days. If bleeding does not occur by end of rest period, cycle repeated. *Vasomotor menopause symptoms —* **Women:** 0.625 mg to 5 mg PO daily in cyclic method of 3 wk on, 1 wk off.	▪ Use cautiously in cerebrovascular disease; CAD; asthma; mental depression; bone dis-ease; migraine; seizures; cardiac, hepatic, or renal dysfunction; and in women with family history of breast or genital tract cancer or who have breast nodules, fibrocystic dis-ease, or abnormal mammographic findings.

Drug	Preparations	Indications & Dosage	Contraindications & Precautions
		Prevention of osteoporosis — **Women:** 0.625 mg PO daily for 25 days of 31-day cycle.	■ Contraindicated in active thrombophlebitis or thromboembolic disorders; in estrogen-dependent neoplasia, breast, reproductive organ, or genital cancer; in undiagnosed genital bleeding; and during pregnancy.
ethacrynate sodium Sodium Edecrin **ethacrynic acid** Edecrit,‡ Edecrin *Loop diuretic* *Diuretic* Preg. Risk Category: B	**ethacrynate sodium** — **inj:** 50 mg (with 62.5 mg of mannitol and 0.1 mg of thimerosal). **ethacrynic acid** — **tab:** 25 mg, 50 mg	*Acute pulmonary edema* — **Adults:** 50 mg or 0.5 to 1 mg/kg IV to max dose of 100 mg of ethacrynate sodium IV slowly over several min. *Edema* — **Adults:** 50 to 200 mg PO qd. Refractory cases may require up to 200 mg PO bid. **Children:** initially, 25 mg PO. Increased in 25-mg increments qd until desired effect is achieved.	■ Use cautiously in electrolyte abnormalities or impaired hepatic function. ■ Contraindicated in anuria or hypersensitivity to drug and in infants.
ethambutol hydrochloride Etibi,† Myambutol *Semisynthetic antitubercular* *Antitubercular agent* Preg. Risk Category: C	**tab:** 100, 400 mg	*Adjunctive treatment in pulmonary TB* — **Adults and children > 13 yr:** initially for patients who have not received previous antitubercular therapy, 15 mg/kg PO as 1 dose qd. Retreatment: 25 mg/kg PO as 1 dose qd for 60 days (or until smears and cultures negative) with at least 1 other antitubercular; then decrease to 15 mg/kg/day as 1 dose.	■ Use cautiously in impaired renal function, cataracts, recurrent eye inflammations, gout, and diabetic retinopathy. ■ Contraindicated in hypersensitivity to drug or optic neuritis and in children < 13 yr.
ethinyl estradiol (ethinyloestradiol) Estinyl, Feminone *Estrogen* *Estrogen replacement/ antineoplastic* Preg. Risk Category: X	**tab:** 0.02, 0.05, 0.5 mg	*Palliative treatment of metastatic breast cancer (at least 5 yr after menopause)* — **Women:** 1 mg PO tid for at least 3 mo. *Female hypogonadism* — **Women:** 0.05 mg PO qd to tid 2 wk per mo, followed by 2 wk of progesterone therapy; continued for 3 to 6 mo dosing cycles, followed by 2 mo off. *Vasomotor menopause symptoms* — **Women:** 0.02 to 0.05 mg PO qd for cycles of 3 wk on and 1 wk off.	■ Use cautiously in cerebrovascular disease; CAD; asthma; mental depression; bone disease; cardiac, hepatic, or renal dysfunction; or in women with family history of breast or genital tract cancer, or who have breast nodules, fibrocystic disease, or abnormal mammographic findings. ■ Contraindicated in patients with thrombophlebitis or thromboembolic disorders, *(continued)*

†Canadian ‡Australian

DRUG / CLASS / CATEGORY	DOSAGE FORMS	INDICATIONS / DOSAGES	KEY PRECAUTIONS
ethinyl estradiol *(continued)*		*Palliative treatment of metastatic inoperable prostate cancer* — **Men:** 0.15 to 2 mg PO qd.	estrogen-dependent neoplasia, breast or reproductive organ cancer (except for palliative treatment), or undiagnosed abnormal genital bleeding and during pregnancy.
ethinyl estradiol *monophasic:* w/desogestrel — Desogen; w/ethynodiol diacetate — Demulen 1/35; w/levonorgestrel — Nordette; w/norethindrone — Genora 1/35; w/norethindrone acetate — Loestrin 21 1/20; w/norgestimate — Ortho Cyclen; w/norgestrel — Ovral; w/norethindrone acetate and ferrous fumarate — Loestrin Fe 1/20; *biphasic:* w/ norethindrone — Jenest-28; *triphasic:* w/levonorgestrel — Triphasil; w/norethindrone — Ortho-Novum 7/7/7; w/norgestimate — Ortho Tri-Cyclen **mestranol** *monophasic:* w/norethindrone — Genora 1/50; w/norethynodrel — Enovid *Estrogen and progestin Oral contraceptive* Preg. Risk Category: X	**Monophasic, biphasic and triphasic oral contraceptives — tab:** strengths vary with phase and combinations in product	*Contraception* — **Adults:** *Monophasic* — 1 tab PO daily, starting on day 5 of menstrual cycle. With 20- and 21-tab pkg, new dosing cycle begins 7 days after last tab taken. With 28-tab pkg, dosage is 1 tab qd without interruption. *Biphasic* — 1 color tab PO daily for 10 days; then next color tab for 11 days. With 21-tab pkg, new dosing cycle begins 7 days after last tab taken. With 28-tab pkg, dosage is 1 tab daily without interruption. *Triphasic* — 1 tab PO qd in sequence specified by brand. With 21-tab pkg, new dosing cycle begins 7 days after last tab taken. With 28-tab pkg, dosage is 1 tab qd without interruption. *Endometriosis* — **Adults:** 1 tab Enovid 5 mg or 10 mg PO daily for 2 wk starting on day 5 of menstrual cycle. Continue without interruption for 6 to 9 mo, increasing by 5 to 10 mg q 2 wk, up to 20 mg daily; up to 40 mg daily as needed and ordered if breakthrough bleeding occurs.	■ Use cautiously in cardiac, renal, or hepatic insufficiency; hyperlipidemia; hypertension; migraine; seizure disorders; or asthma. ■ Contraindicated in thromboembolic disorders, cerebrovascular disease, CAD, diplopia or ocular lesions arising from ophthalmic vascular disease, classical migraine, MI, known or suspected breast cancer, known or suspected estrogen-dependent neoplasia, benign or malignant liver tumors, active liver disease or history of cholestatic jaundice with pregnancy or prior use of oral contraceptives, and undiagnosed abnormal vaginal bleeding; in known or suspected pregnancy; and in breast-feeding patients.

ethosuximide Zarontin *Succinimide derivative* *Anticonvulsant* Preg. Risk Category: NR	*cap:* 250 mg; *syrup:* 250 mg/5 ml	*Absence seizures* — **Adults and children ≥ 6 yr:** 250 mg PO bid. May increase by 250 mg q 4 to 7 days up to 1.5 g daily. **Children 3 to 6 yr:** 250 mg PO daily. Adjust until control achieved. Optimal: 20 mg/kg/day. Dosages > 1.5 g daily require strict supervision.	▪ Use with extreme caution in hepatic or renal disease. ▪ Contraindicated in hypersensitivity to succinimide derivatives.
etidronate disodium Didronel *Pyrophosphate analogue* *Antihypercalcemic* Preg. Risk Category: C	*tab:* 200, 400 mg; *inj:* 50 mg/ml	*Symptomatic Paget's disease of bone* — **Adults:** 5 to 10 mg/kg PO qd (max 6 mo) or 11 to 20 mg/kg PO qd (max 3 mo) in 1 dose 2 hr before meal with water or juice. *Heterotopic ossification after total hip replacement* — **Adults:** 20 mg/kg PO daily for 1 mo before total hip replacement and for 3 mo afterward. *Malignancy-associated hypercalcemia* — **Adults:** 7.5 mg/kg IV daily for 3 consecutive days; period of ≥ 7 days should elapse between courses of IV therapy. Maint dosage 20 mg/kg PO daily for 30 days, initiated day after last IV dosage. May use for max 90 days.	▪ Use cautiously in impaired renal function. ▪ Contraindicated in known hypersensitivity to drug or in clinically overt osteomalacia. IV form contraindicated if serum creatinine 5 mg/dl or greater.
etoposide (VP-16) VePesid **etoposide phosphate** Etopophos *Podophyllotoxin (cell cycle–phase specific, G2 and late S phase)* *Antineoplastic* Preg. Risk Category: D	*cap:* 50 mg; *inj:* 20 mg/ml in 5- and 50-ml vials; *phos.* — *inj:* 113.6-mg vials equiv to 100 mg etoposide	*Testicular cancer* — **Adults:** 50 to 100 mg/m² IV on 5 consecutive days q 3 to 4 wk; or 100 mg/m² on days 1, 3, and 5 q 3 to 4 wk. *Small-cell carcinoma of lung* — **Adults:** 35 mg/m²/ day IV for 4 days; or 50 mg/m²/day IV for 5 days. Oral dosage: twice IV dose, rounded to nearest 50 mg.	▪ Use cautiously in patients who have had cytotoxic or radiation therapy. ▪ Contraindicated in hypersensitivity to drug. ▪ Etoposide phosphate dosage expressed as etoposide equiv.
etretinate Tegison *Retinoid* *Anti-inflammatory/dekeratinizing agent* Preg. Risk Category: X	*cap:* 10, 25 mg	*Severe recalcitrant psoriasis, including erythrodermia and generalized pustular types in patients unresponsive to standard therapy* (topical tar plus UVB light, psoralens plus UVA light, systemic corticosteroids, and methotrexate) — **Adults:** 0.75 to 1 mg/kg PO qd in divided doses. Max initial dosage 1.5 mg/kg PO daily. After initial response, maint 0.5 to 0.75 mg/kg daily.	▪ Contraindicated in patients who are pregnant, intend to become pregnant, or may not use reliable contraception during and after treatment (drug causes severe birth defects).

f

DRUG/CLASS/ CATEGORY	DOSAGE FORMS	INDICATIONS/ DOSAGES	KEY PRECAUTIONS
factor IX (human) AlphaNine, AlphaNine SD, Mononine **factor IX complex** Bebulin VH Immuno, Konyne-80, Profilnine Heat-Treated, Proplex T *Blood derivative* *Systemic hemostatic* Preg. Risk Category: C	*inj:* vials with diluent. Units specified on label.	*Factor IX deficiency (hemophilia B or Christmas disease), anticoagulant overdosage* — **Adults and children:** determine units required factor IX by multiplying 1 unit/kg body weight in kg percentage of desired increase of factor IX level. Infusion rates vary according to product and patient comfort. Dosage highly individualized, depending on degree of deficiency, level of factor IX desired, patient weight, and bleeding severity.	• Use cautiously in neonates and infants. • Contraindicated in hepatic disease with suspected intravascular coagulation or fibrinolysis. Mononine contraindicated in hypersensitivity to murine (mouse) protein.
famciclovir Famvir *Synthetic acyclic guanine derivative* *Antiviral* Preg. Risk Category: B	*tab:* 125, 250, 500 mg	*Acute herpes zoster infection (shingles)* — **Adults:** 500 mg PO q 8 hr for 7 days. *Recurrent episodes of genital herpes* — **Adults:** 125 mg PO bid for 5 days. Start as soon as symptoms occur.	• Use cautiously in renal or hepatic impairment; may require dosage adjustment. • Contraindicated in hypersensitivity to drug.
famotidine Pepcid, Pepcid AC, Pepcidine‡ *Histamine₂-receptor antagonist* *Antiulcer agent* Preg. Risk Category: B	*tab:* 10, 20, 40 mg; *powder for oral susp:* 40 mg/5 ml after reconstitution; *inj:* 10 mg/ml; *premixed inj:* 20 mg/50 ml in 0.9% NaCl	*Duodenal ulcer (short-term treatment)* — **Adults:** Acute therapy: 40 mg PO qd hs or 20 mg PO bid. Maintenance therapy: 20 mg PO qd hs. *Benign gastric ulcer (short-term)* — **Adults:** 40 mg PO daily hs for 8 wk. *Gastroesophageal reflux disease (GERD)* — **Adults:** 20 mg PO bid up to 6 wk. For esophagitis caused by GERD, 20 to 40 mg PO bid up to 12 wk. *Prevention or treatment of heartburn* — **Adults:** 10 mg (Pepcid AC only) PO 1 hr before meals (prevention) or 10 mg (Pepcid AC only) PO with water for symptoms. Max 20 mg daily. Don't take daily for > 2 wk. *Hospitalized patients with intractable ulcerations or hypersecretory conditions* — **Adults:** 20 mg IV q 12 hr.	• Contraindicated in hypersensitivity to drug.

felodipine
Agona, Agon SR‡, Plendil, Plendil
ER‡, Renedil†
Calcium channel blocker
Antihypertensive
Preg. Risk Category: C

tab (ext-release): 2.5, 5, 10 mg

Hypertension — **Adults:** initially, 5 mg PO daily. Adjust according to patient response, generally at intervals not less than 2 wk. Usual dose 5 to 10 mg daily; max recommended 20 mg daily. In elderly patients and impaired hepatic function, 5 mg PO daily; dosage adjusted as for adults. Max recommended 10 mg daily.

- Use cautiously in heart failure, particularly in patients on beta blockers, and in impaired hepatic function.
- Contraindicated in hypersensitivity to drug.

---

fenoprofen calcium
Nalfon, Nalfon 200
Nonsteroidal anti-inflammatory
Non-narcotic
Preg. Risk Category: NR

tab: 600 mg;
cap: 200, 300
mg

Rheumatoid arthritis and osteoarthritis — **Adults:** 300 to 600 mg PO tid to qid. Max 3.2 g daily.
Mild to moderate pain — **Adults:** 200 mg PO q 4 to 6 hr, prn.
Fever — **Adults:** single PO doses up to 400 mg.

- Use cautiously in elderly patients and in history of serious GI events or peptic ulcer disease or compromised cardiac function or hypertension.
- Contraindicated in hypersensitivity to drug, significantly impaired renal function, pregnancy, or history of aspirin- or NSAID-induced asthma, rhinitis, or urticaria.

---

fentanyl citrate
Sublimaze
fentanyl transdermal system
Duragesic-25, Duragesic-50, Duragesic-75, Duragesic-100
fentanyl transmucosal
Fentanyl Oralet
Opioid agonist
Analgesic/adjunct to anesthesia/adjunct to anesthesia/anesthetic
Preg. Risk Category: C
Controlled Sub. Sched.: II

inj: 50 mcg/
ml; *transderm
system:* patches are designed to
release 25, 50,
75, or 100 mcg
of drug/hr;
transmucosal:
200, 300, 400
mcg

Preop — **Adults:** 50 to 100 mcg IM 30 to 60 min before surgery. Or, 5 mcg/kg as oralet unit, 20 to 40 min prior to need.
Adjunct to general anesthetic — **Adults:** low-dose therapy, 2 mcg/kg IV. Moderate-dose therapy, 2 to 20 mcg/kg IV; then 25 to 100 mcg IV prn. High-dose therapy, 20 to 50 mcg/kg IV; then 25 mcg to half of initial loading dose IV, prn.
Adjunct to regional anesthesia — **Adults:** 50 to 100 mcg IM or IV over 1 to 2 min, prn.
Induction and maintenance of anesthesia — **Children 2 to 12 yr:** 2 to 3 mcg/kg IV.
Postop — **Adults:** 50 to 100 mcg IM q 1 to 2 hr, prn.
Management of chronic pain — **Adults:** 1 transdermal system applied to upper torso skin area not irritated or irradiated. Start with 25-mcg/hr system; adjust dosage as needed and tolerated. May wear system for 72 hr; some may need applied q 48 hr.

- Use with caution in head injury, increased CSF pressure, COPD, decreased respiratory reserve, potentially compromised respirations, hepatic or renal disease, and bradyarrhythmias. Also use with caution in elderly or debilitated patients.
- Contraindicated in known intolerance of drug.

DRUG/CLASS/ CATEGORY	DOSAGE FORMS	INDICATIONS/ DOSAGES	KEY PRECAUTIONS
ferrous fumarate Femiron, Feostat, Fumasorb, Fumerin, Novofumar† *Oral iron supplement* *Hematinic* Preg. Risk Category: A	Each 100 mg provides 33 mg elemental iron. **tab:** 63, 195, 200, 300, 324, 325, 350 mg; **tab (chew):** 100 mg; **cap (ext-release):** 325 mg; **oral susp:** 100 mg/5 ml; **drops:** 45 mg/0.6 ml	*Iron deficiency* — **Adults:** 50 to 100 mg elemental iron PO tid. **Children:** 4 to 6 mg/kg/day of elemental iron PO in 3 divided doses.	▪ Use cautiously on long-term basis. ▪ Contraindicated in primary hemochromatosis or hemosiderosis, in hemolytic anemia unless iron deficiency anemia also present, in patients receiving repeated blood transfusions, and in peptic ulcer disease, regional enteritis, or ulcerative colitis.
ferrous gluconate Fergon, Fertinic†, Simron *Oral iron supplement* *Hematinic* Preg. Risk Category: A	Each 100 mg provides 11.6 mg elemental iron. **tab:** 300, 320, 325 mg; **cap:** 86 mg; **elixir:** 300 mg/5 ml	*Iron deficiency* — **Adults:** 50 to 100 mg elemental iron PO tid. **Children:** 4 to 6 mg/kg/ day elemental iron PO in 3 divided doses.	▪ Use cautiously on long-term basis. ▪ Contraindicated in peptic ulceration, regional enteritis, ulcerative colitis, hemosiderosis, and primary hemochromatosis; in hemolytic anemia unless iron-deficiency anemia also present; and in patients receiving repeated blood transfusions.
ferrous sulfate Apo-Ferrous Sulfate†, Feosol, Feritard‡, Mol-Iron Feosol *Oral iron supplement* *Hematinic* Preg. Risk Category: A **ferrous sulfate, dried**	**tab:** 195, 300, 324 mg; 200 mg (dried); **tab (ext-release):** 159 (dried), 525 mg; **cap:** 190 (dried), 250 mg; **cap**	*Iron deficiency* — **Adults:** 50 to 100 mg elemental iron PO tid. **Children:** 4 to 6 mg/kg/day elemental iron PO in 3 divided doses. Ferrous sulfate is 20% elemental iron; dried and powdered, about 32% elemental iron.	▪ Use cautiously on long-term basis. ▪ Contraindicated in hemosiderosis and primary hemochromatosis; in hemolytic anemia unless iron deficiency anemia also present; in peptic ulceration, ulcerative colitis, and regional enteritis; and in patients receiving repeated blood transfusions.

	(ext-release): 150 (dried), 159 mg (dried); **elixir:** 220 mg/5 ml; **syrup:** 90 mg/5 ml; **sol.:** 300 mg/5 ml; **drops:** 125 mg/ml	
fexofenadine hydrochloride Allegra H_1-receptor antagonist Antihistaminic Preg. Risk Category: C	**cap:** 60 mg	*Seasonal allergic rhinitis* — **Adults and children ≥ 12 yr:** 60 mg PO bid; initially 60 mg PO qd in impaired renal function.	• Use cautiously in impaired renal function. • Contraindicated in hypersensitivity to drug or drug components. • Safety and effectiveness in children <12 yr not established.
filgrastim (granulocyte colony-stimulating factor; G-CSF) Neupogen *Biologic response modifier Colony stimulating factor* Preg. Risk Category: C	**inj:** 300 mcg/ml	*To decrease incidence of infection in patients with nonmyeloid malignant disease receiving myelosuppressive antineoplastic agents* — **Adults and children:** 5 mcg/kg/day IV or SC as 1 dose given ≥ 24 hr after cytotoxic chemotherapy. May increase by 5 mcg/kg for each chemotherapy cycle based on duration and severity of absolute neutrophil count nadir. *To decrease incidence of infection in patients with nonmyeloid malignant disease receiving myelosuppressive antineoplastic agents followed by bone marrow transplantation* — **Adults and children:** 10 mcg/kg/day IV or SC ≥ 24 hr after cytotoxic chemotherapy and bone marrow infusion. Adjust dosage according to neutrophil response. *Congenital neutropenia* — **Adults:** 6 mcg/kg SC bid. Dosage adjusted to response.	• Contraindicated in hypersensitivity to proteins derived from *E. coli* or to drug or its components.

DRUG / CLASS / CATEGORY	DOSAGE FORMS	INDICATIONS / DOSAGES	KEY PRECAUTIONS
finasteride Proscar *Steroid (synthetic 4-azasteroid) derivative* *Androgen synthesis inhibitor* Preg. Risk Category: X	**tab:** 5 mg	*Symptomatic benign prostatic hyperplasia* — **Adults:** 5 mg PO daily.	• Contraindicated in hypersensitivity to drug. Although not used in women, manufacturer indicates pregnancy as contraindication.
flecainide acetate Tambocor *Benzamide derivative local anesthetic* *Ventricular antiarrhythmic* Preg. Risk Category: C	**tab:** 50, 100, 150 mg	*PSVT, paroxysmal atrial fibrillation or flutter in patients without structural heart disease; life-threatening ventricular arrhythmias, such as sustained ventricular tachycardia* — **Adults:** for PSVT, 50 mg PO q 12 hr. May increase in increments of 50 mg PO q 4 days until efficacy achieved. Max 300 mg/day. For life-threatening ventricular arrhythmias, 100 mg PO q 12 hr. Increase in increments of 50 mg bid q 4 days until efficacy achieved. Max 400 mg daily.	• Use cautiously in preexisting heart failure, cardiomyopathy, severe renal or hepatic disease, prolonged QT interval, sick sinus syndrome, or blood dyscrasia. • For prevention of ventricular arrhythmias, reserve for patients with documented life-threatening arrhythmias. • Contraindicated in hypersensitivity; preexisting 2nd- or 3rd-degree AV block or right bundle-branch block when associated with left hemiblock (in absence of artificial pacemaker); recent MI; and cardiogenic shock.
fluconazole Diflucan *Bis-triazole derivative* *Antifungal* Preg. Risk Category: C	**tab:** 50, 100, 150, 200 mg; **powder for oral susp:** 10, 40 mg/ml; **susp:** 350 mg/35 ml, 1,400 mg/35 ml; **inj:** 200 mg/100 ml, 400 mg/200 ml	*Oropharyngeal and esophageal candidiasis* — **Adults:** 200 mg PO or IV on first day, then 100 mg qd. Continue for at least 2 wk after symptoms resolve. **Children:** 6 mg/kg on first day, then 3 mg/kg for at least 2 wk. *Vaginal candidiasis* — **Adults:** 150 mg PO as single dose. *Systemic candidiasis* — **Adults:** up to 400 mg PO or IV qd. Continue for at least 2 wk after symptoms resolve. *Cryptococcal meningitis* — **Adults:** 400 mg PO or IV on first day, then 200 mg qd. Continue for 10 to 12 wk after CSF cultures negative.	• Use cautiously in hypersensitivity to other antifungal azole compounds; no information exists regarding cross-sensitivity. • Contraindicated in hypersensitivity to drug.

flucytosine (5-fluoro-cytosine, 5-FC)
Ancobon, Ancotil†
Fluorinated pyrimidine
Antifungal
Preg. Risk Category: C

cap: 250, 500 mg

Severe fungal infections caused by susceptible strains of Candida (including septicemia, endocarditis, UTI, and pulmonary infections) and Cryptococcus (meningitis, pulmonary infection, and possible UTI) — **Adults and children > 50 kg:** 50 to 150 mg/kg daily PO q 6 hr. **Adults and children < 50 kg:** 1.5 to 4.5 g/m²/day PO in 4 divided doses.

- Use with extreme caution in impaired hepatic or renal function or bone marrow suppression.
- Contraindicated in hypersensitivity to drug.

fludarabine phosphate
Fludara
Antimetabolite
Antineoplastic
Preg. Risk Category: D

powder for inj: 50 mg

B-cell chronic lymphocytic leukemia in patients who have not responded or responded inadequately to ≥ 1 standard alkylating agent regimen — **Adults:** 25 mg/m² IV over 30 min for 5 consecutive days. Repeat cycle q 28 days.

- Use cautiously in renal insufficiency.
- Contraindicated in hypersensitivity to drug or its components.

fludrocortisone acetate
Florinef
Mineralocorticoid/glucocorticoid
Mineralocorticoid replacement therapy
Preg. Risk Category: C

tab: 0.1 mg

Adrenal insufficiency (partial replacement), salt-losing adrenogenital syndrome — **Adults:** 0.1 to 0.2 mg PO daily. Decrease to 0.05 mg daily if transient hypertension occurs. **Children:** 0.05 to 0.1 mg PO daily.
Postural hypotension in diabetic patients, orthostatic hypotension — **Adults:** 0.1 to 0.4 mg PO daily.

- Use cautiously in hypothyroidism, cirrhosis, ocular herpes simplex, emotional instability, psychotic tendencies, nonspecific ulcerative colitis, diverticulitis, fresh intestinal anastomoses, active or latent peptic ulcer, renal insufficiency, hypertension, osteoporosis, and myasthenia gravis.
- Contraindicated in hypersensitivity to drug or in systemic fungal infections.

flumazenil
Romazicon
Benzodiazepine antagonist
Antidote
Preg. Risk Category: C

inj: 0.1 mg/ml in 5-, 10-ml multidose vials

Complete or partial reversal of sedative effects of benzodiazepines after anesthesia or short diagnostic procedures (conscious sedation) — **Adults:** 0.2 mg IV over 15 sec. If patient doesn't reach desired LOC after 45 sec, repeat at 1-min intervals until total dose of 1 mg given (initial dose plus 4 additional doses), prn. Most patients respond after 0.6 to 1 mg. In case of resedation, may repeat after 20 min; however, don't give > 1 mg at one time and not > 3 mg/hr.
Suspected benzodiazepine overdose — **Adults:** 0.2 mg IV over 30 sec. If patient doesn't reach desired LOC af-

- Use cautiously in patients at high risk for developing seizures; those who recently received multiple doses of parenteral benzodiazepine; patients displaying signs of seizure activity; those who may be at risk for unrecognized benzodiazepine dependence, such as ICU patients; psychiatric patients; and in head injury or alcohol dependence.
- Contraindicated in hypersensitivity to drug or benzodiazepines, in evidence of serious

(continued)

FLUMAZENIL   101

DRUG/CLASS/CATEGORY	DOSAGE FORMS	INDICATIONS/DOSAGES	KEY PRECAUTIONS
flumazenil (continued)		ter 30 sec, 0.3 mg given over 30 sec. If poor response, 0.5-mg doses over 30 sec; repeat 0.5-mg doses prn at 1-min intervals until total dose of 3 mg given. Most patients respond to total doses between 1 and 3 mg; rarely, patients who respond partially after 3 mg may require additional doses, up to 5 mg total. If patient doesn't respond in 5 min after receiving 5 mg, sedation unlikely to be caused by benzodiazepines. In case of resedation, may repeat dosage after 20 min; however, don't give > 1 mg at one time and not > 3 mg/hr.	tricyclic antidepressant overdose; and in patients who received benzodiazepines to treat potentially life-threatening condition (such as status epilepticus). • Should not be used in mixed overdose, especially in cases where seizures (from any cause) are likely. • Safety and efficacy in children not established.
flunisolide AeroBid, AeroBid-M, Nasalide (nasal inhalant), Rhinalar Nasal Mist‡ *Glucocorticoid* *Anti-inflammatory/antiasthmatic* Preg. Risk Category: C	**oral inhalant:** 250 mcg/metered spray (≥ 100 metered inh/container); **nasal inh:** 25 mcg/metered spray; 200 doses/bottle‡; **nasal sol:** 0.25 mg/ml in pump spray bottle	*Persistent asthma* — **Adults:** 2 inhalations (500 mcg) bid. Max total daily 2,000 mcg (8 inhalations/day). **Children 6 to 15 yr:** 2 inhalations (500 mcg) bid. Don't exceed 4 inhalations/day. *Seasonal or perennial rhinitis* — **Adults:** 2 sprays (50 mcg) in each nostril bid. If needed, increase to 2 sprays in each nostril tid. **Children 6 to 14 yr:** 1 spray in each nostril tid or 2 sprays in each nostril bid.	• Use extremely cautiously in active or quiescent respiratory tract tubercular infections or in untreated fungal, bacterial, or systemic viral or ocular herpes simplex infections. • Use cautiously after recent nasal septal ulcers, nasal surgery, or nasal trauma. • Contraindicated in hypersensitivity and in status asthmaticus or respiratory infections. • Not recommended in asthma controlled by bronchodilators or other noncorticosteroids alone or in nonasthmatic bronchial diseases. Don't use in untreated localized infection involving nasal mucosa.
fluocinolone acetonide Fluocet, Fluonid, Flurosyn, Synalar, Synemol *Topical adrenocorticoid* *Anti-inflammatory* Preg. Risk Category: C	**cream:** 0.01%, 0.025%, 0.2%; **oint:** 0.025%; **topical sol:** 0.01%	*Inflammation associated with corticosteroid-responsive dermatoses* — **Adults and children:** clean area; apply cream, oint, or topical sol sparingly bid to qid. Rub in gently, leaving thin coat.	• Contraindicated in hypersensitivity to drug.

fluocinonide Lidemol†, Lidex, Lidex-E, Topsyn *Topical adrenocorticoid* *Anti-inflammatory* Preg. Risk Category: C	**cream:** 0.05%; **gel:** 0.05%; **oint:** 0.05%; **topical sol:** 0.05%	*Inflammation associated with corticosteroid-responsive dermatoses* — **Adults and children:** clean area; apply cream, gel, oint, or topical sol sparingly bid or qid.	• Contraindicated in hypersensitivity to drug.
fluorescein sodium Fluorescite, Fluor-I-Strip, Fluor-I-Strip A.T., Ful-Glo, Funduscein Injections *Dye* *Diagnostic aid* Preg. Risk Category: C	**ophth sol:** 2%; **ophth strips:** 0.6, 1, 9 mg; **parenteral inj:** 10%, 25%	*Diagnostic aid in corneal abrasions and foreign bodies; fitting hard contact lenses; lacrimal patency; fundus photography; applanation tonometry* — **Adults and children:** 1 or 2 drops 2% sol followed by irrigation; or strip moistened with sterile water, then conjunctiva or fornix touched with moistened tip, and eye flushed with irrigating sol. Patient should blink several times after application. *Retinal angiography* — **Adults:** 5 ml of 10% sol (500 mg) or 3 ml of 25% sol (750 mg) rapidly injected into antecubital vein. **Children:** 7.5 mg/kg injected rapidly into antecubital vein.	• Use cautiously in history of allergy or bronchial asthma. • Contraindicated in hypersensitivity to drug; don't use with soft contact lenses (lenses may become discolored).
fluorometholone Flarex, FML Forte, FML Liquifilm Ophthalmic *Corticosteroid* *Ophth anti-inflammatory* Preg. Risk Category: C	**ophth oint:** 0.1%; **ophth** **susp:** 0.1%, 0.25%	*Inflammatory and allergic conditions of cornea, conjunctiva, sclera, anterior uvea* — **Adults and children:** 1 to 2 drops instilled in conjunctival sac bid to qid. May give q 2 hr during 1st 1 to 2 days if needed. Alternatively, 1.25-cm ribbon of oint applied to conjunctival sac q 4 hr, decreased to 1 to 3 times daily as inflammation subsides.	• Use cautiously in corneal abrasions that may be contaminated (especially with herpes). • Contraindicated in vaccinia, varicella, acute superficial herpes simplex (dendritic keratitis), or other fungal or viral eye diseases; ocular TB; or any acute, purulent, untreated eye infection. • Safety and efficacy in children < 2 yr not established.
fluorouracil **(5-fluorouracil, 5-FU)** Adrucil, Efudex, Fluoroplex *Antimetabolite (cell cycle–phase specific, S phase)* *Antineoplastic*	**inj:** 50 mg/ml; **cream:** 1%, 5%; **topical** **sol:** 1%, 2%, 5%	*Colon, rectal, breast, stomach, and pancreatic cancers* — **Adults:** 12 mg/kg IV daily for 4 days; if no toxicity, 6 mg/kg on 6th, 8th, 10th, and 12th day; then single weekly maintenance dose of 10 to 15 mg/kg IV begun after toxicity from 1st course subsides. Max single dose 800 mg/day.	• Use cautiously after high-dose pelvic radiation therapy, use of alkylating agents, in impaired hepatic or renal function, or widespread neoplastic infiltration of bone marrow.

(continued)

†Canadian ‡Australian

DRUG/CLASS/CATEGORY	DOSAGE FORMS	INDICATIONS/DOSAGES	KEY PRECAUTIONS
fluorouracil *(continued)* Preg. Risk Category: D (injection), X (topical)		*Palliative treatment of advanced colorectal cancer* — **Adults:** 425 mg/m² IV daily for 5 consecutive days. Given with 20 mg/m² of leucovorin IV. Repeat at 4-wk intervals for 2 additional courses; then repeat at intervals of 4 to 5 wk if tolerated. *Multiple actinic (solar) keratoses; superficial basal cell carcinoma* — **Adults:** apply cream or topical sol bid. Usual duration of treatment 2 to 6 wk.	• Contraindicated in hypersensitivity to drug; poor nutritional status; bone marrow suppression (WBC count of ≤ 5,000/mm³ or platelet count of ≤ 100,000/mm³); potentially serious infections; and within 1 mo of major surgery.
fluoxetine hydrochloride Prozac, Prozac-20† *Selective serotonin reuptake inhibitor* *Antidepressant* Preg. Risk Category: B	**cap:** 10, 20 mg; **oral sol:** 20 mg/5 ml	*Depression, obsessive-compulsive disorder* — **Adults:** initially, 20 mg PO in morning; increase dosage according to response. May give bid in morning and at noon. Gradually increase as needed and tolerated to 60 to 80 mg daily. *Treatment of binge-eating and vomiting behavior in moderate to severe bulimia nervosa* — **Adults:** 60 mg/day PO in morning.	• Use cautiously in high risk of suicide or in history of seizures, diabetes mellitus, or renal, hepatic, or CV disease. • Contraindicated in hypersensitivity to drug and within 14 days of MAO inhibitor therapy.
fluoxymesterone Android-F, Halotestin *Androgen* *Androgen replacement/antineoplastic* Preg. Risk Category: X Controlled Sub. Sched.: III	**tab:** 2, 5, 10 mg	*Hypogonadism caused by testicular deficiency* — **Adults:** 5 to 20 mg PO daily, in single dose or in 3 or 4 divided doses. *Delayed puberty* — **Males:** 2.5 to 20 mg daily. *Palliation of breast cancer in women* — **Adults:** 10 to 40 mg PO daily in 3 or 4 divided doses. All dosages individualized and reduced to minimum when effect noted.	• Use cautiously in prepubertal males and patients with benign prostatic hyperplasia or aspirin sensitivity. • Contraindicated in hypersensitivity to drug; in males with breast cancer or prostate cancer; in cardiac, hepatic, or renal decompensation; during pregnancy; and in breast-feeding patients.
fluphenazine decanoate Modecate†‡, Prolixin Decanoate **fluphenazine enanthate** Prolixin Enanthate	**decanoate** — **depot inj:** 25 mg/ml. **enanthate** — **depot inj:** 25 mg/ml.	*Psychotic disorders* — **Adults:** initially, 0.5 to 10 mg HCl PO daily in divided doses q 6 to 8 hr; may increase cautiously to 20 mg. Higher doses (50 to 100 mg) have been given. Maint: 1 to 5 mg PO daily. For IM doses, give third to half of oral doses. Usual IM	• Use cautiously in elderly or debilitated patients and in pheochromocytoma, severe CV disease, respiratory disorders, seizure disorders, peptic ulcer, exposure to extreme heat or cold (including antipyretic therapy) or

fluphenazine hydrochloride
Moditen HCl†, Permitil Concentrate, Prolixin, Prolixin Concentrate

Phenothiazine
Antipsychotic
Preg. Risk Category: NR

hydrochloride — tab: 1, 2.5, 5, 10 mg; **oral conc:** 5 mg/ml; **elixir:** 2.5 mg/5 ml; **IM inj:** 2.5 mg/ml

dose 1.25 mg. Use dosages above 10 mg/day with caution. Use lower dosages for elderly patients (1 to 2.5 mg daily). Or, 12.5 to 25 mg of long-acting esters (decanoate or enanthate) IM or SC q 1 to 6 wk; maint: 25 to 100 mg, prn.

phosphorus insecticides; hypocalcemia; severe reactions to insulin or electroconvulsive therapy; mitral insufficiency; glaucoma; or prostatic hyperplasia. Use parenteral form cautiously in asthma and in sulfite allergy.
- Contraindicated in hypersensitivity, coma, CNS depression, bone marrow suppression or other blood dyscrasia, subcortical damage, or liver damage.

---

flurandrenolide
Cordran, Cordran SP, Cordran Tape, Denison

Topical adrenocorticoid
Anti-inflammatory
Preg. Risk Category: C

cream: 0.025%, 0.05%; **lotion:** 0.05%; **oint:** 0.025%, 0.05%; **tape:** 4 mcg/cm²

Inflammation associated with corticosteroid-responsive dermatoses — **Adults and children:** clean area; apply cream, lotion, or oint sparingly bid or tid. Apply Cordran tape q 12 to 24 hr. Before applying, clean skin carefully, removing scales, crust, and dried exudate. Let skin dry for 1 hr before applying new tape. Shave or clip hair to allow good contact with skin and comfortable removal. If tape ends loosen prematurely, trim off and replace with fresh tape.

- Contraindicated in hypersensitivity to drug.

---

flurazepam hydrochloride
Apo-Flurazepam†, Dalmane, Novoflupam

Benzodiazepine
Sedative-hypnotic
Preg. Risk Category: X
Controlled Sub. Sched.: IV

cap: 15, 30 mg

Insomnia — **Adults:** 15 to 30 mg PO hs. **Adults > 65 yr:** 15 mg PO hs.

- Use cautiously in impaired renal or hepatic function, chronic pulmonary insufficiency, mental depression, suicidal tendencies, or history of drug abuse.
- Contraindicated in hypersensitivity to drug and during pregnancy.

---

flurbiprofen
Ansaid, Apo-Flurbiprofen†, Froben†, Froben SR†

tab: 50, 100 mg; **cap (ext-release)†:** 200 mg

Rheumatoid arthritis and osteoarthritis — **Adults:** 200 to 300 mg PO daily, divided bid, tid or qid. Where available, patients maintained on 200 mg daily may switch to one 200-mg ext-release cap PO daily, taken in evening after food.

- Use cautiously in elderly or debilitated patients and in history of peptic ulcer disease, herpes simplex keratitis, impaired renal or hepatic function, cardiac disease, or conditions associated with fluid retention.

(continued)

†Canadian ‡Australian

DRUG/CLASS/ CATEGORY	DOSAGE FORMS	INDICATIONS/ DOSAGES	KEY PRECAUTIONS
flurbiprofen *(continued)* *Nonsteroidal anti-inflammatory/ phenylalkanoic acid derivative* *Antiarthritic* Preg. Risk Category: B			▪ Contraindicated in hypersensitivity to drug or history of aspirin- or NSAID-induced asthma, urticaria, or other allergic-type reactions. ▪ Safety and efficacy in children not established.
flurbiprofen sodium Ocufen Liquifilm *Nonsteroidal anti-inflammatory* *Ophthalmic anti-inflammatory/ antimiotic* Preg. Risk Category: C	***ophth sol:*** 0.03%	*Inhibition of intraoperative miosis* — **Adults:** 1 drop instilled into affected eye approximately q ½ hr, beginning 2 hr before surgery. Total of 4 drops given.	▪ Use cautiously in possible allergy to aspirin and other NSAIDs. Also use cautiously in bleeding tendencies and in patients receiving medications that may prolong clotting times. ▪ Contraindicated in hypersensitivity to drug.
flutamide Euflex†, Eulexin *Nonsteroidal antiandrogen* *Antineoplastic* Preg. Risk Category: D	***cap:*** 125, 250 mg	*Metastatic prostate cancer (stage B2, C, D2) in combination with LH-releasing hormone analogues such as leuprolide acetate* — **Adults:** 250 mg PO q 8 hr.	▪ Contraindicated in hypersensitivity to drug.
fluticasone propionate Cutivate *Corticosteroid* *Topical anti-inflammatory* Preg. Risk Category: C	***cream:*** 0.05%; ***oint:*** 0.005%	*Inflammatory and pruritic manifestations associated with corticosteroid-responsive dermatoses* — **Adults:** apply sparingly to affected area bid; rub in gently and completely.	▪ Contraindicated in hypersensitivity to drug or components and in viral, fungal, herpetic, or tubercular skin lesions. ▪ Safety in children not established.
fluticasone propionate Flonase *Corticosteroid* *Topical anti-inflammatory* Preg. Risk Category: C	***nasal spray:*** 50 mcg/metered spray (9, 16-g bottles)	*Seasonal and perennial allergic rhinitis* — **Adults:** initially, 2 sprays (50 mcg each spray) in each nostril qd. Alternatively, 1 spray in each nostril bid. After several days, may reduce dosage to 1 spray in each nostril daily. Max daily dosage 2 sprays in each nostril. **Children ≥ 12 yr:** initially, 1 spray (50 mcg) in each	▪ Use cautiously, if at all, in active or quiescent TB infections; glaucoma; untreated fungal, bacterial, or systemic viral infections; or ocular herpes simplex. Also use cautiously in patients already receiving systemic corticosteroids and in breast-feeding patients.

fluvastatin sodium
Lescol
Hydroxymethylglutaryl-coenzyme A (HMG-CoA) reductase inhibitor
Cholesterol-lowering agent/antilipemic
Preg. Risk Category: X

cap: 20, 40 mg

Reduction of LDL and total cholesterol levels in patients with primary hypercholesterolemia (types IIa and IIb) — **Adults:** initially, 20 mg PO hs. Increase prn to max 40 mg daily.

- Contraindicated in hypersensitivity to drug or any component.
- Use cautiously in impaired renal function or history of hepatic disease or heavy alcohol use.
- Contraindicated in hypersensitivity to drug, in active liver disease or conditions associated with unexplained persistent elevations of serum transaminase levels, in pregnant and breast-feeding women, and in women of child-bearing age (unless no risk of pregnancy).

fluvoxamine maleate
Luvox
Selective serotonin reuptake inhibitor
Anticompulsive
Preg. Risk Category: C

tab: 50, 100 mg

Obsessive-compulsive disorder — **Adults:** initially, 50 mg PO daily hs, increased in 50-mg increments q 4 to 7 days until max benefit achieved. Max 300 mg daily. Give total daily doses of more than 100 mg in 2 divided doses.

- Use cautiously in hepatic dysfunction, concomitant conditions that may affect hemo-dynamic responses or metabolism, or history of mania or seizures.
- Contraindicated in hypersensitivity to drug or to other phenylpiperazine antidepressants and within 14 days of MAO inhibitor therapy.

folic acid (vitamin B₉)
Folvite, Novofolacid†
Folic acid derivative
Vitamin supplement
Preg. Risk Category: NR

tab: 0.4, 0.8, 1 mg; **inj:** 10-ml vials (5 mg/ml with 1.5% benzyl alcohol or 10 mg/ml with 1.5% benzyl alcohol and 0.2% EDTA)

RDA — **Neonates and infants to 6 mo:** 25 mcg. **Infants 6 mo to 1 yr:** 35 mcg. **Children 1 to 3 yr:** 50 mcg. **Children 4 to 6 yr:** 75 mcg. **Children 7 to 10 yr:** 100 mcg. **Children 11 to 14 yr:** 150 mcg. **Males ≥ 15 yr:** 200 mcg. **Females ≥ 15 yr:** 180 mcg. **Pregnant women:** 400 mcg. **Breast-feeding women (1st 6 mo):** 280 mcg. **Breast-feeding women (2nd 6 mo):** 260 mcg.
Megaloblastic or macrocytic anemia secondary to folic acid or other nutritional deficiency, hepatic disease, alcoholism, intestinal obstruction, excessive hemolysis — **Adults and children > 4 yr:** 0.4 mg to 1 mg PO, SC, or IM daily. After correction of anemia

- Contraindicated in undiagnosed anemia and vitamin B₁₂ deficiency.
- Safety in pregnancy not established, but pregnant women more prone to develop folate deficiency. Folate-deficient women may be more likely to develop pregnancy-related complications and fetal abnormalities.

(continued)

FOLIC ACID **107**

†Canadian ‡Australian

DRUG/CLASS/ CATEGORY	DOSAGE FORMS	INDICATIONS/ DOSAGES	KEY PRECAUTIONS
folic acid *(continued)*		secondary to folic acid deficiency, proper diet and RDA supplements necessary to prevent recurrence. **Children < 4 yr:** up to 0.3 mg PO, SC, or IM daily. **Pregnant and breast-feeding women:** 0.8 mg PO, SC, or IM daily. *Prevention of megaloblastic anemia during pregnancy to prevent fetal damage* — **Adults:** up to 1 mg PO, SC, or IM daily throughout pregnancy.	
foscarnet sodium (phosphonoformic acid) Foscavir *Pyrophosphate analogue* *Antiviral* Preg. Risk Category: C	*inj:* 24 mg/ml in 250- and 500-ml vials	*CMV retinitis in patients with AIDS* — **Adults:** 60 mg/ kg IV as induction treatment in patients with normal renal function. Give IV over 1 hr q 8 hr for 2 to 3 wk, per response. Then maint. inf of 90 to 120 mg/kg qd, over 2 hr. *Mucocutaneous acyclovir resistant herpes simplex virus (HSV) infection* — **Adults:** 40 mg/kg IV. Give IV infusion over 1 hr q 8 to 12 hr for 2 to 3 wk.	▪ Use cautiously and with reduced dosage in abnormal renal function. Nephrotoxic; may worsen renal impairment. Some degree of nephrotoxicity occurs in most patients. ▪ Contraindicated in hypersensitivity to drug.
fosfomycin tromethamine Monurol *Phosphonic acid derivative* *Antibiotic* Preg. Risk Category: B	*single-dose sachet:* 3 g	*Uncomplicated UTI (acute cystitis) in women caused by susceptible strains of E. coli and E. faecalis* — **Women > 18 yr:** 1 sachet PO mixed with cold water just before ingestion.	▪ Contraindicated in known hypersensitivity to drug and breast-feeding. Avoid use in pregnancy unless clearly needed. ▪ Use cautiously in renal impairment. Safety and effectiveness in children ≤ 12 yr not established.
fosinopril sodium Monopril *ACE inhibitor* *Antihypertensive* Preg. Risk Category: C (D in 2nd and 3rd trimesters)	*tab:* 10, 20 mg	*Hypertension* — **Adults:** initially, 10 mg PO daily. Adjusted based on BP response at peak and trough levels. Usual dosage 20 to 40 mg, up to 80 mg daily. May be divided. *Heart failure* — **Adults:** initially, 10 mg PO qd. Increase over several wk to max 40 mg PO daily.	▪ Use cautiously in impaired renal or hepatic function. ▪ Contraindicated in hypersensitivity to drug or other ACE inhibitors and in breast-feeding patients.

fosphenytoin sodium

Cerebyx
Hydantoin derivative
Anticonvulsant
Preg. Risk Category: D

inj: 2 ml (150 mg fosphenytoin sodium equiv to 100 mg phenytoin sodium), 10 ml (750 mg fosphenytoin sodium equiv to 500 mg phenytoin sodium)

Status epilepticus — **Adults:** 15 to 20 mg phenytoin sodium equiv (PE)/kg IV at 100 to 150 mg PE/min as loading dose; then 4 to 6 mg PE/kg/day IV as maintenance dose. (Phenytoin may be used instead of fosphenytoin as maintenance, using appropriate dose.)
Prevention and treatment of seizures during neurosurgery — **Adults:** loading dose 10 to 20 mg PE/kg IM or IV at infusion rate not exceeding 150 mg PE/min. Maintenance dose: 4 to 6 mg PE/kg/day IV.
Short-term substitution for oral phenytoin — **Adult:** same total daily dosage equivalent as oral phenytoin sodium therapy as single daily dose IM or IV at infusion rate not exceeding 150 mg PE/min. May require more frequent dosing.

- Use cautiously in hypotension, severe myocardial insufficiency, impaired renal or hepatic function, hypoalbuminemia, diabetes mellitus, or porphyria and in history of hypersensitivity to similarly structured drugs, such as barbiturates, oxazolidinediones, and succinimides.
- Contraindicated in hypersensitivity to drug or components or to phenytoin or other hydantoins. Also contraindicated in sinus bradycardia, SA block, second- or third- degree AV block, and Adams-Stokes syndrome.
- Safety and effectiveness in children not established.

furosemide
(frusemide†‡)

Apo-Furosemide†, Furosidet†, Lasix,
Lasix Special†, Myrosemide,
Novosemidet†, Urex‡, Urex-M‡,
Uritol†
Loop diuretic
Diuretic/antihypertensive
Preg. Risk Category: C

tab: 20, 40, 80, 500 mg†‡; **oral sol:** 8 and 10 mg/ml, 40 mg/5 ml; **inj:** 10 mg/ml

Acute pulmonary edema — **Adults:** 40 mg IV slowly over a period of 1 to 2 min; followed by 80 mg IV in 1 to 1½ hr if needed.
Edema — **Adults:** 20 to 80 mg PO daily in morning. Give 2nd dose in 6 to 8 hr. Dosages should be carefully titrated up to 600 mg qd, as needed and tolerated. Alternatively, give 20 to 40 mg IM or IV, increased by 20 mg every 2 hr until desired response achieved. Administer IV slowly over a period of 1 to 2 min.
Infants and children: 2 mg/kg PO daily, increased by 1 to 2 mg/kg in 6 to 8 hr, as needed and tolerated. Dosages should be carefully titrated to 6 mg/kg daily, as needed and tolerated.
Hypertension — **Adults:** 40 mg PO bid. Adjust dosage according to clinical response.

- Use cautiously in hepatic cirrhosis. Use during pregnancy only if potential benefits clearly outweigh possible risks to fetus.
- Contraindicated in anuria or history of hypersensitivity to drug.

DRUG/CLASS/ CATEGORY	DOSAGE FORMS	INDICATIONS/ DOSAGES	KEY PRECAUTIONS
gabapentin Neurontin *1-aminomethyl cyclohexonacetic acid* Anticonvulsant Preg. Risk Category: C	*cap:* 100, 300, 400 mg	*Adjunctive treatment of partial seizures with or without secondary generalization in adults who have epilepsy —* **Adults:** Initially 300 mg PO hs on day 1; 300 mg PO bid on day 2; then 300 mg PO tid on day 3. Increase as needed and tolerated to 1,800 mg daily in 3 divided doses. Dosages up to 3,600 mg daily have been well tolerated.	▪ Contraindicated in hypersensitivity to drug.
gallium nitrate Ganite *Heavy metal* Antihypercalcemic Preg. Risk Category: C	*inj:* 25 mg/ml	*Symptomatic, unresponsive hypercalcemia caused by cancer —* **Adults:** 200 mg/m² as continuous IV infusion daily for 5 consecutive days or until serum calcium is normal. Lower doses (100 mg/m²) may be given in mild hypercalcemia.	▪ Use cautiously in reduced CV function. ▪ Contraindicated in severe renal impairment.
ganciclovir Cytovene *Synthetic nucleoside* Antiviral Preg. Risk Category: C	*cap:* 250 mg; *inj:* 500 mg/ vial	*CMV retinitis in immunocompromised patients, including those with AIDS and normal renal function —* **Adults:** induction: 5 mg/kg IV q 12 hr for 14 to 21 days; maintenance: 5 mg/kg IV qd for 7 days each wk, or 6 mg/kg qd for 5 days each wk. Or, 1,000 mg PO tid with food; or 500 mg PO q 3 hr while awake (6 times daily). Adjust dosage for impaired renal function based on creatinine clearance. *Prevention of CMV disease in advanced HIV infection and normal renal function —* **Adults:** 1,000 mg PO tid with food. *Prevention of CMV disease in transplant recipients with normal renal function —* **Adults:** 5 mg/kg IV q 12 hr for 7 to 14 days, then 5 mg/kg qd for 7 days each wk, or 6 mg/kg qd for 5 days each wk.	▪ Use cautiously and at reduced dosage in renal dysfunction. Adjust dosage if creatinine clearance < 70 ml/min. ▪ Contraindicated in hypersensitivity to drug or acyclovir and in absolute neutrophil count < 500/mm³ or platelet count < 25,000/mm³.

gemcitabine hydrochloride	powder for inj: 200-mg, 1-g vials	Locally advanced or metastatic adenocarcinoma of pancreas and patients treated previously with fluorouracil — **Adults:** 1,000 mg/m² IV over 30 min q wk for ≤ 7 wk, unless toxicity occurs. Patients should be monitored before each dose with CBC (including differential) and platelet count. If bone marrow suppression detected, adjust therapy. Give full dose if absolute granulocyte count (AGC) ≥ 1,000/mm³ and platelet count ≥ 100,000/mm³. If AGC 500/mm³ to 999/mm³ or platelet count 50,000/mm³ to 99,999/mm³, give 75% of dose. Withhold dose if AGC < 500/mm³ or platelet count < 50,000/mm³. Follow treatment course of 7 wk with 1 wk rest. Subsequent dosage cycles consist of 1 infusion q wk for 3 out of 4 consecutive wk. Base dosage adjustments for subsequent cycles on AGC and platelet count nadirs and degree of nonhematologic toxicity.	▪ Use cautiously in renal or hepatic impairment. ▪ Not recommended for pregnant or breast-feeding women. ▪ Safety in children not established. ▪ Contraindicated in hypersensitivity to drug.
Gemzar *Nucleoside analogue (cell cycle–phase specific, S and G1 phase)* *Antineoplastic* Preg. Risk Category: D			
gemfibrozil	tab: 600 mg; cap: 300 mg	*Types IV and V hyperlipidemia unresponsive to diet and other drugs; reduction of CAD risk in patients with type IIb hyperlipidemia who can't tolerate or are refractory to bile acid sequestrants or niacin* — **Adults:** 1,200 mg PO daily in 2 divided doses, 30 min before morning and evening meals.	▪ Contraindicated in hypersensitivity to drug, hepatic or severe renal dysfunction (including primary biliary cirrhosis), or preexisting gallbladder disease.
Lopid *Fibric acid derivative* *Antilipemic* Preg. Risk Category: C			
gentamicin sulfate	inj: 40 mg/ml (adult), 10 mg/ml (ped), 2 mg/ml (intrathecal); IV infusion (premixed): 40, 60, 70, 80, 90, 100 mg, avail in 0.9% NaCl sol	*Serious infections caused by susceptible organisms* — **Adults:** 3 mg/kg qd in divided doses IM or IV infusion q 8 hr. For life-threatening infections, up to 5 mg/kg qd in 3 to 4 divided doses; reduce to 3 mg/kg qd as soon as indicated. **Children:** 2 to 2.5 mg/kg q 8 hr IM or by IV infusion. **Neonates > 1 wk or infants:** 7.5 mg/kg qd in divided doses q 8 hr. *Meningitis* — **Adults:** systemic therapy as above; or 4 to 8 mg intrathecally qd. **Children and infants > 3 mo:** systemic therapy as above; or 1 to 2 mg intrathecally qd.	▪ Use cautiously in neonates, infants, elderly patients, impaired renal function, and neuromuscular disorders. ▪ Contraindicated in hypersensitivity to drug or other aminoglycosides.
Cidomycin†, Garamycin, Gentamicin Sulfate ADD-Vantage, Jenamicin *Aminoglycoside* *Antibiotic* Preg. Risk Category: NR			

(continued)

†Canadian ‡Australian

DRUG / CLASS / CATEGORY	DOSAGE FORMS	INDICATIONS / DOSAGES	KEY PRECAUTIONS
gentamicin sulfate *(continued)*		*Endocarditis prophylaxis for GI or GU procedure or surgery* — **Adults:** 1.5 mg/kg IM or IV 30 to 60 min before procedure or surgery. Max 80 mg. Repeat in 8 hr. **Children:** 2 mg/kg IM or IV 30 min before procedure or surgery. Max 80 mg. After 8 hr, give half of initial dose.	▪ Contraindicated in hypersensitivity to drug or in cross-sensitivity with other aminoglycosides such as neomycin.
gentamicin sulfate Garamycin Ophthalmic, Genoptic, Gentacidin, Gentak, Ocu-Mycin *Aminoglycoside* *Ophthalmic antibiotic* Preg. Risk Category: C	***ophth oint:*** 0.3% (base); ***ophth sol:*** 0.3% (base)	*External ocular infections (conjunctivitis, keratoconjunctivitis, corneal ulcers, blepharitis, blepharoconjunctivitis, meibomianitis, and dacryocystitis) caused by susceptible organisms, especially P. aeruginosa, Proteus, K. pneumoniae, E. coli, and other gram-neg organisms* — **Adults and children:** 1 to 2 drops instilled in eye q 4 hr. In severe infections, up to 2 drops q 1hr. Alternatively, apply oint to lower conjunctival sac bid or tid.	▪ Contraindicated in hypersensitivity to drug or in cross-sensitivity with other aminoglycosides such as neomycin.
gentamicin sulfate Garamycin, G-Myticin *Aminoglycoside* *Topical antibiotic* Preg. Risk Category: C	***cream:*** 0.1%; ***oint:*** 0.1%	*Treatment and prophylaxis of superficial skin infections caused by susceptible bacteria* — **Adults and children > 1 yr:** rub in small amount gently tid or qid, with or without gauze dressing.	▪ Restrict use to selected patients; widespread use may lead to resistant organisms. ▪ Contraindicated in hypersensitivity to drug or in cross-sensitivity with other aminoglycosides such as neomycin. ▪ Avoid use on large skin lesions or over wide area.
glimepiride Amaryl *Sulfonylurea* *Antidiabetic* Preg. Risk Category: C	***tab:*** 1, 2, 4 mg	*Adjunct to diet and exercise to lower blood glucose in type 2 diabetes mellitus when hyperglycemia can't be managed by diet and exercise alone* — **Adults:** initially, 1 to 2 mg PO qd with first main meal of day; usual maintenance: 1 to 4 mg PO qd. After reaching 2 mg, increase dosage in increments not exceeding 2 mg q 1 to 2 wk, based on blood glucose response. Max 8 mg/day.	▪ Use cautiously in debilitated or malnourished patients and in adrenal, pituitary, hepatic, or renal insufficiency. ▪ Not recommended in elderly patients. ▪ Contraindicated in hypersensitivity to drug and in diabetic ketoacidosis, which should be treated with insulin.

		▪ Safety and effectiveness in children not established. ▪ Not known if drug excreted in breast milk. Don't give to breast-feeding women.

Adjunct to insulin therapy in type 2 diabetes mellitus when hyperglycemia can't be managed by diet and exercise in conjunction with oral hypoglycemic agents — **Adults:** 8 mg PO qd with first main meal of day; used in combination with low-dose insulin.

glipizide Glucotrol, Glucotrol XL, Minidiab‡ *Sulfonylurea* *Antidiabetic* Preg. Risk Category: C	**tab:** 5, 10 mg; **tab (ext-release):** 5, 10 mg	*Adjunct to diet to lower blood glucose in type 2 diabetes mellitus* — **Adults:** initially, 5 mg PO daily 30 min before breakfast. Elderly patients or those with liver disease may start at 2.5 mg. Usual maintenance: 10 to 15 mg. Max recommended daily dose 40 mg. Divide doses above 15 mg, except when using ext-release tablets. For ext-release tablets, initially, 5 mg PO daily. Titrate in 5-mg increments q 3 mo depending on level of glycemic control. Max daily dosage 20 mg. *To replace insulin therapy* — **Adults:** if insulin dosage > 20 units daily, start at usual dosage plus 50% of insulin. If insulin dosage < 20 units, may discontinue insulin on initiating glipizide.	▪ Use cautiously in renal and hepatic disease and in debilitated, malnourished, or elderly patients. ▪ Contraindicated in hypersensitivity to drug, diabetic ketoacidosis with or without coma, and in pregnant or breast-feeding patients.
glucagon *Antihypoglycemic* *Antidiabetic/diagnostic aid* Preg. Risk Category: B	**powder for inj:** 1 mg (1 unit)-vial, 10 mg (10 unit)-vial	*Hypoglycemia* — **Adults and children > 20 kg:** 0.5 to 1 mg SC, IM, or IV; may repeat q 20 min for 2 doses, if necessary. In deep coma, also give glucose 10% to 50% IV. When patient responds, give more carbohydrate immediately. **Children ≤ 20 kg:** 0.025 mg SC, IM, or IV; may repeat within 25 min. In deep coma, also give glucose 10% to 50% IV. When patient responds, give more carbohydrate immediately. *Note:* May repeat in 15 min. if necessary. Must give IV glucose if patient fails to respond. When patient responds, must give supplemental carbohydrate immediately. *Diagnostic aid for radiologic examination* — **Adults:** 0.25 to 2 mg IV or IM before radiologic procedure.	▪ Use cautiously in history of insulinoma or pheochromocytoma. ▪ Contraindicated in hypersensitivity to drug or pheochromocytoma.

DRUG/CLASS/CATEGORY	DOSAGE FORMS	INDICATIONS/DOSAGES	KEY PRECAUTIONS
glyburide (glibenclamide) DiaBeta, Euglucon†, Glynase PresTab, Micronase *Sulfonylurea* *Antidiabetic* Preg. Risk Category: C	*tab:* 1.25, 2.5, 5 mg; *tab (micronized):* 1.5, 3, 6 mg	*Adjunct to diet to lower glucose in type 2 diabetes mellitus* — **Adults:** initially, 2.5 to 5 mg regular tabs PO qd with breakfast. In sensitive patients, start at 1.25 mg qd. Usual maintenance: 1.25 to 20 mg qd as single dose or in divided doses or may use micronized formulation. Initial dosage 1.5 to 3 mg qd. In sensitive patients, started at 0.75 mg qd. Usual maintenance: 0.75 to 12 mg/day. Patients receiving > 6 mg/day may respond better with bid dosing. *To replace insulin therapy* — **Adults:** if insulin dosage > 40 units/day, may start at 5 mg daily plus 50% of insulin dose; if < 20 units/day, should receive 2.5 to 5 mg/day; if 20 to 40 units/day, should receive 5 mg/day. In all patients, substitute glyburide and discontinue insulin immediately. For micronized tablets, if insulin dosage > 40 units/day, give 3 mg PO with 50% reduction in insulin; if 20 to 40 units/day, should receive 3 mg PO as single daily dose; if < 20 units/day, should receive 1.5 to 3 mg/day as single dose.	▪ Use cautiously in hepatic or renal impairment or in debilitated, malnourished, or elderly patients. ▪ Contraindicated in hypersensitivity to drug or diabetic ketoacidosis with or without coma and in pregnant or breast-feeding patients.
glycerin Fleet Babylax, Sani-Supp *Trihydric alcohol* *Laxative (osmotic)/lubricant* Preg. Risk Category: C	*enema (ped):* 4 ml/applicator; *supp:* adult, children, and infant sizes	*Constipation* — **Adults and children ≥ 6 yr:** 2 to 3 g as rectal supp or 5 to 15 ml as enema. **Children 2 to 6 yr:** 1 to 1.7 g as rectal supp or 2 to 5 ml as enema.	▪ Use oral form cautiously in elderly or dehydrated patients, diabetes, and cardiac, renal, or hepatic disease. ▪ Contraindicated in hypersensitivity to drug and in intestinal obstruction, undiagnosed abdominal pain, vomiting or other signs of appendicitis, fecal impaction, and acute surgical abdomen.

glycopyrrolate
Robinul, Robinul Forte
Anticholinergic
Antimuscarinic/GI antispasmodic
Preg. Risk Category: B

tab: 1, 2 mg; **inj:** 0.2 mg/ml in 1, 2, 5, and 20-ml vials

Blockade of adverse cholinergic effects caused by anticholinesterase agents used to reverse neuromuscular blockade — **Adults and children:** 0.2 mg IV for each 1 mg neostigmine or 5 mg pyridostigmine. May give IV without dilution or may add to dextrose injection and give by infusion.

Prep to diminish secretions and block cardiac vagal reflexes — **Adults and children ≥ 2 yr:** 0.0044 mg/kg of body weight IM 30 to 60 min before anesthesia. **Children < 2 yr:** 0.0088 mg/kg IM 30 to 60 min before anesthesia.

Adjunctive therapy in peptic ulcer and other GI disorders — **Adults:** 1 to 2 mg PO tid or 0.1 to 0.2 mg IM or IV tid or qid. Must individualize dosage. Max oral dosage 8 mg/day.

- Use cautiously in autonomic neuropathy, hyperthyroidism, CAD, arrhythmias, heart failure, hypertension, hiatal hernia, hepatic or renal disease, and ulcerative colitis. Also use cautiously in hot or humid environment to avoid drug-induced heatstroke.
- Contraindicated in hypersensitivity to drug and in glaucoma, obstructive uropathy, obstructive disease of GI tract, myasthenia gravis, paralytic ileus, intestinal atony, unstable CV status in acute hemorrhage, severe ulcerative colitis, or toxic megacolon.

gonadorelin acetate
Lutrepulse
Gonadotropin-releasing hormone
Fertility agent
Preg. Risk Category: B

inj: 0.8 mg/10 ml, 3.2 mg/10 ml vials; supplied as kit with IV supplies and ambulatory infusion pump

Induction of ovulation in women with primary hypothalamic amenorrhea — **Adults:** 5 mcg IV q 90 min for 21 days. If no response follows 3 treatment intervals, increase dosage. Usual dose 1 to 20 mcg.

- Contraindicated in hypersensitivity to drug, in women with conditions that could be complicated by pregnancy (such as prolactinoma), in patients anovulatory from other than hypothalamic disorders, and in ovarian cysts.

granisetron hydrochloride
Kytril
Selective 5-hydroxytryptamine (5-HT3) receptor antagonist
Antiemetic/antinauseant
Preg. Risk Category: B

inj: 1 mg/ml; **tab:** 1 mg

Prevention of nausea and vomiting associated with emetogenic cancer chemotherapy — **Adults and children 2 to 16 yr:** 10 mcg/kg IV infused over 5 min. Begin infusion within 30 min before chemotherapy administration. Alternatively, 1 mg PO up to 1 hr before chemotherapy, and repeated 12 hr later.

- Contraindicated in hypersensitivity to drug.

DRUG / CLASS / CATEGORY	DOSAGE FORMS	INDICATIONS / DOSAGES	KEY PRECAUTIONS
griseofulvin microsize Fulcin‡, Fulvicin-U/F, Grifulvin V, Grisactin, Grisovin‡, Grisovin 500‡, Grisovin-FP **griseofulvin ultramicrosize** Fulvicin P/G, Grisactin Ultra, Griseostatin‡, Gris-PEG *Penicillin antibiotic* *Antifungal* Preg. Risk Category: C	microsize — *tab:* 250, 500 mg; *cap:* 250 mg; *oral susp:* 125 mg/5 ml. ultramicrosize — *tab:* 125, 165, 250, 330 mg	*Ringworm infections of skin, hair, nails* — **Adults:** 500 mg microsize PO qd in single or divided doses. Severe infections may require up to 1 g qd. Or, 330 to 375 mg ultramicrosize PO qd in single or divided doses. **Children > 2 yr:** 11 mg/kg/day ultramicrosize PO qd or 125 to 250 mg microsize PO qd for child 13.1 to 22.7 kg; or 250 to 500 mg microsize PO qd for child > 22.7 kg. *Tinea pedis and tinea unguium* — **Adults:** 0.75 to 1 g microsize PO daily. Or, 660 to 750 mg ultramicrosize PO qd in divided doses. **Children > age 2:** 11 mg/kg/ day ultramicrosize PO qd or 125 to 250 mg microsize PO qd for child 13.1 to 22.7 kg; or 250 to 500 mg microsize PO qd for child > 22.7 kg.	▪ Use cautiously in penicillin sensitivity. ▪ Contraindicated in hypersensitivity to drug, in porphyria or hepatocellular failure, in pregnant patients, and in women who intend to become pregnant during therapy. ▪ Ultramicrosize absorbed more rapidly and completely than microsize preparations; effective at half to two-thirds of usual griseofulvin dose.
guaifenesin (glyceryl guaiacolate) Anti-Tuss, Glytuss, Halotussin, Humibid L.A., Neo-Spect, Robitussin *Propanediol derivative* *Expectorant* Preg. Risk Category: C	*tab:* 100, 200 mg; *tab (ext-release):* 600 mg; *cap:* 200 mg; *cap (ext-release):* 300 mg; *sol:* 100, 200 mg/5 ml	*Expectorant* — **Adults and children ≥ 12 yr:** 100 to 400 mg PO q 4 hr, max 2.4 g/day; or 600 to 1,200 mg ext-release caps q 12 hr. Max 2,400 mg daily. **Children 6 to 12 yr:** 100 to 200 mg PO q 4 hr, max 1,200 mg daily. For ext-release caps, 600 mg q 12 hr, not to exceed 1,200 mg in 24 hr. **Children 2 to 6 yr:** 50 to 100 mg PO q 4 hr. Max 600 mg daily. For ext-release cap, 300 mg q 12 hr, not to exceed 600 mg in 24 hr.	▪ Contraindicated in hypersensitivity to drug.
guanethidine monosulfate Apo-Guanethidine†, Ismelin *Adrenergic neuron blocker* *Antihypertensive* Preg. Risk Category: C	*tab:* 10, 25 mg	*Moderate to severe hypertension and renal hypertension* — **Adults:** initially, 10 mg PO daily. Increase by 10 mg at weekly to monthly intervals, prn. Usual dosage 25 to 50 mg daily. Some patients may need up to 300 mg daily.	▪ Use cautiously in severe cardiac disease, recent MI, cerebrovascular disease, peptic ulceration, impaired renal function, and bronchial asthma and in patients taking other antihypertensives. ▪ Contraindicated in pheochromocytoma, frank heart failure, and hypersensitivity to drug and concurrent MAO inhibitor therapy.

h

haloperidol
Apo-Haloperidol†, Haldol, Novo-Peridol†, Peridol†, Serenace‡
haloperidol decanoate
Haldol Decanoate, Haldol LA‡
haloperidol lactate
Haldol
Butyrophenone
Antipsychotic
Preg. Risk Category: C

haloperidol —
tab: 0.5, 1, 2, 5, 10, 20 mg; *decanoate —*
inj: 50, 100 mg/ml.
lactate — oral conc: 2 mg/ml; *inj:* 5 mg/ml

Psychotic disorders — **Adults and children ≥ 12 yr:** dosage varies. Initial range 0.5 to 5 mg PO bid or tid; or 2 to 5 mg IM q 4 to 8 hr. Max 100 mg PO qd. **Children 3 to 12 yr:** 0.05 mg/kg to 0.15 mg/kg PO qd.
Chronic psychotic patients who require prolonged therapy — **Adults:** 50 to 100 mg IM haloperidol decanoate q 4 wk.
Nonpsychotic behavior disorders — **Children 3 to 12 yr:** 0.05 mg/kg PO qd. Max 6 mg qd.

▪ Use cautiously in elderly and debilitated patients; in history of seizures or EEG abnormalities, severe CV disorders, allergies, glaucoma, or urine retention; and with concurrent anticonvulsant, anticoagulant, antiparkinsonian, or lithium therapy.
▪ Contraindicated in hypersensitivity, parkinsonism, coma, or CNS depression.

heparin calcium
Calcilean†, Calciparine, Caprin‡
heparin sodium
Hepalean†, Liquaemin Sodium, Uniparin‡
Anticoagulant
Anticoagulant
Preg. Risk Category: C

Products are derived from beef lung or porcine intestinal mucosa.
calcium —
ampule: 12,500 units/0.5 ml, 20,000 units/0.8 ml; *syringe:* 5,000 units/0.2 ml. **sodium —**
Carpuject: 5,000 units/ml; *disp syringes:* from 1,000 to 40,000 units/ml; *premixed IV sol:* 1,000; 2,000; 12,500; 20,000 or 25,000 units/ml

Dosage highly individualized, depending on disease state, age, and renal and hepatic status.
Full-dose continuous IV infusion therapy for DVT, MI, pulmonary embolism — **Adults:** initially, 5,000 units by IV bolus, followed by 750 to 1,500 units/hr by IV infusion with pump. Adjust hourly rate 8 hr after bolus dose and according to PTT. **Children:** initially, 50 units/kg IV followed by 25 units/kg/hr or 20,000 units/m² daily by IV infusion pump. Adjust dosage according to PTT.
Full-dose SC therapy for DVT, MI, pulmonary embolism — **Adults:** initially, 5,000 units IV bolus and 10,000 to 20,000 units in conc sol SC, followed by 8,000 to 10,000 units SC q 8 hr or 15,000 to 20,000 units in conc sol q 12 hr.
Fixed low-dose therapy for venous thrombosis, pulmonary embolism, atrial fibrillation with embolism, postop DVT, and embolism prevention — **Adults:** 5,000 units SC q 12 hr. In surgical patients, give 1st

▪ Use cautiously during menses; in mild hepatic or renal disease, alcoholism, occupations with high risk of physical injury, or immediately postpartum; and in history of allergies, asthma, or GI ulcerations.
▪ Contraindicated in hypersensitivity to drug. Conditionally contraindicated in active bleeding, blood dyscrasia, bleeding tendencies, suppurative thrombophlebitis, inaccessible ulcerative lesions (especially of GI tract) and open ulcerative wounds, extensive skin denudation, ascorbic acid deficiency and other conditions that increase capillary permeability, subacute bacterial endocarditis, shock, advanced renal disease, threatened abortion, and severe hypertension; and during or after brain, eye, or spinal cord surgery; during spinal tap or spinal anesthesia; during continuous tube drainage of stomach or small intestine. Although

(continued)

HEPARIN   117

†Canadian ‡Australian

DRUG / CLASS / CATEGORY	DOSAGE FORMS	INDICATIONS / DOSAGES	KEY PRECAUTIONS
heparin *(continued)*	in varying vols of 0.45%, 0.9% NaCl; D₅W sol. *unit-dose ampules*: 1,000, 5,000, 10,000 units/ml; *vials*: 1,000 to 40,000 units/ml	dose 2 hr before procedure, then 5,000 units SC q 8 to 12 hr for 5 to 7 days or until patient can walk. *Consumptive coagulopathy (such as DIC)* — **Adults:** 50 to 100 units/kg by IV bolus or continuous IV infusion q 4 hr. **Children:** 25 to 50 units/kg by IV bolus or continuous IV infusion q 4 hr. If no improvement within 4 to 8 hr, discontinue.	heparin use clearly hazardous in these conditions, risks and benefits must be evaluated.
hepatitis B immune globulin, human H-BIG, Hep-B-Gammagee, HyperHep *Immune serum* *Hepatitis B prophylaxis product* Preg. Risk Category: C	*inj*: 1-, 4-, 5-ml vials; 0.5-ml neonatal single-dose syringe	*Hepatitis B exposure in high-risk patients* — **Adults and children:** 0.06 ml/kg IM within 7 days after exposure. Repeat dosage 28 days after exposure if patient refuses hepatitis B vaccine. **Neonates born to women who test positive for hepatitis B surface antigen (HbsAg):** 0.5 ml within 12 hr of birth.	▪ Contraindicated in history of anaphylactic reaction to immune serum.
hetastarch Hespan *Amylopectin derivative* *Plasma volume expander* Preg. Risk Category: C	*inj*: 500 ml (6 g/100 ml in 0.9% NaCl sol)	*Plasma expander* — **Adults:** 500 to 1,000 ml IV, depending on amount of blood lost and resultant hemoconcentration. Total dosage usually ≤ 1,500 ml/day. Up to 20 ml/kg hourly may be used in hemorrhagic shock.	▪ Contraindicated in known hypersensitivity, severe bleeding disorders, severe heart failure, or renal failure with oliguria and anuria.
histrelin acetate Supprelin *Gonadotropin-releasing hormone* *Posterior pituitary hormone* Preg. Risk Category: X	*inj*: 120, 300, 600 mcg/0.6 ml	*Centrally mediated (idiopathic or neurogenic) precocious puberty* — **Children (girls 2 to 8 yr; boys 2 to 9 yr):** 10 mcg/kg SC daily as single injection.	▪ Indicated only for patients who will comply with daily schedule ▪ Contraindicated in hypersensitivity to any drug component and in pregnant or breast-feeding patients. ▪ Safety and efficacy not established in children < 2 yr.

homatropine hydrobromide
Homatrine, Homatropine, Isopto Homatropine
Anticholinergic
Cycloplegic/mydriatic
Preg. Risk Category: C

ophth sol: 2%, 5%

Cycloplegic refraction — **Adults and children:** 1 to 2 drops instilled into eyes; if needed, repeat in 5 to 10 min for 2 or 3 doses.
Uveitis — **Adults and children:** 1 to 2 drops instilled into eyes q 3 to 4 hr.
Note: Use only 2% sol with children. Patients with heavily pigmented irises may require larger doses.

- Use cautiously in elderly patients and others who may have increased IOP.
- Contraindicated in glaucoma, hypersensitivity to drug or other belladonna alkaloids such as atropine, and patients with adhesions between iris and lens.

hydralazine hydrochloride
Alphapress‡, Apresoline, Novo-Hylazin‡, Supres‡
Peripheral vasodilator
Antihypertensive
Preg. Risk Category: C

tab: 10, 25, 50, 100 mg; **inj:** 20 mg/ml

Essential hypertension (orally); severe essential hypertension (parenterally) — **Adults:** *PO:* 10 mg qid; increase gradually to 50 mg qid prn. Max 200 mg qd, but some patients may require 300 to 400 mg qd. *IV:* 10 to 20 mg repeated prn; switch to PO as soon as possible. *IM:* 10 to 50 mg, repeated prn; switch to PO form as soon as possible.
Children: *PO:* 0.75 mg/kg/day divided into 4 doses; increase gradually over 3 to 4 wk to max 7.5 mg/kg or 200 mg qd. *IV or IM:* 1.7 to 3.5 mg/kg qd or 50 to 100 mg/m² qd in 4 to 6 divided doses. Initial parenteral dose shouldn't exceed 20 mg.

- Use cautiously in suspected cardiac disease, CVA, or severe renal impairment and in patients taking other antihypertensives.
- Contraindicated in hypersensitivity to drug, CAD, or mitral valvular rheumatic heart disease.

hydrochlorothiazide
Apo-Hydro‡, Aquazide-H, Diaqua, Dichlotride‡, HydroDIURIL
Thiazide diuretic
Diuretic/antihypertensive
Preg. Risk Category: B

tab: 25, 50, 100 mg; **oral sol:** 10 mg/ml, 50 mg/5 ml, 100 mg/ml

Edema — **Adults:** 25 to 100 mg PO daily or intermittently. **Children 2 to 12 yr:** 37.5 to 100 mg PO daily in 2 divided doses. **Children 6 mo to 2 yr:** 12.5 to 37.5 mg PO daily in 2 divided doses. **Infants < 6 mo:** up to 3 mg/kg PO daily in 2 divided doses. Max dosage may range from 12.5 to 37.5 mg qd.
Hypertension — **Adults:** 25 to 50 mg PO daily as single dose or divided bid. Increase or decrease daily dosage according to BP. Doses > 50 mg/day not required when combined with other antihypertensives.

- Use cautiously in children and in severe renal disease, impaired hepatic function, and progressive hepatic disease.
- Contraindicated in anuria and hypersensitivity to other thiazides or other sulfonamide derivatives.

hydrocortisone
Acticort, CaldeCort, Cortef, Cortizone 5, Squibb-HC‡

aerosol: 0.5%; **cream:** 0.25% to 2.5%; **gel:**

Inflammation associated with corticosteroid-responsive dermatoses; adjunctive topical management of seborrheic dermatitis of scalp — **Adults and children:**

- Contraindicated in hypersensitivity to drug.

(continued)

‡Canadian †Australian

HYDROCORTISONE 119

DRUG/CLASS/ CATEGORY	DOSAGE FORMS	INDICATIONS/ DOSAGES	KEY PRECAUTIONS
hydrocortisone (continued) CortaGel, Cortaid, Cortamed†, Dermacort‡, Hydrocortisone Acetate **hydrocortisone butyrate** Locoid **hydrocortisone valerate** Westcort Cream *Glucocorticoid Antiinflammatory* Preg. Risk Category: C	0.5%, 1%; *lotion:* 0.125% to 2.5%; *oint:* 0.5%, 1%, 2.5%; *pledgets:* 0.5%; *topical sol:* 0.5%, 1%, 2.5%. **acetate** — *cream, lotion:* 0.5%; *oint:* 0.5%, 1%; *paste:* 0.5%; *sol:* 1%. **butyrate** — *cream, oint, sol:* 0.1%. **valerate** — *cream, oint:* 0.2%	clean area: apply cream, gel, lotion, oint, or topical sol sparingly daily to qid. Spray aerosol onto affected area daily to qid until acute phase controlled; then reduce dosage to 1 to 3 times weekly prn.	
hydrocortisone Cortef, Cortenem‡, Hydrocortone **hydrocortisone acetate** Cortifoam, Hydrocortone Acetate **hydrocortisone sodium phosphate** Hydrocortone Phosphate	**hydrocortisone** — *tab:* 5, 10, 20 mg; *enema:* 100 mg/60 ml; *inj:* 25 mg/ml susp. **acetate** — *inj:* 25 mg/ml, 50	*Severe inflammation, adrenal insufficiency* — **Adults:** 5 to 30 mg PO bid, tid, or qid (up to 80 mg qid in acute situations); or initially, 100 to 500 mg succinate IM or IV, and then 50 to 100 mg IM; or 15 to 240 mg phosphate IM or IV daily in divided doses q 12 hr; or 5 to 75 mg acetate into joints or soft tissue. Dosage varies with size of joint. Local anesthetics often injected with dose.	▪ Use with extreme caution in recent MI. Use cautiously in GI ulcer, renal disease, hypertension, osteoporosis, diabetes mellitus, hypothyroidism, cirrhosis, diverticulitis, nonspecific ulcerative colitis, recent intestinal anastomoses, thromboembolic disorders, seizures, myasthenia gravis, heart failure, tuberculosis, ocular herpes simplex, emotional instability, and psychotic tendencies.

Drug	Forms	Indications & Dosages	Cautions
hydrocortisone sodium succinate A-hydroCort, Solu-Cortef *Glucocorticoid/mineralocorticoid* *Adrenocorticoid replacement/anti-inflammatory* Preg. Risk Category: C	mg/ml susp; *enema:* 10% *enema aerosol* foam (provides 90 mg/application); *supp:* 25 mg. **sodium phosphate** — *inj:* 50 mg/ml sol. **sodium succinate** — *inj:* 100-, 250-, 500-, 1,000-mg vials	*Shock* — **Adults:** initially, 50 mg/kg succinate IV, repeated q 24 hr prn. Or, 100 to 500 mg to 2 g q 2 to 6 hr; continue until patient stabilized (usually not longer than 48 to 72 hr). **Children:** phosphate (IM) or succinate (IM or IV) 0.16 to 1 mg/kg or 6 to 30 mg/m² qd or bid. *Adjunct for ulcerative colitis and proctitis* — **Adults:** 1 enema (100 mg) PR nightly for 21 days. Or, 1 applicator (90-mg foam) PR daily or bid for 14 to 21 days.	• Contraindicated in allergy to any component of formulation, systemic fungal infections, and premature infants (succinate).
hydromorphone hydrochloride (dihydromorphinone hydrochloride) Dilaudid, Dilaudid-HP *Opioid* *Analgesic/antitussive* Preg. Risk Category: C Controlled Sub. Sched.: II	*tab:* 1, 2, 3, 4, 8 mg; *inj:* 1, 2, 3, 4, 10 mg/ml; *supp:* 3 mg; *syrup:* 5 mg/5 ml	*Moderate to severe pain* — **Adults:** 2 to 10 mg PO q 3 to 6 hr, prn or around the clock; or 2 to 4 mg IM, SC, or IV (slowly over at least 3 to 5 min) q 4 to 6 hr prn or around the clock; or 3 mg rectal supp hs, prn or around the clock. (Give 1 to 14 mg Dilaudid-HP SC or IM q 4 to 6 hr.) *Cough* — **Adults and children > 12 yr:** 1 mg PO q 3 to 4 hr. **Children 6 to 12 yr:** 0.5 mg PO q 3 to 4 hr, prn.	■ Use with extreme caution in hepatic or renal disease, hypothyroidism, Addison's disease, prostatic hyperplasia, or urethral stricture. Also use with caution in elderly or debilitated patients. • Contraindicated in hypersensitivity to drug, in intracranial lesions associated with increased ICP, and depression of ventilator function.
hydroxychloroquine sulfate Plaquenil *4-aminoquinoline* *Antimalarial/anti-inflammatory* Preg. Risk Category: C	*tab:* 200 mg (155-mg base)	*Suppressive prophylaxis of malarial attacks* — **Adults:** 400 mg sulfate (310 mg base) PO weekly on exactly same day each wk (begin 2 wk before entering endemic area and continue for 8 wk after leaving endemic area). If not started before exposure, initial dose doubled (10 mg/kg) in 2 divided doses PO 6 hr apart. **Infants and children:** 5 mg, calculated as base/kg of body weight (shouldn't exceed adult dose regardless of weight) on exactly same day each week.	■ Use with extreme caution in severe GI, neurologic, or blood disorders. Use cautiously in hepatic disease, alcoholism, G6PD deficiency, or psoriasis. • Contraindicated in hypersensitivity to drug, in long-term therapy for children, and in retinal or visual field changes or porphyria.

(continued)

HYDROXYCHLOROQUINE SULFATE 121

†Canadian ‡Australian

DRUG/CLASS/CATEGORY	DOSAGE FORMS	INDICATIONS/DOSAGES	KEY PRECAUTIONS
hydroxychloroquine sulfate *(continued)*		Start 2 wk prior to exposure. If unable, give 10 mg base/kg in 2 divided doses 6 hr apart. *Acute malarial attacks* — **Adults:** initially, 800 mg (sulfate: 620 mg base) PO, then 400 mg (310-mg base) in 6 to 8 hr, and 400 mg daily for 2 days (total 2 g sulfate salt). **Infants and children:** initially, 10 mg base/kg (but not exceeding single dose of 620-mg base). Second dose 5 mg base/kg (but not exceeding single dose of 310-mg base) 6 hr after first dose; third dose 5 mg base/kg 18 hr after second; fourth dose 5 mg base/kg 24 hr after third. *Lupus erythematosus (chronic discoid and systemic)* — **Adults:** 400 mg (sulfate) PO daily or bid, continued for several weeks or months, depending on response. Prolonged maintenance dosage 200 to 400 mg (sulfate) daily.	
hydroxyprogesterone caproate Delta-Lutin, Duralutin, Gesterol L.A. 250, Hy/Gestrone, Hylutin, Hyprogest 250, Pro-Depo, Prodrox 250, Pro-Span *Progestin* *Progestin/antineoplastic* Preg. Risk Category: X	*inj:* 125, 250 mg/ml	*Amenorrhea, uterine bleeding* — **Adults:** 375 mg IM. May repeat at 4-wk intervals if needed. After 4 days of desquamation or if no bleeding occurs within 21 days after administration, start cyclic therapy with estrogen. *Palliative treatment of advanced inoperable endometrial cancer* — **Adults:** 1 g IM up to 7 times/wk for 12 wk or as indicated. Therapy discontinued if relapse occurs or no objective response seen after 12 wk.	• Use cautiously in diabetes mellitus, seizures, migraine, cardiac or renal disease, asthma, mental depression, or impaired liver function. • Contraindicated in hypersensitivity to drug, thromboembolic disorders, cerebral apoplexy, breast or genital organ cancer, undiagnosed abnormal vaginal bleeding, severe hepatic disease, and missed abortion and during pregnancy. • Shouldn't be used to induce withdrawal bleeding or as test for pregnancy; may cause birth defects and masculinization of female fetus.

hydroxyurea
Hydrea
Antimetabolite (cell cycle–phase specific, S phase)
Antineoplastic
Preg. Risk Category: NR

cap: 500 mg

Melanoma: resistant chronic myelocytic leukemia; recurrent, metastatic, or inoperable ovarian cancer; head and neck cancers — **Adults:** 80 mg/kg PO as single dose q 3 days; or 20 to 30 mg/kg PO as single daily dose.

- Use cautiously in renal dysfunction.
- Contraindicated in hypersensitivity to drug and marked bone marrow depression (leukopenia [< 2,500/mm³ WBCs], thrombocytopenia [< 100,000/mm³ platelets], or severe anemia).
- Don't give to women who are or may become pregnant unless benefit outweighs risk.

hydroxyzine embonate‡
Atarax‡
hydroxyzine hydrochloride
Apo-Hydroxyzine†, Atarax, Hyzine-50, Multipax†, Vistaquel, Vistaril, Vistazine 50
hydroxyzine pamoate
Hy-Pam, Vamate, Vistaril
Antihistamine (piperazine derivative)
Antianxiety agent/sedative/antipruritic/antiemetic/antispasmodic
Preg. Risk Category: C

embonate‡ — cap: 25, 50 mg. hydrochloride — tab: 10, 25, 50, 100 mg; cap: 10, 25, 50 mg; syrup: 10 mg/5 ml; inj: 25, 50 mg/ml. pamoate — cap: 25, 50, 100 mg; oral susp: 25 mg/5 ml

Anxiety, tension, hyperkinesia — **Adults:** 50 to 100 mg PO qid. **Children ≥ 6 yr:** 50 to 100 mg PO daily in divided doses. **Children < 6 yr:** 50 mg PO daily in divided doses.
Preop and postop adjunctive sedation, to control vomiting (excluding pregnancy), or as adjunct to asthma treatment — **Adults:** 25 to 100 mg IM q 4 to 6 hr. **Children:** 1.1 mg/kg IM q 4 to 6 hr.
Pruritus due to allergies — **Adults:** 25 mg PO tid or qid. **Children ≥ 6 yr:** 50 to 100 mg PO daily in divided doses. **Children < 6 yr:** 50 mg PO daily in divided doses.

- Use cautiously with dosage adjustments in elderly or debilitated patients.
- Contraindicated in hypersensitivity to drug, during early pregnancy, and in breast-feeding patients.

hyoscyamine
Cystospaz
hyoscyamine sulfate
Anaspaz, Bellaspaz, Levsin, Levsin S/L, Neoquess
Belladonna alkaloid
Anticholinergic
Preg. Risk Category: C

hyoscyamine — tab: 0.15 mg. sulfate — tab: 0.125, 0.13, 0.15 mg; cap (ext-release): 0.375 mg; elixir: 0.125 mg/5 ml; oral sol: 0.125 mg/ml; inj: 0.5 mg/ml

GI tract disorders caused by spasm; to diminish secretions and block cardiac vagal reflexes preop; adjunctive therapy for peptic ulcerations — **Adults and children ≥ 12 yr:** 0.125 to 0.25 mg PO or SL tid or qid before meals and hs; 0.375 to 0.75 mg PO (ext-release form) q 12 hr; or 0.25 to 0.5 mg (1 or 2 ml) IM, IV, or SC q 4 hr bid to qid. Max 1.5 mg daily. **Children < 12 yr:** dosage individualized according to weight.

- Use cautiously in autonomic neuropathy, hyperthyroidism, CAD, arrhythmias, heart failure, hypertension, hiatal hernia with reflux esophagitis, hepatic or renal disease, ulcerative colitis, and in hot or humid environment.
- Contraindicated in glaucoma, obstructive uropathy, obstructive GI tract disease, severe ulcerative colitis, myasthenia gravis, hypersensitivity to anticholinergics, paralytic ileus, intestinal atony, unstable CV status in acute hemorrhage, and toxic megacolon.

†Canadian ‡Australian

DRUG / CLASS / CATEGORY	DOSAGE FORMS	INDICATIONS / DOSAGES	KEY PRECAUTIONS
ibuprofen Aches-N-Pain, ACT-3‡, Advil, Children's Advil, Children's Motrin, Motrin, Motrin IB Caplets, Motrin IB Tablets, Nuprin Caplets, Nuprin Tablets, PediaProfen *Nonsteroidal anti-inflammatory* *Nonnarcotic analgesic/antipyretic/anti-inflammatory* Preg. Risk Category: B	**tab:** 100, 200, 300, 400, 600, 800 mg; **tab (chew):** 50, 100 mg; **cap:** 200 mg; **oral susp:** 100 mg/5 ml	*Rheumatoid arthritis, osteoarthritis, arthritis* — **Adults:** 300 to 800 mg PO tid or qid, not to exceed 3.2 g/day. *Mild to moderate pain, dysmenorrhea* — **Adults:** 400 mg PO q 4 to 6 hr, prn. *Fever* — **Adults:** 200 to 400 mg PO q 4 to 6 hr. Don't exceed 1.2 g daily or give > 3 days. **6 mo to 12 yr:** if fever < 102.5° F (39.2° C), 5 mg/kg PO q 6 to 8 hr. Max 40 mg/kg/day. Treat higher fevers with 10 mg/kg q 6 to 8 hr. Max 40 mg/kg/day. *Juvenile arthritis* — **Children:** 30 to 70 mg/kg/day in 3 or 4 divided doses.	• Use cautiously in GI disorders, history of peptic ulcer disease, hepatic or renal disease, cardiac decompensation, hypertension, or known intrinsic coagulation defects. • Contraindicated in hypersensitivity to drug or in syndrome of nasal polyps, angioedema, and bronchospastic reaction to aspirin or other NSAIDs. • Not recommended during pregnancy.
ibutilide fumarate Corvert *Ibutilide derivative* *Supraventricular antiarrhythmic* Preg. Risk Category: C	**inj:** 0.1 mg/ml in 10-ml vials	*Rapid conversion of fibrillation or atrial flutter of recent onset to sinus rhythm* — **Adults > 60 kg (132 lb):** 1 mg IV over 10 min. **Adults < 60 kg:** 0.01 mg/kg IV over 10 min. Stop infusion if arrhythmia ends or if ventricular tachycardia or marked prolongation of QT or QTc occurs. If arrhythmia doesn't end 10 min after infusion ends, may give second 10-min infusion of equal strength.	• Use cautiously in hepatic or renal dysfunction. • Contraindicated in hypersensitivity to drug or its components, in history of polymorphic ventricular tachycardia, and in breast-feeding patients. • Safety in children not established.
idarubicin hydrochloride Idamycin *Antibiotic/antineoplastic* *Antineoplastic* Preg. Risk Category: D	**powder for inj:** 5, 10, 20 mg	Dosage and indications vary. Check treatment protocol. *Acute myeloid leukemia, including FAB (French-American-British) classifications M1 through M7, in combination with other approved antileukemic agents* — **Adults:** 12 mg/m²/day for 3 days by slow IV injection (over 10 to 15 min) in combination with 100 mg/m²/day of cytarabine for 7 days by continuous IV infusion; or as 25 mg/m² bolus (cytarabine),	• Use with extreme caution in bone marrow suppression induced by previous drug therapy or radiotherapy, impaired hepatic or renal function, prior treatment with anthracyclines or cardiotoxic agents, or preexisting cardiac condition.

followed by 200 mg/m²/day (cytarabine) for 5 days by continuous infusion. Second course may be given prn. If patient experiences severe mucositis, delay until recovery complete, and reduce dosage by 25%. Also reduce dosage in hepatic or renal impairment. Don't give if bilirubin > 5 mg/dl.

ifosfamide
IFEX
Alkylating agent (cell cycle–phase nonspecific)
Antineoplastic
Preg. Risk Category: D

inj: 1, 2, 3 g

Testicular cancer — **Adults:** 1.2 g/m²/day IV for 5 consecutive days. Infuse each dose over ≥ 30 min. Repeat treatment q 3 wk or after patient recovers from hematologic toxicity. Administer with protecting agent (mesna) to prevent hemorrhagic cystitis.

- Use cautiously in renal or hepatic impairment or compromised bone marrow reserve as indicated by leukopenia, granulocytopenia, extensive bone marrow metastases, prior radiation therapy, or prior therapy with cytotoxic agents.
- Contraindicated in hypersensitivity to drug and in severe bone marrow suppression.

imiglucerase
Cerezyme
Glycosidase
Replacement enzyme
Preg. Risk Category: C

inj: 200 units/vial

Long-term endogenous enzyme (glucosylceramidase) replacement therapy in confirmed type I Gaucher's disease — **Adults and children:** dosage individualized; initially, give 2.5 to 60 U/kg IV over 1 to 2 hr. Typical dosing frequency once q 2 wk, but may range from 3 times weekly to once monthly, depending on disease severity. May reduce dosage for maintenance therapy, at intervals of 3 to 6 mo, while response parameters carefully monitored.

- Use with caution in symptoms of hypersensitivity to drug or in patients who have developed antibody to alglucerase during previous treatment with that drug or have shown symptoms of hypersensitivity.

imipenem/cilastatin sodium
Primaxin IM, Primaxin IV
Carbapenem (thienamycin class)
beta-lactam antibiotic
Antibiotic
Preg. Risk Category: C

powder for inj: 250, 500 mg

Serious lower respiratory, urinary tract, intra-abdominal, gyn, bone and joint, and skin and soft-tissue infections; bacterial septicemia and endocarditis — **Adults and children > 40 kg:** 250 mg to 1 g by IV infusion q 6 to 8 hr. Max 50 mg/kg/day or 4 g/day, whichever is less. Alternatively, 500 to 750 mg IM q 12 hr. Max 1,500 mg/day. **Children < 40 kg:** 60 mg/kg IV daily in divided doses. **Premature infants < 36 wk gestational age:** 20 mg/kg IV q 12 hr.

- Use cautiously in allergy to penicillins or cephalosporins, in history of seizure disorder, and in children < 3 mo.
- Contraindicated in hypersensitivity to drug. If reconstituted with lidocaine hydrochloride for IM injection, contraindicated in known hypersensitivity to local anesthetics of amide type and in severe heart block or shock.

IMIPENEM/CILASTATIN SODIUM   125

DRUG/CLASS/CATEGORY	DOSAGE FORMS	INDICATIONS/DOSAGES	KEY PRECAUTIONS
imipramine hydrochloride Apo-Imipramine†, Imprilt, Janimine, Melipramine‡, Norfranil, Tipramine, Tofranil **imipramine pamoate** Tofranil-PM *Dibenzazepine tricyclic antidepressant* Preg. Risk Category: B	**hydrochloride — tab:** 10, 25, 50 mg; **inj:** 12.5 mg/ml. **pamoate — cap:** 75, 100, 125, 150 mg	*Depression* — **Adults:** 75 to 100 mg PO or IM daily in divided doses, increased in 25- to 50-mg increments. Max for outpatients 200 mg daily; 300 mg daily may be used for hospital patients. Entire dosage may be given hs. **Elderly and adolescent patients:** initially, 30 to 40 mg daily; usually not necessary to exceed 100 mg daily. *Childhood enuresis* — **Children ≥ 6 yr:** 25 mg PO 1 hr before bedtime. If no response within 1 wk, increase to 50 mg if child < 12 yr; 75 mg for children ≥ 12 yr. In either case, max 2.5 mg/kg/day.	• Use with extreme caution in risk for suicide; in history of urine retention or angle-closure glaucoma, increased intraocular pressure, CV disease, impaired hepatic function, hyperthyroidism, history of seizure disorders, or impaired renal function; in patients receiving thyroid medications; and in allergy to sulfites (injectible form only). • Contraindicated during acute recovery phase of MI, in hypersensitivity to drug, and during concurrent MAO inhibitor therapy.
immune globulin intramuscular (IGIM, IG, gamma globulin) Gammar **immune globulin intravenous (IGIV)** Gamimune N, Gammagard S/D, Iveegam, Sandoglobulin, Venoglobulin-I, Venoglobulin-S *Immune serum* *Immune serum* Preg. Risk Category: C	**IGIM — inj:** 2-, 10-ml vials. **IGIV — inj:** 5% in 10-, 50-, 100-, 250-ml vials (Gami. N); 5% in 2.5-, 5-, 10-g vials; 10% in 5-, 10-, 20-g vials (Veno.-S); **powder for inj:** 500-mg, 1-, 2.5-, 5-g vials (Iveegam); 1-, 3-, 6-g vials (Sando.); 500-mg, 2.5-, 5-, 10-g vials (Veno.-I)	*Agammaglobulinemia or hypogammaglobulinemia* — **Adults:** initially, 1.2 ml/kg IM, then 0.6 ml/kg once q 2 to 4 wk. Max single dose 30 to 50 ml. Alternatively, 100 to 400 mg/kg IV q 2 to 4 wk. Infuse at 0.01 to 0.02 ml/kg/min for 30 min. If no discomfort, increase rate to max 0.06 ml/kg/min. For Sandoglobulin, 200 mg/kg IV monthly. Infuse at 0.5 to 1 ml/min. After 15 to 30 min, increase rate to 1.5 to 2.5 ml/min. **Children:** 20 to 40 ml IM monthly. *Hepatitis A exposure* — **Adults and children:** 0.02 ml/kg IM as soon as possible after exposure. May give up to 0.06 ml/kg q 4 to 6 mo if exposure will be ≥ 3 mo. *Idiopathic thrombocytopenic purpura* — **Adults:** 0.4 g/kg Gamimune N for 5 consecutive days or Sandoglobulin IV for 2 to 5 consecutive days. May give additional doses based on response. May give up to 3 doses of Gammagard 1,000 mg/kg (qod) if necessary. Or, Venoglobulin-I 500 mg/kg (up to 2,000 mg/kg) daily for 2 to 7 days.	• Contraindicated in hypersensitivity to drug.

indapamide
Lozide†, Lozol, Natrilix‡
Thiazide-like diuretic
Diuretic/antihypertensive
Preg. Risk Category: B

tab: 1.25, 2.5 mg

Edema — **Adults:** initially, 2.5 mg PO daily in morning. Increase to 5 mg daily after 1 wk, if needed.
Hypertension — **Adults:** initially, 1.25 mg PO daily in morning. Increase to 2.5 mg daily after 4 wk, if needed. Increase to 5 mg daily after 4 more wk, if needed.

- Use cautiously in severe renal disease, impaired hepatic function, and progressive hepatic disease.
- Contraindicated in anuria or hypersensitivity to other sulfonamide-derived drugs.

indinavir sulfate
Crixivan
HIV protease inhibitor
Antiviral
Preg. Risk Category: C

cap: 200, 400 mg

Treatment of HIV infection when antiretroviral therapy warranted — **Adults:** 800 mg PO q 8 hr. Reduce to 600 mg PO q 8 hr in mild to moderate hepatic insufficiency due to cirrhosis.

- Use cautiously in hepatic insufficiency due to cirrhosis.
- Contraindicated in hypersensitivity to any drug component.
- Safety and efficacy in children not established.

indomethacin
Apo-Indomethacin†, Indochron E-R, Indocid SR†, Indocin, Indocin SR, Novomethacin†, Rheumacin†
indomethacin sodium trihydrate
Apo-Indomethacin†, Indocid PDA†, Indocin IV, Novomethacin†
Nonsteroidal anti-inflammatory
Nonnarcotic analgesic/antipyretic/anti-inflammatory
Preg. Risk Category: NR

indomethacin — *cap:* 25, 50 mg; *cap (sust-release):* 75 mg; *oral susp:* 25 mg/5 ml; *supp:* 50 mg. **sodium trihydrate** — *inj:* 1-mg vials

Moderate to severe rheumatoid arthritis or osteoarthritis, ankylosing spondylitis — **Adults:** 25 mg PO or PR bid or tid with food or antacids; increase daily dosage 25 or 50 mg q 7 days, up to 200 mg daily. Or, sust-release cap (75 mg): 75 mg PO to start, in morning or hs, followed, if necessary, by 75 mg bid.
Acute gouty arthritis — **Adults:** 50 mg PO tid. Reduce as soon as possible; then stop.
Acute painful shoulders (bursitis or tendinitis) — **Adults:** 75 to 150 mg PO daily in divided doses tid or qid for 7 to 14 days.
To close hemodynamically significant PDA in premature infants (IV form only) — **Neonates < 48 hr:** 0.2 mg/kg IV followed by 2 doses of 0.1 mg/kg at 12- to 24-hr intervals. **Neonates 2 to 7 days:** 0.2 mg/kg IV followed by 2 doses of 0.2 mg/kg at 12- to 24-hr intervals. **Neonates > 7 days:** 0.2 mg/kg IV followed by 2 doses of 0.25 mg/kg at 12- to 24-hr intervals.

- Use cautiously in epilepsy, parkinsonism, hepatic or renal disease, CV disease, infection, and mental illness or depression. Also use cautiously in elderly patients and in history of GI disease.
- Contraindicated in hypersensitivity to drug; history of aspirin- or NSAID-induced asthma, rhinitis, or urticaria; and in pregnant or breast-feeding patients. Also contraindicated in infants with untreated infection, active bleeding, coagulation defects or thrombocytopenia, congenital heart disease in which PDA patency necessary, necrotizing enterocolitis, or impaired renal function. Suppositories contraindicated in history of proctitis or recent rectal bleeding.

†Canadian ‡Australian

DRUG/CLASS/CATEGORY	DOSAGE FORMS	INDICATIONS/DOSAGES	KEY PRECAUTIONS
insulin inj (regular insulin, crystalline zinc insulin) Humulin R, Novolin R, Regular (Conc.) Iletin II **insulin zinc susp, prompt (semilente)** Semilente MC‡ **isophane insulin susp (NPH)** Humulin N, Humulin NPH‡, Novolin N, NPH Insulin **isophane insulin susp with insulin inj** Humulin 50/50, Humulin 70/30, Novolin 70/30 **insulin zinc susp (lente)** Humulin L, Lente Insulin, Lente MC‡, Novolin L **protamine zinc susp (PZI)** Protamine Zinc Insulin MC‡ **insulin zinc susp, ext (ultralente)** Humulin U, Ultralente Insulin *Pancreatic hormone* *Antidiabetic agent* Preg. Risk Category: NR	**prep for inj:** range from 100 to 500 units/ml; from human, pork, and beef sources; from vials to cartridge systems, and from slow to fast-acting	*Diabetic ketoacidosis (use reg insulin only)* — **Adults:** 0.33 units/kg as IV bolus, followed by 0.1 units/kg/hr by continuous infusion. Continue infusion until blood glucose drops to 250 mg/dl; then begin SC insulin with dosage and intervals adjusted according to blood glucose level. Or, 50 to 100 units IV and 50 to 100 units SC stat; then additional doses q 2 to 6 hr based on blood glucose levels. To prepare infusion, add 100 units reg insulin and 1 g albumin to 100 ml 0.9% NaCl. Insulin concentration will be 1 unit/ml. **Children:** 0.1 unit/kg as IV bolus, then 0.1 unit/kg/hr by continuous infusion until blood glucose drops to 250 mg/dl; then start SC insulin. Alternatively, 1 to 2 units/kg in 2 divided doses, one IV and other SC, followed by 0.5 to 1 unit/kg IV q 1 to 2 hr based on blood glucose levels. *Type 1 diabetes, adjunct to type 2 diabetes* — **Adults and children:** therapeutic regimen adjusted according to blood glucose levels.	▪ Contraindicated in history of systemic allergic reaction to pork. ▪ Only give reg insulin IV. Intermittent infusion not recommended. ▪ Some patients may develop insulin resistance and require large doses. U-500 insulin available as Regular (Concentrated) Iletin II for such patients. However, not every pharmacy may stock it. Give hospital pharmacy sufficient notice before requesting refill of in-house prescription. ▪ Drug of choice to treat diabetes in pregnancy. Insulin requirements rise in pregnant diabetics, and then decline immediately postpartum. Monitor closely.

interferon alfa-2a, recombinant (rIFN-A)
Roferon-A
Biological response modifier
Antineoplastic
Preg. Risk Category: C

inj: 3 million IU/vial; 18 and 36 million IU/multidose vial

Hairy-cell leukemia — **Adults:** for induction, 3 million IU SC or IM daily for 16 to 24 wk. For maintenance, 3 million IU SC or IM 3 times weekly.
AIDS-related Kaposi's sarcoma — **Adults:** for induction, 36 million IU SC or IM daily for 10 to 12 wk. For maintenance, 36 million IU SC or IM 3 times/wk.
Philadelphia chromosome-positive chronic myelogenous leukemia — **Adults:** initially, 3 million IU daily for 3 days; then 6 million IU for 3 days, then 9 million IU for duration of treatment.

- Use cautiously in CV or pulmonary disease, diabetes mellitus, coagulation disorders, or myelosuppression.
- Contraindicated in hypersensitivity to drug or to murine (mouse) immunoglobulin.

---

interferon alfa-2b, recombinant (IFN-alpha 2)
Intron A
Biological response modifier
Antineoplastic
Preg. Risk Category: C

powder for inj: 3, 5, 10, 18, 25, 50 million IU/vial with diluent; *inj:* 10 million IU/2-ml, 18 million IU/3-ml, 25 million IU/5-ml vials

Hairy-cell leukemia — **Adults:** 2 million IU/m² IM or SC, 3 times/wk.
AIDS-related Kaposi's sarcoma — **Adults:** 30 million IU/m² SC or IM 3 times/wk.
Chronic hepatitis B — **Adults:** 30 to 35 million IU weekly IM or SC, given either as 5 million IU daily or 10 million IU 3 times/wk for 16 wk.

- Use cautiously in history of CV disease, pulmonary disease, diabetes mellitus, coagulation disorders, or severe myelosuppression.
- Contraindicated in hypersensitivity to drug.

---

interferon alfa-n3
Alferon N
Biological response modifier
Antineoplastic
Preg. Risk Category: C

inj: 5 million units/ml in 1-ml vials

Condylomata acuminata (genital or venereal warts) — **Adults:** 0.05 ml (250,000 units) for each wart by intralesional injection. Treatment usually continues twice weekly for up to 8 wk. Dosage shouldn't exceed 0.5 ml (2.5 million units) per session.

- Use cautiously in debilitating illness (uncontrolled heart failure, unstable angina, severe pulmonary disease, coagulation disorders, seizure disorders, severe myelosuppression, or diabetes mellitus with ketoacidosis).
- Contraindicated in hypersensitivity to interferon alfa and in history of anaphylactic reactions to murine (mouse) immunoglobulin, egg protein, or neomycin.

INTERFERON ALFA-N3 129

DRUG/CLASS/ CATEGORY	DOSAGE FORMS	INDICATIONS/ DOSAGES	KEY PRECAUTIONS
interferon beta-1a Avonex *Biological response modifier Antiviral immunoregulator* Preg. Risk Category: C	*lyoph powder for inj:* 33 mcg (6.6 million IU)	*Treatment of relapsing forms of multiple sclerosis to slow accumulation of physical disability and decrease frequency of clinical exacerbation* — **Adults:** 30 mcg IM q wk.	▪ Use cautiously in depression, seizure disorders, or severe cardiac conditions. ▪ Contraindicated in history of hypersensitivity to natural or recombinant interferon beta, human albumin, or other component of formulation. ▪ Safety and efficacy in chronic progressive multiple sclerosis or in children < 18 yr not established. ▪ Not known if excreted in breast milk. Potential for serious adverse reactions in breast-fed infants; must decide whether to discontinue breast-feeding or drug.
interferon beta-1b, recombinant Betaseron *Biological response modifier Antiviral immunoregulator* Preg. Risk Category: C	*powder for inj:* 9.6 million IU (0.3 mg)	*To reduce frequency of exacerbations in relapsing-remitting multiple sclerosis* — **Adults:** 8 million IU (0.25 mg) SC qod.	▪ Use cautiously in women of childbearing age. ▪ Contraindicated in hypersensitivity to interferon beta or human albumin.
interferon gamma-1b Actimmune *Biological response modifier Antineoplastic* Preg. Risk Category: C	*inj:* 100 mcg (3 million units)/0.5-ml vial	*Chronic granulomatous disease* — **Adults with BSA > 0.5 m²:** 50 mcg/m² (1.5 million units/m²) SC 3 times weekly, preferably at hs. Preferred injection site deltoid or anterior thigh muscle. **Adults with BSA ≤ 0.5 m²:** 1.5 mcg/kg 3 times weekly.	▪ Use cautiously in cardiac disease (including arrhythmias, ischemia, or heart failure), compromised CNS function, or seizure disorders and in patients receiving myelosuppression. ▪ Contraindicated in hypersensitivity to drug or to genetically engineered products derived from *E. coli.*

Drug	Form	Indications/Dosage	Contraindications

ipecac syrup
Alkaloid emetic
Emetic
Preg. Risk Category: C

syrup: 70 mg powdered ipecac/ml (contains glycerin 10% and alcohol 1% to 2.5%)

To induce vomiting in poisoning — **Adults and children > 12 yr:** 15 to 30 ml PO, followed by 3 to 4 glasses of water. **Children 1 to 12 yr:** 15 ml PO, followed by 240 to 480 ml water. **Children 6 mo to 1 yr:** 5 to 10 ml PO, followed by 120 to 240 ml water. May repeat dose in patients > 1 yr if vomiting doesn't occur within 20 min. If no vomiting occurs within 30 to 35 min after 2nd dose, gastric lavage should be performed.

- Contraindicated in semicomatose or unconscious patients and in severe inebriation, seizures, shock, or loss of gag reflex. Unless advised otherwise by poison control center, don't give after ingestion of petroleum distillates (for example, kerosene, gasoline) or volatile oils.

---

ipratropium bromide
Atrovent
Anticholinergic
Bronchodilator
Preg. Risk Category: B

inhaler: each metered dose supplies 18 mcg; **sol (for inh):** 0.02% (500 mcg/vial); **sol (for nebulizer):** 0.025% (250 mcg/ ml)‡; **nasal spray:** 0.03% (each metered dose supplies 21 mcg), 0.06% (each metered dose supplies 42 mcg)

Bronchospasm associated with COPD — **Adults:** 1 to 2 inhalations qid. More may be needed. Total inhalations shouldn't exceed 12 in 24 hr. Or, use inhalation sol. Give 500 mcg dissolved in 0.9% NaCl and administer by nebulizer q 6 to 8 hr. **Children 5 to 12 yr:** 125 to 250 mcg nebulizer sol dissolved in 0.9% NaCl and administer by nebulizer q 6 to 8 hr.
Perennial rhinitis — **Adults and children > 12 yr:** 2 sprays (42 mcg) of 0.03% nasal spray per nostril 2 to 3 times qd.
Common cold-induced rhinorrhea — **Adults and children > 12 yr:** 2 sprays (84 mcg) of 0.06% nasal spray per nostril 3 or 4 times qd

- Use cautiously in angle-closure glaucoma, prostatic hyperplasia, and bladder-neck obstruction.
- Contraindicated in hypersensitivity to drug or to atropine or any derivative, and in history of hypersensitivity to soyalecithin or related food products, such as soybeans and peanuts.

---

irinotecan hydrochloride
Camptosar
Topoisomerase inhibitor
Antineoplastic
Preg. Risk Category: D

inj: 100-mg/5-ml vial

Treatment of metastatic carcinoma of colon or rectum that has recurred or progressed after fluorouracil (5-FU) therapy — **Adults:** initially, 125 mg/m2 IV infusion over 90 min. Recommended treatment 125 mg/m2 IV q wk for 4 wk followed by 2-wk rest period. Thereafter, may repeat additional treatment course q

- Use cautiously in elderly patients and in history of pelvic or abdominal irradiation.
- Contraindicated in hypersensitivity to drug.

(continued)

IRINOTECAN HYDROCHLORIDE 131

†Canadian ‡Australian

DRUG / CLASS / CATEGORY	DOSAGE FORMS	INDICATIONS / DOSAGES	KEY PRECAUTIONS
irinotecan hydrochloride (continued)		6 wk (4 wk on therapy, followed by 2 wk off). May adjust subsequent doses to low of 50 mg/m² or to max 150 mg/m² in 25- to 50-mg/m² increments, depending on tolerance. Treatment with additional courses may continue indefinitely if patient responds favorably or if disease remains stable, unless intolerable toxicity occurs.	
iron dextran Imferon†, InFeD *Parenteral iron supplement* *Hematinic* Preg. Risk Category: C	1 ml iron dextran provides 50 mg elemental iron; *inj:* 50 mg elemental iron/ml	*Iron deficiency anemia* — **Adults and children:** IM or IV test dose required before administration. IM *(by Z-track method):* 0.5 ml test dose injected. If no reactions in 1 hr, give remainder of dose. Daily dosage ordinarily shouldn't exceed 0.5 ml (25 mg) for infants < 5 kg; 1 ml (50 mg) for children < 10 kg; 2 ml (100 mg) for heavier children and adults. IV: 0.5 ml test dose injected over 30 sec. If no reactions in 1 hr, give remainder of therapeutic IV dose. Repeat therapeutic dose IV daily. Single dose shouldn't exceed 100 mg. Give slowly (1 ml/min).	▪ Use cautiously in hepatic impairment, rheumatoid arthritis, and other inflammatory diseases. ▪ Contraindicated in hypersensitivity to drug, in all anemias except iron deficiency, and in acute infectious renal disease.
isoetharine hydrochloride Arm-a-Med Isoetharine, Bronkosol, Dey-Dose Isoetharine, Dispos-a-Med Isoetharine **isoetharine mesylate** Bronkometer *Adrenergic* *Bronchodilator* Preg. Risk Category: C	*aerosol inhaler:* 340 mcg/metered spray; *nebulizer inhaler:* 0.062, 0.08, 0.1, 0.125, 0.167, 0.17, .2, 0.25, 1% sol	*Bronchial asthma and reversible bronchospasm that may occur with bronchitis and emphysema* — **Adults:** *hydrochloride form* — given by hand nebulizer, oxygen aerosolization, or IPPB. Adjust dosage carefully according to individual tolerance and response. Usual adult dose given through oxygen aerosolization 0.5 ml (range: 0.25 to 0.5 ml) of 1% solution, diluted 1:3. Alternatively, may give undiluted solutions through oxygen aerosolization; usual adult dose 4 ml (range: 2 to 4 ml) of 0.125% solution, 2.5 ml of 0.2% solution, or 2 ml of 0.25% solution. Usual	▪ Use cautiously in hyperthyroidism, hypertension, or CAD; in hypersensitivity to sympathomimetics; or in patients receiving general anesthetics that sensitize myocardium to sympathomimetics. ▪ Contraindicated in hypersensitivity to drug.

Drug	Forms	Indications & Dosage	Nursing Considerations
		adult dosage through hand-bulb nebulizer of undiluted 1% solution 4 inhalations (range: 3 to 7 inhalations). *Mesylate form* — 1 to 2 inhalations. Occasionally, more may be required.	
isoniazid (isonicotinic acid hydride, INH) Isotamine†, Laniazid, Nydrazid, PMS Isoniazid† *Isonicotinic acid hydrazine* *Antitubercular agent* Preg. Risk Category: C	**tab:** 50, 100, 300 mg; **oral sol:** 50 mg/5 ml; **inj:** 100 mg/ml	*Actively growing tubercle bacilli* — **Adults:** 5 mg/kg PO or IM daily in single dose, up to 300 mg/day for 9 mo to 2 yr. **Infants and children:** 10 mg/kg PO or IM daily in single dose, up to 300 mg/day, for 18 mo to 2 yr. Give with one other antitubercular. *Prevention of tubercle bacilli in those exposed to TB or those with tests consistent with nonprogressive TB* — **Adults:** 300 mg PO daily in single dose, continued for 6 mo to 1 yr. **Infants and children:** 10 mg/kg PO daily in single dose, up to 300 mg/day, continued for 6 mo to 1 yr.	▪ Use cautiously in chronic non-isoniazid-associated liver disease, seizure disorders (especially in patients taking phenytoin), severe renal impairment, and chronic alcoholism and in elderly patients. ▪ Contraindicated in acute hepatic disease or isoniazid-associated liver damage.
isoproterenol (isoprenaline) Dey-Dose Isoproterenol, Isuprel, Vapo-Iso **isoproterenol hydrochloride** Isuprel, Norisodrine Aerotrol **isoproterenol sulfate** Medihaler-Iso *Adrenergic* *Bronchodilator/cardiac stimulant* Preg. Risk Category: C	**nebulizer inhaler:** 0.25%, 0.5%, 1%; **hydrochloride — tab (SL):** 10, 15 mg; **aerosol inhaler:** 120 mcg or 131 mcg/metered spray; **inj:** 200 mcg/ml. **sulfate — aerosol inhaler:** 80 mcg/metered spray	*Shock* — **Adults and children:** (hydrochloride) 0.5 to 5 mcg/min by continuous IV infusion titrated to response. Usual concentration 1 mg (5 ml) in 500 ml D₅W. *Bronchodilation* — **Adults:** 10 to 15 mg hydrochloride SL tid or qid. Max daily SL 60 mg. **Children:** 5 to 10 mg hydrochloride SL tid. Max daily SL 30 mg. *Bronchospasm during acute asthma attacks* — **Adults and children:** 1 inhalation of sulfate form initially; repeat if needed after 2 to 5 min, with max 6 inhalations daily. *Bronchospasm in COPD* — **Adults and children:** (hydrochloride) by hand-held nebulizer; 5 to 15 deep inhalations of 0.5% sol. In adults requiring stronger sol, 3 to 7 deep inhalations of 1% sol no more frequently than q 3 to 4 hr. *Heart block and ventricular arrhythmias* — **Adults:** (hydrochloride) 0.02 to 0.06 mg IV. Subsequent dos-	▪ Use cautiously in elderly patients and in renal or CV disease, coronary insufficiency, diabetes, hyperthyroidism, or history of sensitivity to sympathomimetic amines. ▪ Contraindicated in tachycardia caused by digitalis intoxication, preexisting arrhythmias (other than those that may respond to isoproterenol), and angina pectoris.

(continued)

ISOPROTERENOL 133

DRUG/CLASS/ CATEGORY	DOSAGE FORMS	INDICATIONS/ DOSAGES	KEY PRECAUTIONS
isoproterenol *(continued)*	*oral sol:* 45% (100 g/225 ml) in 220-ml containers	es 0.01 to 0.2 mg IV or 5 mcg/min IV titrated to response; or 0.2 mg IM, then 0.02 to 1 mg IM prn. **Children:** (hydrochloride): IV infusion of 2.5 mcg/min to 0.1 mcg/kg/min. Dosage based on response.	■ Use cautiously in diseases associated with sodium retention, such as heart failure. ■ Contraindicated in anuria caused by severe renal disease, severe dehydration, acute pulmonary edema, severe cardiac decompensation, and hemorrhagic glaucoma.
isosorbide Ismotic *Osmotic diuretic* *Antiglaucoma agent* Preg. Risk Category: B		*Short-term reduction of IOP caused by glaucoma* — **Adults:** initially, 1.5 g/kg PO. Usual dosage range 1 to 3 g/kg bid to qid.	■ Use cautiously in blood volume depletion (such as from diuretic therapy) or mild hypotension. ■ Contraindicated in hypersensitivity or idiosyncrasy to nitrates, severe hypotension, shock, or acute MI with low left ventricular filling pressure.
isosorbide dinitrate Apo-ISDN†, Dilatrate-SR, Isonate, Isorbid, Isordil, Isordil Tembids, Isotrate, Sorbitrate **isosorbide mononitrate** Imdur, ISMO, Monoket *Nitrate* *Antianginal agent/vasodilator* Preg. Risk Category: C	*tab:* 5, 10, 20, 30, 40 mg; *tab (chew):* 5, 10 mg; *tab (SL):* 2.5, 5, 10 mg; *tab (sust-release):* 40 mg; *cap:* 40 mg; *cap (sust-release):* 40 mg. **mononitrate — tab:** 10, 20 mg; *tab (ext-release):* 30, 60, 120 mg	*Acute anginal attacks (SL and chew tab of isosorbide dinitrate only), prophylaxis in situations likely to cause anginal attacks* — **Adults:** *SL form* — 2.5 to 5 mg under tongue, repeated q 5 to 10 min (max 3 doses for each 30-min period). For prophylaxis, 2.5 to 10 mg q 2 to 3 hr. *Chewable form* — 5 to 10 mg prn for acute attack or q 2 to 3 hr for prophylaxis, but only after initial test dose of 5 mg. *Oral form (dinitrate)* — 5 to 30 mg PO tid or qid for prophylaxis (use smallest effective dose); 20 to 40 mg PO (SR form) q 6 to 12 hr. *Oral form (mononitrate, using Imdur)* — 30 to 60 mg PO qd on arising; increased to 120 mg qd after several days, prn. *Oral form (mononitrate, using ISMO or Monoket)* — 20 mg PO bid with 2 doses given 7 hr apart.	

isotretinoin
Accutane, Roaccutane‡
Retinoic acid derivative
Antiacne agent/keratinization stabilizer
Preg. Risk Category: X

cap: 10, 20, 40 mg

Severe recalcitrant nodular acne unresponsive to conventional therapy — **Adults and adolescents:** 0.5 to 2 mg/kg PO daily in 2 divided doses for 15 to 20 wk.

- Contraindicated in women of childbearing age unless serum pregnancy test within 2 wk before starting therapy is negative; begin therapy on 2nd or 3rd day of next menstrual period; must comply with stringent contraceptive measures for 1 mo before therapy, during therapy, and for ≥ 1 mo after. *Severe fetal abnormalities may occur if used during pregnancy.* Also contraindicated in hypersensitivity to parabens.

isoxsuprine hydrochloride
Duvadilan‡, Vasodilan
Adrenergic stimulator
Vasodilator
Preg. Risk Category: NR

tab: 10, 20 mg

Adjunct for relief of symptoms associated with cerebrovascular insufficiency, peripheral vascular diseases (such as arteriosclerosis obliterans, thromboangiitis obliterans, Raynaud's disease) — **Adults:** 10 to 20 mg PO tid or qid.

- Use cautiously in CV or cerebrovascular disease.
- Contraindicated in immediate postpartum period and in arterial bleeding.
- Safety during pregnancy and breast-feeding not established.

isradipine
DynaCirc
Calcium channel blocker
Antihypertensive
Preg. Risk Category: C

cap: 2.5, 5 mg

Hypertension — **Adults:** initially, 2.5 mg PO bid, alone or with thiazide diuretic. If response inadequate after first 2 to 4 wk, make dosage adjustments of 5 mg daily at 2- to 4-wk intervals to max 20 mg daily.

- Use cautiously in heart failure, especially if combined with beta blocker.
- Contraindicated in hypersensitivity to drug.

itraconazole
Sporanox
Synthetic triazole
Antifungal
Preg. Risk Category: C

cap: 100 mg

Pulmonary and extrapulmonary blastomycosis; nonmeningeal histoplasmosis — **Adults:** 200 mg PO daily. Increase dosage as needed and tolerated in 100-mg increments to max 400 mg daily. Give dosages > 200 mg daily in 2 divided doses.
Aspergillosis — **Adults:** 200 to 400 mg PO daily.

- Use cautiously in hypochlorhydria or HIV infection and in patients receiving other highly protein-bound medications.
- Contraindicated in hypersensitivity to drug, in patients receiving astemizole or cisapride, and in breast-feeding patients.

k

DRUG/CLASS/CATEGORY	DOSAGE FORMS	INDICATIONS/DOSAGES	KEY PRECAUTIONS
kaolin and pectin mixtures Kaolin with Pectin, Kao-Spen, Kaodene Non-Narcotic, Kapectolin, K-C *Adsorbent* *Antidiarrheal* Preg. Risk Category: C	**oral susp:** 5.2 mg kaolin and 260 mg pectin/30 ml (Kao-Spen); 90 g kaolin, 2 g pectin/30 ml (Kaolin with Pectin, Kapectolin)	*Mild, nonspecific diarrhea* — **Adults and children ≥ 12 yr:** 60 to 120 ml PO after each bowel movement. **Children 3 to 6 yr:** 15 to 30 ml PO after each bowel movement. **Children 6 to 12 yr:** 30 to 60 ml PO after each bowel movement.	▪ No known contraindications.
ketoconazole Nizoral *Imidazole derivative* *Antifungal* Preg. Risk Category: C	**tab:** 200 mg; **cream:** 2%; **shampoo:** 2%	*Fungal infections caused by susceptible organisms* — **Adults:** 200 mg PO qd in single dose. Max 400 mg qd. **Children ≥ 2 yr:** 3.3 to 6.6 mg/kg PO qd as single dose. *Topical treatment of tinea infestations* — **Adults and children:** Apply qd or bid for about 2 wk; for tinea pedis, apply for 4 wk.	▪ Use cautiously in hepatic disease and in patients taking other hepatotoxic drugs. ▪ Contraindicated in hypersensitivity to drug and in patients taking astemizole or cisapride.
ketoprofen Actron, Orudis *Nonsteroidal anti-inflammatory* *Nonnarcotic analgesic/antipyretic/ anti-inflammatory* Preg. Risk Category: B	**tab:** 12.5 mg; **cap (ext-release):** 100, 150, 200 mg; **cap:** 25, 50, 75 mg; **supp:** 100 mg	*Rheumatoid arthritis and osteoarthritis* — **Adults:** 75 mg tid or 50 mg qid or 200 mg as ext-release qd. Max 300 mg/day. *Mild to moderate pain; dysmenorrhea* — **Adults:** 25 to 50 mg PO q 6 to 8 hr, prn. *Minor aches and pain or fever* — **Adults:** 12.5 mg PO q 4 to 6 hr. Don't exceed 75 mg in 24 hr.	▪ Use cautiously in history of peptic ulcer disease, impaired renal or hepatic function, hypertension, heart failure, or fluid retention. ▪ Contraindicated in hypersensitivity to drug and in history of aspirin- or NSAID-induced asthma, urticaria, or other allergic-type reactions. ▪ Avoid during last trimester of pregnancy and in pediatric patients.

ketorolac tromethamine
Toradol
Nonsteroidal anti-inflammatory
Analgesic
Preg. Risk Category: C

tab: 10 mg;
inj: 15, 30 mg

Short-term management of pain — **Adults < 65 yr:** 60 mg IM or 30 mg IV as single dose, or multiple doses of 30 mg IM or IV q 6 hr; max 120 mg daily. **Adults ≥ 65 yr, renally impaired patients, or patients < 50 kg:** 30 mg IM or 15 mg IV as single dose, or multiple doses of 15 mg IM or IV q 6 hr; max 60 mg daily.
Short-term management of moderately severe, acute pain when switching from parenteral to oral therapy — **Adults < 65 yr:** 20 mg PO as a single dose, then 10 mg PO q 4 to 6 hr, not to exceed 40 mg/day. **Adults ≥ 65 yr, renally impaired patients, or patients < 50 kg:** 10 mg PO as single dose followed by 10 mg PO q 4 to 6 hr, not to exceed 40 mg/day.

- Use cautiously in hepatic or renal impairment.
- Contraindicated in hypersensitivity to drug, active peptic ulcer disease, recent GI bleeding or perforation, advanced renal impairment, risk for renal impairment due to volume depletion, suspected or confirmed cerebrovascular bleeding, hemorrhagic diathesis, incomplete hemostasis, high risk of bleeding, history of peptic ulcer disease, GI bleeding, or allergic reactions to aspirin or other NSAIDs and during labor and delivery or breast-feeding. Contraindicated as prophylactic analgesic before major surgery or intraop when hemostasis is critical and in patients currently receiving aspirin, NSAIDs, or probenecid or requiring epidural or intrathecal analgesic administration.
- Not recommended in pediatric patients.

ketorolac tromethamine
Acular
Nonsteroidal anti-inflammatory
Ophthalmic anti-inflammatory
Preg. Risk Category: C

ophth sol:
0.5%

Relief of ocular itching caused by seasonal allergic conjunctivitis — **Adults:** 1 drop instilled into conjunctival sac of each eye qid.

- Use cautiously in hypersensitivity to other NSAIDs or aspirin and in bleeding disorders.
- Contraindicated in hypersensitivity to any component of formulation and in wearers of soft contact lenses.

█

labetalol hydrochloride
Normodyne, Presolol‡, Trandate
Alpha- and beta-adrenergic blocker
Antihypertensive

tab: 100, 200, 300 mg; **inj:** 5 mg/ml

Hypertension — **Adults:** 100 mg PO bid with or without diuretic. May increase by 100 mg bid q 2 or 4 days until optimum response reached. Usual maint 200 to 400 mg bid; max 2,400 mg daily.

- Use cautiously in heart failure, hepatic failure, chronic bronchitis, emphysema, preexisting peripheral vascular disease, and pheochromocytoma.

(continued)

LABETALOL HYDROCHLORIDE   137

DRUG / CLASS / CATEGORY	DOSAGE FORMS	INDICATIONS / DOSAGES	KEY PRECAUTIONS
labetalol hydrochloride *(continued)* Preg. Risk Category: C		*Hypertensive emergencies* — **Adults:** infuse 2 mg/min and titrate; usual cumulative dose 50 to 200 mg. Or, by repeated IV injection: initially, 20 mg IV slowly over 2 min. Then repeat injections of 40 to 80 mg q 10 min to max 300 mg.	▪ Contraindicated in bronchial asthma, overt cardiac failure, > first-degree heart block, cardiogenic shock, severe bradycardia, other conditions associated with severe and prolonged hypotension, and hypersensitivity to drug.
lactulose Chronulac, Constulose, Enulose, Lactulax†, Lactulose, Portalac *Disaccharide Laxative* Preg. Risk Category: B	***syrup:*** 10 g/15 ml; ***rect sol:*** 3.33 g/5 ml	*Constipation* — **Adults:** 10 to 20 g (15 to 30 ml) PO daily, increased to 60 ml/day, if needed. *Hepatic encephalopathy* — **Adults:** 20 to 30 g PO tid or qid, until 2 or 3 soft stools qd. Or, 300 ml diluted with 700 ml water or saline solution PR and retained for 40 to 60 min q 4 to 6 hr, prn.	▪ Use cautiously in diabetes mellitus. ▪ Contraindicated in low-galactose diet.
lamivudine Epivir *Synthetic nucleoside analogue Antiviral* Preg. Risk Category: C	***tab:*** 150 mg; ***oral sol:*** 10 mg/ml	*Treatment of HIV infection concomitantly with zidovudine* — **Adults ≥ 50 kg and children ≥ 12 yr:** 150 mg PO bid. **Adults < 50 kg:** 2 mg/kg PO bid. **Children 3 mo to 12 yr:** 4 mg/kg PO bid. Max 150 mg bid.	▪ Use cautiously in renal impairment; reduce dosage. Use with extreme caution, if at all, in pediatric patients with history of pancreatitis or other significant risk factors for pancreatitis. ▪ Must give concomitantly with zidovudine. Not currently indicated for use alone. ▪ Contraindicated in hypersensitivity to drug. ▪ Breast-feeding should be discontinued.
lamotrigine Lamictal Phenyltriazine *Anticonvulsant* Preg. Risk Category: C	***tab:*** 25, 100, 150, 200 mg	*Adjunct therapy in treatment of partial seizures caused by epilepsy* — **Adults:** 50 mg PO qd for 2 wk, then 100 mg qd in 2 divided doses for 2 wk. Usual maint dosage 300 to 500 mg PO qd in 2 divided doses. For patients also taking valproic acid, 25 mg PO qod for 2 wk, then 25 mg PO qd for 2 wk. Max 150 mg PO qd in 2 divided doses.	▪ Use cautiously in renal, hepatic, or cardiac impairment. ▪ Contraindicated in hypersensitivity to drug.

lansoprazole
Prevacid
Acid (proton) pump inhibitor
Antiulcer agent
Preg. Risk Category: B

cap (del-re-lease): 15, 30 mg

Short-term treatment of active duodenal ulcer —
Adults: 15 mg PO daily before meals for 4 wk.
Short-term treatment of erosive esophagitis —
Adults: 30 mg PO daily before meals for up to 8 wk. If healing doesn't occur, may give for 8 more wk.
Long-term treatment of pathologic hypersecretory conditions, including Zollinger-Ellison syndrome —
Adults: initially, 60 mg PO qd. Increase dosage prn. Give daily dosages of > 120 mg in divided doses.

- Dosage adjustment may be necessary in severe liver disease. No dosage adjustment needed in renal insufficiency or elderly patients.
- Contraindicated in hypersensitivity to drug.
- Unknown if lansoprazole excreted in breast milk.

---

latanoprost
Xalatan
Prostaglandin analogue
Antiglaucoma/ocular antihypertensive
Preg. Risk Category: C

ophth sol: 0.005% (50 mcg/ml)

Treatment of increased IOP in patients with ocular hypertension or open-angle glaucoma who can't tolerate or who respond insufficiently to other IOP-lowering medications — **Adults:** 1 drop in conjunctival sac of affected eye qd in evening.

- Use cautiously in impaired renal or hepatic function.
- Contraindicated in hypersensitivity to latanoprost, benzalkonium chloride, or other ingredients in product.

---

leucovorin calcium (citrovorum factor, folinic acid)
Wellcovorin
Formyl derivative (active reduced form of folic acid)
Vitamin/antidote
Preg. Risk Category: C

tab: 5, 10, 15, 25 mg; *inj*: 1-ml ampule (3 mg/ml with 0.9% benzyl alcohol); *powder for inj*: 50-, 100-, 350-mg vial

Overdose of folic acid antagonist — **Adults and children:** IM or IV dose equiv to weight of antagonist given.
Leucovorin rescue after high methotrexate dose —
Adults and children: 10 mg/m² PO, IM, or IV q 6 hr until methotrexate levels < 5 × 10^{-8} M.
Megaloblastic anemia caused by congenital enzyme deficiency — **Adults and children:** 3 to 6 mg IM qd.
Folate-deficient megaloblastic anemia — **Adults and children:** up to 1 mg IM qd.

- Contraindicated in pernicious anemia and other megaloblastic anemias secondary to lack of vitamin B_{12}.

---

leuprolide acetate
Lucrin†, Lupron, Lupron Depot, Lupron Depot-Ped, Lupron Depot-3 Month
Gonadotropic-releasing hormone

inj: 1 mg/0.2 ml (5 mg/ml) in 2.8-ml multidose vials; *depot inj*: 3.75, 7.5, 11.5, 15, 22.5 mg

Advanced prostate cancer — **Adults:** 1 mg SC daily. Alternatively, 7.5 mg IM (depot inj) monthly or 22.5 mg IM q 3 mo (depot inj).
Endometriosis — **Adults:** 3.75 mg IM (depot inj only) as single inj q mo for up to 6 mo.
Central precocious puberty — **Children:** initially, 0.3 mg/kg (min 7.5 mg) IM (depot inj only) as single inj q

- Use cautiously in hypersensitivity to benzyl alcohol.
- Contraindicated in hypersensitivity to drug or other GnRH analogues, during pregnancy or breast-feeding, and in undiagnosed vaginal bleeding.

(continued)

LEUPROLIDE ACETATE 139

†Canadian ‡Australian

DRUG/CLASS/ CATEGORY	DOSAGE FORMS	INDICATIONS/ DOSAGES	KEY PRECAUTIONS
leuprolide acetate *(continued)* *Antineoplastic/luteinizing hormone-releasing hormone (LHRH) analogue* Preg. Risk Category: X		4 wk. May increase dosage in increments of 3.75 mg q 4 wk, if needed. Discontinue before female reaches 11 yr or before male reaches 12 yr.	• Contraindicated in hypersensitivity to drug.
levamisole hydrochloride Ergamisol *Immunomodulator* *Antineoplastic* Preg. Risk Category: C	**tab:** 50 mg (base)	*Adjuvant treatment of Dukes' stage C colon cancer (with fluorouracil) after surgical resection —* **Adults:** 50 mg PO q 8 hr for 3 days, starting ≥ 7 days and ≤ 30 days after surgery, if patient out of hospital, ambulating, and maintaining normal oral nutrition; has well-healed wounds; and has recovered from postop complications. Fluorouracil (450 mg/m²/day IV) given for 5 days with 3-day course of levamisole starting 21 to 34 days after surgery. Maint dosage 50 mg PO q 8 hr for 3 days q 2 wk for 1 yr. Given in conjunction with fluorouracil maintenance therapy (450 mg/m²/day by rapid IV push q wk, starting 28 days after initial 5-day course) for 1 yr.	
levobunolol hydrochloride Betagan *Beta-adrenergic blocker* *Antiglaucoma* Preg. Risk Category: C	**ophth sol:** 0.25%, 0.5%	*Chronic open-angle glaucoma and ocular hypertension —* **Adults:** 1 to 2 drop qd (0.5%) or bid (0.25%).	• Use cautiously in chronic bronchitis and emphysema, diabetes mellitus, hyperthyroidism, and myasthenia gravis. • Contraindicated in hypersensitivity to drug, bronchial asthma, history of bronchial asthma or severe COPD, sinus bradycardia, 2nd- or 3rd-degree AV block, cardiac failure, and cardiogenic shock.

levocarnitine (L-carnitine)
Carnitor, VitaCarn
Amino acid derivative
Nutritional supplement
Preg. Risk Category: B

tab: 330 mg; **cap:** 250 mg; **oral liq:** 100 mg/ml; **inj:** 1 g/5 ml

Primary and secondary systemic carnitine deficiency — **Adults:** 990 mg PO bid or tid. Alternatively, 10 to 30 ml (1 to 3 g) of oral liq daily. **Children:** 50 to 100 mg/kg/day PO in divided doses. All dosages depend on clinical response. Higher dosages may be given. However, for children, max 3 g/day.
Acute and chronic treatment of secondary carnitine deficiency — **Adults:** 50 mg/kg IV slowly over 2 to 3 min q 3 to 4 hr.

- No known contraindications.

levodopa
Dopar, Larodopa
Dopamine precursor
Antiparkinsonism agent
Preg. Risk Category: C

tab: 100, 250, 500 mg; **cap:** 100, 250, 500 mg

Parkinsonism — **Adults:** initially, 0.5 to 1 g PO daily, bid, tid, or qid with food; increase by no more than 0.75 g daily q 3 to 7 days as tolerated; usual optimal dose 3 to 6 g daily divided into 3 doses. Don't exceed 8 g/day. Significant therapeutic response may not occur for 6 mo. Higher dosage requires close supervision.

- Use cautiously in severe CV, renal, liver, and pulmonary disorders; peptic ulcer; psychiatric illness; MI with residual arrhythmias; bronchial asthma; emphysema; and endocrine disease.
- Contraindicated within 14 days of MAO inhibitor use and in hypersensitivity to drug, acute angle-closure glaucoma, melanoma, and undiagnosed skin lesions.

levofloxacin
Levaquin
Fluoroquinolone antibiotic
Antibiotic
Preg. Risk Category: C

tab: 250, 500 mg; **single-use vials:** 500 mg; **infusion (premixed):** 250 mg in 50 ml D₅W, 500 mg in 100 ml D₅W

Acute maxillary sinusitis caused by susceptible organisms — **Adults:** 500 mg PO or IV qd for 10 to 14 days.
Acute exacerbation of chronic bronchitis caused by susceptible organisms — **Adults:** 500 mg PO or IV qd for 7 days.
Community-acquired pneumonia caused by susceptible organisms — **Adults:** 500 mg PO or IV qd for 7 to 14 days.
Mild to moderate skin and skin structure infections caused by susceptible organisms — **Adults:** 500 mg PO or IV qd for 7 to 10 days.
UTI caused by susceptible organisms — **Adults:** 250 mg PO or IV qd for 10 days.
Acute pyelonephritis caused by E. coli — **Adults:** 250 mg PO or IV qd for 10 days.

- Use cautiously in history of seizure disorders or other CNS diseases such as cerebral arteriosclerosis.
- Contraindicated in hypersensitivity to drug, drug components, or other fluoroquinolones.
- Safety and efficacy in children < 18 yr and in pregnant and breast-feeding women not established.

DRUG / CLASS / CATEGORY	DOSAGE FORMS	INDICATIONS / DOSAGES	KEY PRECAUTIONS
levomethadyl acetate hydrochloride ORLAAM *Synthetic diphenylheptane derivative* *Opiate agonist* Preg. Risk Category: C Controlled Sub. Sched.: II	*oral sol:* 10 mg/ml	*Opiate addiction* — **Adults:** dosage highly individualized. Initially, 20 to 40 mg 48 to 72 hr. Subsequent doses increased in increments of 5 to 10 mg at 48- to 72-hr intervals until steady state reached, usually within 1 to 2 wk. Most patients stable on 60 to 90 mg 3 times/wk.	■ Use cautiously in cardiac conduction defects or in hepatic or renal failure. ■ Contraindicated in hypersensitivity to drug.
levonorgestrel Norplant System *Progestin* *Contraceptive* Preg. Risk Category: X	*implants:* 36 mg/cap (each kit contains 6 caps)	*Prevention of pregnancy* — **Women:** 6 caps implanted subdermally in midportion of upper arm, about 8 cm above elbow crease, during first 7 days of onset of menses. Caps placed in fanlike position, 15 degrees (total of 75 degrees). Contraceptive efficacy lasts for 5 yr.	■ Use cautiously in history of depression, diabetes, prediabetes, and in hyperlipidemia. ■ Contraindicated in active thrombophlebitis, thromboembolic disorders, undiagnosed abnormal genital bleeding, acute liver disease, malignant or benign liver tumors, known or suspected breast cancer, and known or suspected pregnancy.
levothyroxine sodium (T₄ or L-thyroxine sodium) Eltroxint, Levo-T, Levothroid, Levoxine, Levoxyl, Synthroid *Thyroid hormone* *Thyroid hormone replacement* Preg. Risk Category: A	*tab:* 25, 50, 75, 88, 100, 112, 125, 137, 150, 175, 200, 300 mcg; *inj:* 200-500-mcg vial	*Myxedema coma* — **Adults:** 200 to 500 mcg IV; if no response in 24 hr, give 100 to 300 mcg IV. Maint 50 to 200 mcg IV qd. *Thyroid hormone replacement* — **Adults ≤ 65 yr:** initially, 25 to 50 mcg PO qd, increased by 25 mcg PO q 2 to 4 wk. May give IV or IM with dose adjustment. **Adults > 65 yr:** 12.5 to 50 mcg PO qd. Increase by 12.5 to 25 mcg at 3- to 8-wk intervals prn. **Children > 12 yr:** over 150 mcg or 2 to 3 mcg/kg/day. **Children 6 to 12 yr:** 100 to 150 mcg or 4 to 5 mcg/kg/day. **Children 1 to 5 yr:** 75 to 100 mcg or 5 to 6 mcg/kg/day. **Children 6 to 12 mo:** 50 to 75 mcg or 6 to 8 mcg/kg/day. **Children < 6 mo:** 25 to 50 mcg or 8 to 10 mcg/kg/day.	■ Use cautiously in elderly patients and in angina pectoris, hypertension, other CV disorders, renal insufficiency, ischemia, diabetes mellitus or insipidus, and myxedema. ■ Contraindicated in hypersensitivity to drug, acute MI uncomplicated by hypothyroidism, untreated thyrotoxicosis, and uncorrected adrenal insufficiency.

lidocaine hydrochloride (lignocaine hydrochloride)

LidoPen Auto-Injector, Xylocaine

Amide derivative
Ventricular antiarrhythmic
Preg. Risk Category: B

inj: 5, 10, 15, 20, 40, 100, 200 mg/ml; **infusion (premixed):** D₅W as 2, 4, 8 mg/ml

Ventricular arrhythmias resulting from MI, cardiac manipulation, or cardiac glycosides — **Adults:** 50 to 100 mg (1 to 1.5 mg/kg) by IV bolus at 25 to 50 mg/min. Give half this amount to elderly patients or patients < 50 kg and to those with heart failure or hepatic disease. Repeat bolus dose q 3 to 5 min until arrhythmias subside or adverse reactions develop. Don't exceed 300-mg total bolus over 1-hr period. Simultaneously, begin constant infusion of 20 to 50 mcg/kg/min (1 to 4 mg/min). **Children:** 0.5 to 1 mg/kg by IV bolus, followed by infusion of 10 to 50 mcg/kg/min.

- Use cautiously in complete or second-degree heart block, sinus bradycardia, elderly patients, heart failure, renal or hepatic disease, and patients < 50 kg. Reduce dosage in these patients.
- Contraindicated in hypersensitivity to amide-type local anesthetics, Adams-Stokes syndrome, Wolff-Parkinson-White syndrome, and severe degrees of SA, AV, or intraventricular block in absence of artificial pacemaker.

lindane

gBH†, G-Well, Kwell, Kwellada†, Scabene

Chlorinated hydrocarbon insecticide
Scabicide/pediculicide
Preg. Risk Category: B

cream: 1%; **lotion:** 1%; **shampoo:** 1%

Parasitic infestation (scabies, pediculosis) — **Adults and children:** CDC recommends avoiding bathing before skin application. If patient bathes, let skin dry and cool thoroughly before using. Apply thin layer of cream or lotion over entire skin surface (with special attention to folds, creases, interdigital spaces, and genital area) for scabies, or to hairy areas for pediculosis. After 8 to 12 hr, wash off drug. Repeat in 1 wk if mites appear or new lesions develop. Apply shampoo undiluted to affected area and work into lather for 4 to 5 min; small amount of water may enhance lathering. Apply 30 ml shampoo for short hair, 45 ml for medium-length hair, or 60 ml for long hair. Rinse thoroughly and rub dry with towel.

- Use cautiously in infants and young children; greater risk for CNS toxicity.
- Contraindicated in hypersensitivity to drug, if skin raw or inflamed, or in seizure disorders. Lotion is contraindicated in premature infants.

liothyronine sodium (T₃)

Cyronine, Cytomel, Tertroxin‡, Triostat

Thyroid hormone
Thyroid hormone replacement
Preg. Risk Category: A

tab: 5, 25, 50 mcg; **inj:** 10 mcg/ml

Cretinism — **Children:** 5 mcg PO daily with 5-mcg increases q 3 to 4 days prn.
Myxedema — **Adults:** initially, 5 mcg PO daily, increased by 5 to 10 mcg daily q 1 or 2 wk. Maintenance dose 50 to 100 mcg daily.
Myxedema coma, premyxedema coma — **Adults:** initially, 10 to 20 mcg IV for known or suspected CV

- Use with extreme caution in elderly patients and in angina pectoris, hypertension, other CV disorders, renal insufficiency, ischemia, diabetes mellitus or insipidus, and myxedema.

(continued)

LIOTHYRONINE SODIUM 143

†Canadian ‡Australian

DRUG/CLASS/CATEGORY	DOSAGE FORMS	INDICATIONS/DOSAGES	KEY PRECAUTIONS
liothyronine sodium *(continued)*		disease; 25 to 50 mcg IV for patients without known CV disease. *Nontoxic goiter* — **Adults:** initially, 5 mcg PO daily; increase by 12.5 to 25 mcg daily q 1 to 2 wk. Maintenance dose 75 mcg qd. *Thyroid hormone replacement* — **Adults:** initially, 25 mcg PO daily, increased by 12.5 to 25 mcg q 1 to 2 wk prn. Maintenance dose 25 to 75 mcg qd. **Elderly patients:** 5 mcg daily, increased in 5-mcg daily increments.	• Contraindicated in hypersensitivity to drug, acute MI uncomplicated by hypothyroidism, untreated thyrotoxicosis, or uncorrected adrenal insufficiency.
lisinopril Prinivil, Zestril *ACE inhibitor* *Antihypertensive* Preg. Risk Category: C (D in 2nd and 3rd trimesters)	*tab:* 2.5, 5, 10, 20, 40 mg	*Hypertension* — **Adults:** initially, 10 mg PO daily. Most patients well controlled on 20 to 40 mg daily as single dose. *Treatment adjunct in heart failure (with diuretics and cardiac glycosides)* — **Adults:** initially, 5 mg PO daily. Most patients well controlled on 5 to 20 mg daily as single dose. *Acute MI* — **Adults:** initially 5 mg PO, followed by 5 mg in 24 hr, 10 mg in 48 hr, and then 10 mg daily for 6 wk. In patients with low systolic BP (≤ 120) when treatment starts or during first 3 days after MI, reduce to 2.5 mg PO. If systolic BP ≤ 100, may reduce daily maintenance dose of 5 mg to 2.5 mg.	• Use cautiously in impaired renal function and in patients at risk for hyperkalemia. • Contraindicated in hypersensitivity to ACE inhibitors, and history of angioedema related to previous ACE inhibitor therapy.
lithium carbonate Carbolith‡, Eskalith CR, Lithane, Lithicarb‡, Lithobid, Lithonate, Lithotabs	carbonate — *tab:* 300 mg; *tab (contr-release):* 300, 450 mg; *cap:* 150, 300, 600	*Prevention or control of mania* — **Adults:** 300 to 600 mg PO up to qid or 900 mg PO q 12 hr of contr-release; increase on basis of blood levels to achieve optimal dosage.	• Use with extreme caution in patients receiving neuroleptics, neuromuscular blockers, and diuretics; elderly or debilitated patients; thyroid disease; seizure disorder; renal or CV disease; severe debilitation; and dehydration and sodium depletion.

lithium citrate
Cibalith-S
Alkali metal
Antimanic/antipsychotic
Preg. Risk Category: D

mg. citrate — *syrup (sugarless):* 300 mg/5 ml (with 0.3% alcohol)

- Contraindicated if therapy can't be closely monitored.
- Shouldn't be used during pregnancy.

iodoxamide tromethamine
Alomide
Cromolyn-like mast cell stabilizer
Antiallergic ophthalmic
Preg. Risk Category: B

ophth sol: 0.1%

Vernal conjunctivitis, vernal keratoconjunctivitis, vernal keratitis — **Adults and children ≥ 2 yr:** 1 to 2 drops in affected eye qid for up to 3 mo.

- Contraindicated in hypersensitivity to drug or components.

lomefloxacin hydrochloride
Maxaquin
Fluoroquinolone
Broad-spectrum antibiotic
Preg. Risk Category: C

tab (film-coated): 400 mg

Acute bacterial exacerbations of chronic bronchitis caused by susceptible organisms — **Adults:** 400 mg PO daily for 10 days.
Uncomplicated UTI (cystitis) caused by susceptible organisms — **Adults:** 400 mg PO daily for 10 days.
Complicated UTI caused by susceptible organisms — **Adults:** 400 mg PO daily for 14 days.
Prophylaxis of UTI after transrectal prostate biopsy — **Adults:** 400 mg PO as single dose 1 to 6 hr before procedure.

- Use cautiously in known or suspected CNS disorders, such as seizure disorder or cerebral arteriosclerosis, that may predispose to seizures.
- Safety in children < 18 yr not established.
- Contraindicated in hypersensitivity to lomefloxacin or other fluoroquinolones.

lomustine (CCNU)
CeeNU
Alkylating agent/nitrosourea (cell cycle-phase nonspecific)
Antineoplastic
Preg. Risk Category: D

cap: 10, 40, 100 mg; *dose pack:* two 10-, two 40-, two 100-mg cap

Brain tumor, Hodgkin's disease — **Adults and children:** 100 to 130 mg/m² PO as single dose q 6 wk. Reduce dosage according to degree of bone marrow suppression. Don't give repeat doses until WBC count > 4,000/mm³ and platelet count > 100,000/mm³.

- Use cautiously in decreased platelet, WBC, or RBC counts and in patients receiving other myelosuppressants.
- Contraindicated in hypersensitivity to drug.

loperamide
Imodium, Kaopectate II Caplets‡
Piperadine derivative

cap: 2 mg; *tab:* 2 mg; *oral liq:* 1 mg/5 ml

Acute, nonspecific diarrhea — **Adults and children > 12 yr:** initially, 4 mg PO, then 2 mg after each unformed stool. Max 16 mg daily. **Children 9 to 11 yr:** 2

- Use cautiously in hepatic disease.
- Contraindicated in hypersensitivity, when constipation must be avoided, and in

(continued)

†Canadian   ‡Australian

DRUG / CLASS / CATEGORY	DOSAGE FORMS	INDICATIONS / DOSAGES	KEY PRECAUTIONS
loperamide *(continued)* *Antidiarrheal* Preg. Risk Category: B		mg tid on first day. **Children 6 to 8 yr:** 2 mg bid on first day. **Children 2 to 5 yr:** 1 mg tid on first day. Maintenance dose ⅓ to ½ of initial dose.	children < 2 yr. OTC use contraindicated in fever > 101° F (38.3° C) or if blood in stool.
loracarbef Lorabid *Synthetic beta-lactam antibiotic of carbacephem class* *Antibiotic* Preg. Risk Category: B	**pulvules:** 200 mg; **powder for oral susp:** 100, 200 mg/5 ml	*Secondary bacterial infections of acute bronchitis —* **Adults:** 200 to 400 mg PO q 12 hr for 7 days. *Acute bacterial exacerbations of chronic bronchitis —* **Adults:** 400 mg PO q 12 hr for 7 days. *Pneumonia —* **Adults:** 400 mg PO q 12 hr for 14 days. *Pharyngitis, sinusitis, or tonsillitis —* **Adults:** 200 mg PO q 12 hr for 10 days. **Children:** 15 mg/kg PO daily in divided doses q 12 hr for 10 days. *Acute otitis media —* **Children:** 30 mg/kg (oral susp) PO daily in divided doses q 12 hr for 10 days.	▪ Use cautiously in pregnant or breast-feeding women. ▪ Contraindicated in hypersensitivity to drug or other cephalosporins and in diarrhea caused by pseudomembranous colitis. ▪ Safety and efficacy in infants < 6 mo not established.
loratadine Claratyne‡, Claritin *Tricyclic antihistamine* *Antihistaminic* Preg. Risk Category: B	**tab:** 10 mg	*Symptomatic treatment of seasonal allergic rhinitis —* **Adults and children ≥ 12 yr:** 10 mg PO daily.	▪ Use cautiously in liver impairment and in breast-feeding patients. ▪ Contraindicated in hypersensitivity to drug.
lorazepam Alzapam, Apo-Lorazepam†, Ativan, Lorazepam Intensol, Novo-Lorazem†, Nu-Loraz† *Benzodiazepine* *Antianxiety agent/sedative-hypnotic* Preg. Risk Category: D Controlled Sub. Sched.: IV	**tab:** 0.5, 1, 2 mg; **tab (SL):** 1, 2 mg; **inj:** 2, 4 mg/ml	*Anxiety, agitation, irritability —* **Adults:** 2 to 6 mg PO daily in divided doses. Max 10 mg daily. Or, 0.05 mg/kg up to 4 mg IM daily in divided doses or 0.044 to 0.05 mg/kg up to 4 mg IV daily in divided doses. *Insomnia due to anxiety —* **Adults:** 2 to 4 mg PO hs. *Preop sedation —* **Adults:** 0.05 mg/kg IM 2 hr before procedure. Max 4 mg. Or, 0.044 mg/kg (max total dose 2 mg) IV, 15 to 20 min before surgery. In adults	▪ Use cautiously in pulmonary, renal, or hepatic impairment and in elderly, acutely ill, or debilitated patients. ▪ Contraindicated in acute angle-closure glaucoma; hypersensitivity to drug, other benzodiazepines, or its vehicle (used in parenteral form). Also contraindicated pregnant patients (especially in first trimester).

< 50 yr, may give 0.05 mg/kg (max 4 mg) if increased lack of recall of preop events desired.

losartan potassium
Cozaar
Angiotensin II receptor antagonist
Antihypertensive
Preg. Risk Category: C (D in 2nd and 3rd trimesters)

tab: 25, 50 mg

Hypertension — **Adults:** initially, 25 to 50 mg PO daily. Max 100 mg daily, given qd or bid.

- Use cautiously in impaired renal or hepatic function.
- Contraindicated in hypersensitivity to drug.
- Breast-feeding not recommended.
- Can cause fetal and neonatal morbidity and death when given to pregnant women. These problems not detected when exposure limited to first trimester.

lovastatin (mevinolin)
Mevacor
Lactone
Cholesterol-lowering agent
Preg. Risk Category: X

tab: 10, 20, 40 mg

Reduction of LDL and total cholesterol levels in primary hypercholesterolemia (types IIa and IIb) — **Adults:** initially, 20 mg PO qd with evening meal. For patients with severely elevated cholesterol (for example, > 300 mg/dl), initial dose 40 mg. Recommended daily dosage 20 to 80 mg in single or divided doses.

- Use cautiously in patients who consume substantial amounts of alcohol or in history of liver disease.
- Contraindicated in hypersensitivity to drug, active liver disease or conditions associated with unexplained persistent elevations of serum transaminase levels, pregnant and breast-feeding patients, and women of childbearing age unless no risk of pregnancy.

loxapine hydrochloride
Loxapac†, Loxitane C, Loxitane IM
loxapine succinate
Loxapac†, Loxitane
Dibenzoxazepine
Antipsychotic
Preg. Risk Category: NR

hydrochloride — oral conc: 25 mg/ml; **inj:** 50 mg/ml. **succinate — cap:** 5, 10, 25, 50 mg; **tab:** 5 mg†, 10 mg†, 25 mg†, 50 mg†

Psychotic disorders — **Adults:** 10 mg PO bid to qid, rapidly increasing to 60 to 100 mg PO daily for most patients; dosage varies among individuals. If patient can't take oral dose, 12.5 to 50 mg IM q 4 to 6 hr or longer, both dose and interval depending on patient response. Dosages > 250 mg/day not recommended.

- Use cautiously in seizure disorder, CV disorder, glaucoma, or history of urine retention.
- Contraindicated in hypersensitivity to dibenzoxazepines, coma, severe CNS depression, and drug-induced depressed states.

LOXAPINE SUCCINATE   147

DRUG/CLASS/CATEGORY	DOSAGE FORMS	INDICATIONS/DOSAGES	KEY PRECAUTIONS
magaldrate (aluminum-magnesium complex) Antiflux, Iosopan, Lowsium, Riopan *Aluminum magnesium salt* *Antacid* Preg. Risk Category: C	*tab:* 480 mg; *tab (chew):* 480 mg; *oral susp:* 540 mg/5 ml	*Antacid* — **Adults:** 480 to 960 mg PO (or 5 to 10 ml PO of susp) with water between meals and hs; or 1 to 2 chew tab (chewed before swallowing) between meals and hs.	▪ Use cautiously in mild kidney impairment. ▪ Contraindicated in severe renal disease.
magnesium chloride Slow-Mag **magnesium sulfate** *Mineral/electrolyte* *Antiarrhythmic/anticonvulsant/mineral supplement* Preg. Risk Category: A	**chloride** — *tab (delayed-release):* 64 mg. **sulfate** — *inj sol:* 10, 12.5, 25, 50% in 2-, 5-, 10-, 20-ml, and 30-ml ampules, vials, and pre-filled syringes	*Management of paroxysmal atrial tachycardia* — **Adults:** 3 to 4 g IV over 30 sec. *Management of life-threatening ventricular arrhythmias, such as sustained ventricular tachycardia or torsades de pointes* — **Adults:** 2 to 6 g IV over several min, then IV infusion of 3 to 20 mg/min for 5 to 48 hr. Dosage and duration of therapy based on response and serum magnesium levels. *Prevention or control of seizures in preeclampsia or eclampsia* — **Adults:** 4 g IV in 250 ml D5W and 4 to 5 g deep IM each buttock; then 4 g deep IM alternate buttock q 4 hr, prn. Or, 4 g IV loading dose, then 1 to 2 g hourly as IV infusion. Max 40 g daily. *Seizures* — **Adults:** 1 to 2 g (as 10% sol) IV over 15 min, then 1 g IM q 4 to 6 hr per response and drug levels. *Seizures, hypomagnesemia associated with acute nephritis in children* — **Children:** 0.2 ml/kg of 50% sol IM q 4 to 6 hr, prn, or 100 to 200 mg/kg of 1% to 3% sol IV slowly. Titrate dosage according to blood magnesium levels and seizure response. *Mild hypomagnesemia* — **Adults:** 1 g IV by piggyback or IM q 6 hr for 4 doses, depending on serum	▪ Use cautiously in impaired renal function and during labor. ▪ Parenteral administration contraindicated in heart block or myocardial damage.

magnesium level. Or, 3 g PO q 6 hr for 4 doses.
Severe hypomagnesemia (serum magnesium 0.8 mEq/L or less, with symptoms) — **Adults:** 2 to 5 g IV in 1 L sol over 3 hr. Subsequent doses depend on serum magnesium levels.
Magnesium supplementation — **Adults:** 64 mg (1 tab) PO tid.

magnesium citrate (citrate of magnesia) Citroma, Citro-Mag , Citro-Nesia, Evac-Q-Mag **magnesium hydroxide (milk of magnesia)** Milk of Magnesia, Phillips' Milk of Magnesia **magnesium sulfate (epsom salts)** Magnesium salt *Antacid/antiulcer agent/laxative* Preg. Risk Category: NR	**citrate** — *oral sol:* approx 168 mEq magnesium/240 ml. **hydroxide** — *oral susp:* 7% to 8.5% (approximately 80 mEq magnesium/30 ml). **sulfate** — **granules:** approx 40 mEq magnesium/5 g	*Constipation: to evacuate bowel before surgery* — **Adults and children ≥ 12 yr:** 11 to 25 g citrate PO qd; 2.4 to 4.8 g (30 to 60 ml) hydroxide PO qd; 10 to 30 g sulfate PO qd. **Children 6 to 12 yr:** 5.5 to 12.5 g citrate PO qd; 1.2 to 2.4 g (15 to 30 ml) hydroxide PO qd; 5 to 10 g sulfate PO qd. **Children 2 to 6 yr:** 2.7 to 6.25 g citrate PO qd; 0.4 to 1.2 g (5 to 15 ml) hydroxide PO qd; 2.5 to 5 g sulfate PO qd. *Note:* All doses may be single or divided. *Antacid* — **Adults:** 5 to 15 ml milk of magnesia PO tid or qid.	▪ Use cautiously in rectal bleeding. ▪ Contraindicated in abdominal pain, nausea, vomiting, or other symptoms of appendicitis or acute surgical abdomen and in myocardial damage, heart block, fecal impaction, rectal fissures, intestinal obstruction or perforation, or renal disease. Also contraindicated in patients about to deliver.
magnesium oxide Mag-Ox 400, Maox-420, Uro-Mag *Magnesium salt* *Antacid/laxative* Preg. Risk Category: NR	*tab:* 400, 420 mg; *cap:* 140 mg	*Antacid* — **Adults:** 140 mg PO with water or milk after meals and hs. *Laxative* — **Adults:** 4 g PO with water or milk hs. *Oral replacement therapy in mild hypomagnesemia* — **Adults:** 400 to 840 mg PO daily.	▪ Use cautiously in mild renal impairment. ▪ Contraindicated in severe renal disease.

DRUG / CLASS / CATEGORY	DOSAGE FORMS	INDICATIONS / DOSAGES	KEY PRECAUTIONS
mannitol Osmitrol Osmotic diuretic Diuretic/prevention and management of acute renal failure or oliguria Preg. Risk Category: B	*inj:* 5, 10, 15, 20, 25%	*Test dose for marked oliguria or suspected inadequate renal function* — **Adults and children > 12 yr:** 200 mg/kg or 12.5 g as 25% IV sol over 3 to 5 min. Response adequate if 30 to 50 ml urine/hr excreted over 2 to 3 hr; if response inadequate, give 2nd test dose. If still no response, discontinue. *Oliguria* — **Adults and children > 12 yr:** 50 to 100 g IV as 5% to 25% sol over 1½ to several hr.	■ Use cautiously in pregnant patients and in compromised renal function. ■ Contraindicated in hypersensitivity to drug and in anuria, severe pulmonary congestion, frank pulmonary edema, severe heart failure, severe dehydration, metabolic edema, progressive renal disease or dysfunction, or active intracranial bleeding (except during craniotomy).
maprotiline hydrochloride Ludiomil Tetracyclic antidepressant Antidepressant Preg. Risk Category: B	*tab:* 25, 50, 75 mg	*Depression* — **Adults:** initially, 75 mg PO daily in single or divided doses for mild to moderate depression, increased gradually in increments to 150 mg daily, if needed. Max 225 mg daily. Maintain initial dose for 2 wk before increasing; increase by 25-mg increments.	■ Use with extreme caution in history of MI or CV disease. Use cautiously in suicidal tendencies, increased IOP, or history of urine retention or angle-closure glaucoma. ■ Contraindicated during acute recovery phase of MI and in hypersensitivity to drug, seizure disorders, or within 14 days of MAO inhibitor therapy.
mebendazole Vermox Benzimidazole Anthelmintic Preg. Risk Category: C	*tab (chew):* 100 mg	*Pinworm* — **Adults and children > 2 yr:** 100 mg PO as single dose; repeat if infection persists 2 to 3 wk later. *Roundworm, whipworm, hookworm* — **Adults and children > 2 yr:** 100 mg PO bid for 3 days; repeat if infection persists 3 wk later.	■ Contraindicated in hypersensitivity to drug.

meclizine hydrochloride
Antivert, Bonamine†, D-Vert, Meni-D, Vergon
Piperazine-derivative antihistamine
Antiemetic/antivertigo agent
Preg. Risk Category: B

Vertigo — **Adults:** 25 to 100 mg PO daily in divided doses. Dosage varies with response.
Motion sickness — **Adults:** 25 to 50 mg PO 1 hr before travel, then daily for duration of trip.

tab: 12.5, 25, 50 mg; **tab (chew):** 25 mg; **cap:** 15, 25, 30 mg

- Use cautiously in asthma, glaucoma, or prostatic hyperplasia.
- Contraindicated in hypersensitivity to drug.

---

meclofenamate
Meclomen
Nonsteroidal anti-inflammatory
Nonnarcotic analgesic/antipyretic/anti-inflammatory
Preg. Risk Category: NR

Rheumatoid arthritis and osteoarthritis — **Adults:** 200 to 400 mg/day PO in 3 or 4 equally divided doses.
Mild to moderate pain — **Adults:** 50 to 100 mg PO q 4 to 6 hr. Max 400 mg/day.
Dysmenorrhea — **Adults:** 100 mg PO tid.

cap: 50, 100 mg

- Use cautiously in hepatic or renal disease, CV disease, blood dyscrasia, or history of peptic ulcer disease and in elderly patients.
- Avoid in pregnant patients.
- Contraindicated in hypersensitivity to drug or in history of aspirin- or NSAID-induced bronchospasm, urticaria, or rhinitis.

---

medroxyprogesterone acetate
Amen, Curretab, Cycrin, Depo-Provera, Provera
Progestin
Progestin/antineoplastic
Preg. Risk Category: X

Abnormal uterine bleeding caused by hormonal imbalance — **Adults:** 5 to 10 mg PO daily for 5 to 10 days starting on 16th day of menstrual cycle. If patient also has received estrogen, 10 mg PO daily for 10 days starting on 16th day of cycle.
Secondary amenorrhea — **Adults:** 5 to 10 mg PO daily for 5 to 10 days.
Endometrial or renal cancer — **Adults:** 400 to 1,000 mg IM weekly.
Contraception in women — **Adults:** 150 mg IM q 3 mo; give first injection during first 5 days of menstrual cycle.

tab: 2.5, 5, 10 mg; **inj (susp):** 100, 150, 400 mg/ml

- Use cautiously in diabetes mellitus, seizures, migraine, cardiac or renal disease, asthma, and mental depression.
- Contraindicated in hypersensitivity to drug, active thromboembolic disorders, or history of thromboembolic disorders or of cerebrovascular disease or apoplexy, breast cancer, undiagnosed abnormal vaginal bleeding, missed abortion, or hepatic dysfunction and during pregnancy. Tablets also contraindicated in liver dysfunction or known or suspected malignant disease of genital organs.

---

mefloquine hydrochloride
Lariam
Quinine derivative
Antimalarial
Preg. Risk Category: C

Acute malaria infections caused by mefloquine-sensitive strains of P. falciparum or P. vivax — **Adults:** 1,250 mg PO (5 tab) as single dose.
Malaria prophylaxis — **Adults:** 250 mg PO q wk. Initiate 1 wk before entering endemic area and continue 4 wk after returning.

tab: 250 mg

- Use cautiously in cardiac disease or seizure disorders.
- Contraindicated in hypersensitivity to drug or related compounds.

†Canadian ‡Australian

MEFLOQUINE HYDROCHLORIDE   151

DRUG/CLASS/ CATEGORY	DOSAGE FORMS	INDICATIONS/ DOSAGES	KEY PRECAUTIONS
megestrol acetate Megace, Megostat† *Progestin Antineoplastic* Preg. Risk Category: D	*tab:* 20, 40 mg; *oral susp:* 40 mg/ml	*Breast cancer* — **Adults:** 40 mg qid. *Endometrial cancer* — **Adults:** 40 to 320 mg PO daily in divided doses. *Treatment of unexplained significant weight loss* — **Adults:** 800 mg PO (oral susp) daily.	▪ Use cautiously in history of thrombophlebitis. ▪ Contraindicated in hypersensitivity to drug or as diagnostic test for pregnancy.
melphalan (L-phenylalanine mustard) Alkeran *Alkylating agent (cell cycle-phase nonspecific) Antineoplastic* Preg. Risk Category: D	*tab (scored):* 2 mg; *inj:* 50 mg	*Multiple myeloma* — **Adults:** 6 mg PO qd for 2 to 3 wk; then drug stopped for up to 4 wk, or until WBC and platelet counts stop decreasing and begin to rise again; then maint dosage of 2 mg daily. Or, 16 mg/m^2 by IV infusion over 15 to 20 min at 2-wk intervals for 4 doses. After recovery from toxicity, give at 4-wk intervals. May reduce dose up to 50% in renal insufficiency. *Nonresectable advanced ovarian cancer* — **Adults:** 0.2 mg/kg PO daily for 5 days. Repeat q 4 to 5 wk.	▪ Use cautiously in patients receiving concurrent radiation and chemotherapy. ▪ Not recommended in severe leukopenia, thrombocytopenia, anemia, or chronic lymphocytic leukemia. ▪ Contraindicated in hypersensitivity to drug or when disease known to be drug resistant. Patients hypersensitive to chlorambucil may have cross-sensitivity to melphalan.
menotropins Pergonal *Gonadotropin Ovulation stimulant/spermatogenesis stimulant* Preg. Risk Category: X	*inj:* 75 IU of LH and 75 IU of FSH activity per ampule; 150 IU of LH and 150 IU of FSH activity per ampule	*Production of follicular maturation* — **Women:** 75 IU each of FSH and LH IM qd for 7 to 12 days, then 5,000 to 10,000 USP units human chorionic gonadotropin (HCG) IM 1 day after last dose of menotropins; repeat for 2 more menstrual cycles. May increase to 150 IU each of FSH and LH IM qd for 7 to 12 days, then 5,000 to 10,000 USP units HCG IM 1 day after last dose of menotropins; repeat for 2 menstrual cycles. *Stimulation of spermatogenesis* — **Adults:** 75 IU IM 3 times weekly (with 2,000 USP units HCG twice weekly) for 4 mo. After 4 mo, may continue with 75 IU FSH/LH 3 times weekly or 150 IU FSH/LH 3 times weekly prn.	▪ Contraindicated in hypersensitivity to drug; in women with primary ovarian failure, uncontrolled thyroid or adrenal dysfunction, pituitary tumor, abnormal uterine bleeding, uterine fibromas, or ovarian cysts or enlargement; in pregnant patients; and in men with normal pituitary function, primary testicular failure, or infertility disorders other than hypogonadotropic hypogonadism.

meperidine hydrochloride (pethidine hydrochloride)
Demerol
Opioid
Analgesic/adjunct to anesthesia
Preg. Risk Category: C
Controlled Sub. Sched.: II

tab: 50, 100 mg; **syrup:** 50 mg/5 ml; **inj:** 10, 25, 50, 75, 100 mg/ml

Moderate to severe pain — **Adults:** 50 to 150 mg PO, IM, IV, or SC q 3 to 4 hr. **Children:** 0.5 to 0.8 mg/lb PO, IM, IV, or SC q 3 to 4 hr or 175 mg/m² daily in 6 divided doses. Max single dose 100 mg.
Preoperatively — **Adults:** 50 to 100 mg IM, IV, or SC 30 to 90 min before surgery. **Children:** 0.5 to 1 mg/lb IM, IV, or SC up to adult dose 30 to 90 min before surgery. Don't exceed adult dosage.

- Use with extreme caution in increased ICP, head injury, asthma and other respiratory conditions; in SVTs, seizures, acute abdominal conditions, hepatic or renal disease, hypothyroidism, Addison's disease, urethral stricture, and prostatic hyperplasia; and in elderly or debilitated patients.
- Contraindicated in hypersensitivity to drug and within 14 days of MAO inhibitor use.

mephobarbital
Mebaral
Barbiturate
Anticonvulsant/nonspecific CNS depressant
Preg. Risk Category: D
Controlled Sub. Sched.: IV

tab: 32, 50, 100 mg

Generalized tonic-clonic or absence seizures —
Adults: 400 to 600 mg PO qd or in divided doses. **Children < 5 yr:** 16 to 32 mg PO tid or qid. **Children ≥ 5 yr:** 32 to 64 mg PO tid or qid.
Sedation — **Adults:** 32 to 100 mg PO tid or qid. **Children:** 16 to 32 mg PO tid or qid.

- Use cautiously in acute or chronic pain; depression; suicidal tendencies; history of drug abuse; hepatic, renal, cardiac, or respiratory impairment; myasthenia gravis; myxedema; and elderly or debilitated patients.
- Contraindicated in barbiturate hypersensitivity or porphyria.

meprobamate
Apo-Meprobamate†, Equanil, Meprospan 200, Miltown-200, Miltown-400, Probate
Carbamate
Antianxiety agent
Preg. Risk Category: D
Controlled Sub. Sched.: IV

tab: 200, 400, 600 mg; **cap (sust-re-lease):** 200, 400 mg

Anxiety — **Adults:** 1.2 to 1.6 g PO daily in 3 or 4 equally divided doses. Max 2.4 g daily. Alternatively, 400 to 800 mg sust-release cap PO bid. **Children 6 to 12 yr:** 100 to 200 mg PO bid or tid. Or, 200 mg sust-release cap PO bid. Not recommended for children < 6 yr.

- Use cautiously in impaired hepatic or renal function, seizure disorders, or suicidal tendencies.
- Contraindicated in hypersensitivity to drug or related compounds and in porphyria.
- Avoid use during pregnancy, especially first trimester.

MEPROBAMATE   **153**

†Canadian   ‡Australian

DRUG/CLASS/CATEGORY	DOSAGE FORMS	INDICATIONS/DOSAGES	KEY PRECAUTIONS
mercaptopurine (6-mercaptopurine, 6-MP) Purinethol *Antimetabolite (cell cycle–phase specific, S phase)* *Antineoplastic* Preg. Risk Category: D	**tab (scored):** 50 mg	*Acute myeloblastic leukemia, chronic myelocytic leukemia* — **Adults:** 80 to 100 mg/m² (rounded to nearest 25 mg) PO daily as single dose up to 5 mg/kg/day. **Children:** 70 mg/m² (rounded to nearest 25 mg) PO daily. *Acute lymphoblastic leukemia* — **Children:** 70 mg/m² (rounded to nearest 25 mg) PO daily. **Usual maintenance for adults and children:** 1.5 to 2.5 mg/kg/day.	▪ Use cautiously after chemotherapy or radiation therapy in patients with depressed neutrophil or platelet count, and in impaired renal or hepatic function. ▪ Contraindicated in disease with known resistance to drug.
meropenem Merrem IV *Carbapenem derivative* *Antibiotic* Preg. Risk Category: B	**powder for inj:** 500 mg/15 ml, 500 mg/20 ml, 500 mg/100 ml, 1 g/15 ml, 1 g/30 ml, 1 g/100 ml	*Complicated appendicitis and peritonitis caused by susceptible organisms; bacterial meningitis (pediatric patients only) caused by susceptible organisms* — **Adults:** 1 g IV q 8 hr over 15 to 30 min as IV infusion or over about 3 to 5 min as IV bolus injection (5 to 20 ml). **Children ≥ 3 mo:** 20 to 40 mg/kg q 8 hr over 15 to 30 min as IV infusion or over about 3 to 5 min as IV bolus injection (5 to 20 ml). Max 2 g IV q 8 hr. **Children > 50 kg:** 1 to 2 g IV q 8 hr for meningitis.	▪ Use cautiously in elderly patients, in history of seizure disorders or impaired renal function, and in breast-feeding patients. ▪ Contraindicated in hypersensitivity to component of drug or other drugs in same class and in history of anaphylactic reactions to beta-lactams. ▪ Safety and effectiveness in children < 3 mo not established.
mesalamine Asacol, Salofalk, Mesasal, Pentasa, Rowasa *Salicylate* *Anti-inflammatory* Preg. Risk Category: B	**tab (delayed-release):** 400 mg; **cap (contr-release):** 250 mg; **rectal susp:** 4 g/60 ml; **supp:** 500 mg	*Active mild to moderate distal ulcerative colitis, proctitis, or proctosigmoiditis* — **Adults:** 800 mg PO (tab) tid for total dose of 2.4 g/day for 6 wk; 1 g PO (cap) qid for total dose of 4 g up to 8 wk; 500 mg PR (supp) bid, or 4 g as retention enema qd (preferably hs). Rectal dosage form should be retained overnight (for about 8 hr).	▪ Use cautiously in renal impairment. ▪ Contraindicated in hypersensitivity to drug, its components, or salicylates.

mesna
Mesnex, Dromitexan
Thiol derivative
Uroprotectant
Preg. Risk Category: B

inj: 100 mg/ml

Prophylaxis of hemorrhagic cystitis in patients receiving ifosfamide — **Adults:** dosage varies with amount of ifosfamide administered; calculated as 20% (w/w) of ifosfamide dose at time of ifosfamide administration. Usual dosage 240 mg/m² as IV bolus with ifosfamide administration; repeat at 4 and 8 hr after ifosfamide given.

- Contraindicated in hypersensitivity to mesna or thiol-containing compounds.
- Although formulated to prevent hemorrhagic cystitis from ifosfamide, won't protect against other toxicities associated with drug.

---

mesoridazine besylate
Serentil, Serentil Concentrate
Phenothiazine (piperidine derivative)
Antipsychotic
Preg. Risk Category: NR

tab: 10, 25, 50, 100 mg; *oral conc:* 25 mg/ml (0.6% alcohol); *inj:* 25 mg/ml

Alcoholism — **Adults and children > 12 yr:** 25 mg PO bid up to max 200 mg daily.
Behavioral problems associated with chronic organic mental syndrome — **Adults and children > 12 yr:** 25 mg PO tid to max 300 mg daily.
Psychoneurotic manifestations (anxiety) — **Adults and children > 12 yr:** 10 mg PO tid to max 150 mg daily.
Schizophrenia — **Adults and children > 12 yr:** initially, 50 mg PO tid or 25 mg IM, repeated in 30 to 60 min, prn. Max oral dosage 400 mg daily; max IM dosage 200 mg.

- Contraindicated in hypersensitivity to drug or in severe CNS depression or comatose states.

---

metaproterenol sulfate
Alupent, Dey-Dose Metaproterenol, Dey-Lute Metaproterenol, Metaprel
Adrenergic
Bronchodilator
Preg. Risk Category: C

tab: 10, 20 mg; *syrup:* 10 mg/5 ml; *aerosol inhaler:* 0.65 mg/metered spray; *neb inhaler:* 0.4%, 0.6%, 5% sol

Acute episodes of bronchial asthma — **Adults and children ≥ 12 yr:** 2 to 3 inhalations. Don't repeat inhalation more often than q 3 to 4 hr. Max 12 inhalations/day.
Bronchial asthma and reversible bronchospasm — **Adults and children > 9 yr or > 27 kg:** 20 mg PO q 6 to 8 hr. **Children 6 to 9 yr or < 27 kg:** 10 mg PO q 6 to 8 hr. Or, via IPPB or nebulizer: **Adults and children ≥ 12 yr:** 0.2 to 0.3 ml of 5% sol diluted in approx 2.5 ml of 0.45% or 0.9% NaCl or 2.5 ml commercially available 0.4% or 0.6% solution q 4 hr prn. **Children 6 to 12 yr:** 0.1 to 0.2 ml of 5% sol diluted in 0.9% NaCl to final volume of 3 ml q 4 hr prn.

- Use cautiously in hypertension, hyperthyroidism, heart disease, diabetes, or cirrhosis and in patients receiving cardiac glycosides.
- Contraindicated in hypersensitivity to drug or any ingredient; during anesthesia with cyclopropane or halogenated hydrocarbon general anesthetics; in tachycardia and arrhythmias associated with tachycardia; or in peripheral or mesenteric vascular thrombosis, profound hypoxia, or hypercapnia.

DRUG/CLASS/CATEGORY	DOSAGE FORMS	INDICATIONS/DOSAGES	KEY PRECAUTIONS
metaraminol bitartrate Aramine *Adrenergic* *Vasopressor* Preg. Risk Category: C	**inj:** 10 mg/ml	*Prevention of hypotension* — **Adults:** 2 to 10 mg IM or SC. **Children:** 0.1 mg/kg or 3 mg/m² IM or SC. *Hypotension in severe shock* — **Adults:** 0.5 to 5 mg by direct IV injection, followed by IV infusion titrated to maintain BP. If necessary, mix 15 to 100 mg (up to 500 mg has been used) in 500 ml of 0.9% NaCl solution or D₅W. **Children:** 0.01 mg/kg or 0.3 mg/m² IV bolus followed by IV infusion, if necessary, of 0.4 mg/kg or 12 mg/m² diluted and titrated to maintain desired BP.	• Use cautiously in heart disease, hypertension, peripheral vascular disease, thyroid disease, diabetes, cirrhosis, history of malaria, or sulfite sensitivity and in patients receiving cardiac glycosides. • Contraindicated in hypersensitivity to drug and in patients receiving anesthesia with cyclopropane and halogenated hydrocarbon anesthetics.
metformin hydrochloride Glucophage *Biguanide* *Antidiabetic agent* Preg. Risk Category: B	**tab:** 500, 850 mg	*Adjunct to diet to lower blood glucose in type 2 diabetes* — **Adults:** initially, 500 mg PO bid with morning and evening meals, or 850 mg PO qd with morning meal. When 500-mg dose form used, increase dosage 500 mg weekly to max 2,500 mg PO daily in divided doses prn. When 850-mg dose form used, increase dosage 850 mg every other wk to max 2,550 mg PO daily in divided doses prn. Use conservative dose in elderly and debilitated patients.	• Use cautiously in elderly, debilitated, or malnourished patients and in adrenal or pituitary insufficiency. • Contraindicated in hypersensitivity to drug, renal disease, or metabolic acidosis. • Temporarily withhold in patients undergoing radiologic studies involving parenteral administration of iodinated contrast materials. • Stop if patient enters hypoxic state. • Avoid in hepatic disease.
methadone hydrochloride Dolophine, Methadose, Physeptone‡ *Opioid* *Analgesic/narcotic detoxification adjunct* Preg. Risk Category: C Controlled Sub. Sched.: II	**tab:** 5, 10 mg; ***dispers tab (for maintenance therapy):** 40 mg; **oral sol:** 5 mg/5 ml, 10 mg/10 ml, 10 mg/ml (conc); **inj:** 10 mg/ml	*Severe pain* — **Adults:** 2.5 to 10 mg PO, IM, or SC q 3 to 4 hr, prn. *Narcotic withdrawal syndrome* — **Adults:** 15 to 40 mg PO daily (highly individualized). Maintenance 20 to 120 mg PO daily. Adjust dosage prn. Daily dosages >120 mg require special state and federal approval.	• Use with extreme caution in acute abdominal conditions, severe hepatic or renal impairment, hypothyroidism, Addison's disease, prostatic hyperplasia, urethral stricture, head injury, increased ICP, asthma, and other respiratory conditions. Also use with caution in elderly or debilitated patients. • Contraindicated in hypersensitivity to drug.

methamphetamine hydrochloride Desoxyn *CNS stimulant/adjunctive anorexigenic/sympathomimetic amine* Preg. Risk Category: C Controlled Sub. Sched.: II	*tab:* 5 mg; *tab (long-acting):* 5, 10, 15 mg	*Attention deficit disorder with hyperactivity —* **Children ≥ 6 yr:** 2.5 to 5 mg PO qd or bid, with 5-mg increments weekly, prn. Usual effective dosage 20 to 25 mg daily. *Short-term adjunct in exogenous obesity —* **Adults:** 2.5 to 5 mg PO bid to tid, 30 min before meals; or 10 to 15 mg long-acting tab PO daily before breakfast.	■ Use cautiously in elderly, debilitated, asthenic, or psychopathic patients and in history of suicidal or homicidal tendencies. ■ Contraindicated in agitation, moderate to severe hypertension, hyperthyroidism, symptomatic CV disease, advanced arteriosclerosis, glaucoma, hypersensitivity or idiosyncrasy to sympathomimetic amines, history of drug abuse, or within 14 days of MAO inhibitor therapy.
methazolamide Neptazane *Carbonic anhydrase inhibitor* *Adjunctive treatment for open-angle glaucoma/preop for acute angle-closure glaucoma* Preg. Risk Category: C	*tab:* 25, 50 mg	*Glaucoma (chronic open-angle or secondary, or preop in obstructive or acute angle-closure) —* **Adults:** 50 to 100 mg PO bid or tid.	■ Use cautiously in emphysema and pulmonary obstruction. ■ Contraindicated for long-term use in angle-closure glaucoma, depressed serum sodium or potassium levels, renal or hepatic disease or dysfunction, adrenal gland dysfunction, or hyperchloremic acidosis.
methenamine hippurate Hiprex, Hip-Rex†, Urex **methenamine mandelate** Mandelamine, Sterine† *Formaldehyde prodrug* *Urinary tract anti-infective* Preg. Risk Category: C	hippurate — *tab:* 1 g. mandelate — *tab:* 500 mg, 1 g; *tab (enteric-coated):* 500 mg, 1 g; *tab (film-coated):* 500 mg, 1 g; *susp:* 500 mg/5 ml	*Long-term prophylaxis or suppression of chronic UTIs —* **Adults and children > 12 yr:** 1 g (hippurate) PO q 12 hr; or 1 g (mandelate) PO qid after meals and hs. **Children 6 to 12 yr:** 500 mg to 1 g (hippurate) PO q 12 hr, or 500 mg (mandelate) PO qid after meals and hs. **Children < 6 yr:** 18.4 mg/kg (mandelate) PO qid.	■ Use cautiously in elderly or debilitated patients. Oral susp contains vegetable oil. ■ Contraindicated in renal insufficiency, severe hepatic disease, or severe dehydration.

†Canadian ‡Australian

DRUG/CLASS/ CATEGORY	DOSAGE FORMS	INDICATIONS/ DOSAGES	KEY PRECAUTIONS
methimazole Tapazole *Thyroid hormone antagonist* *Antihyperthyroid agent* Preg. Risk Category: D	**tab:** 5, 10 mg	*Hyperthyroidism* — **Adults:** if mild, 15 mg PO daily; if moderately severe, 30 to 45 mg daily; if severe, 60 mg daily. All given in 3 equally divided doses q 8 hr. Maintenance 5 to 15 mg daily. **Children:** 0.4 mg/kg/day PO divided q 8 hr. Maintenance 0.2 mg/kg/day divided q 8 hr.	▪ Use with extreme caution during pregnancy. Pregnant women may require less drug as pregnancy progresses. Monitor thyroid function studies closely. Thyroid may be added to regimen. Drug may be stopped during last few weeks of pregnancy. ▪ Contraindicated in hypersensitivity to drug and in breast-feeding patients.
methocarbamol Robaxin, Robaxin-750 *Carbamate derivative of guaifenesin* *Skeletal muscle relaxant* Preg. Risk Category: NR	**tab:** 500, 750 mg; **inj:** 100 mg/ml	*Adjunct in acute, painful musculoskeletal conditions* — **Adults:** 1.5 g PO qid for 2 to 3 days. Maintenance 4 to 4.5 g PO daily in 3 to 6 divided doses. Or, 1 g IM or IV. Max 3 g daily IM or IV for 3 consecutive days. *Supportive therapy in tetanus management* — **Adults:** 1 to 2 g IV push or 1 to 3 g as infusion q 6 hr. **Children:** 15 mg/kg IV q 6 hr.	▪ Contraindicated in hypersensitivity to drug, impaired renal function (injectable form), or seizure disorder (injectable form).
methotrexate (amethopterin, MTX) **methotrexate sodium** Folex, Folex PFS, Mexate-AQ, Rheumatrex *Antimetabolite (cell cycle-phase specific, S phase)* *Antineoplastic* Preg. Risk Category: X	**tab (scored):** 2.5 mg; **inj:** 20-, 25-, 50-, 100-, 250 mg vials, lyoph powder, preserv-free; 25 mg/ml vials, preserv-free sol; 2.5, 25 mg/ml vials, lyoph powder, preserved	*Trophoblastic tumors (choriocarcinoma, hydatidiform mole)* — **Adults:** 15 to 30 mg PO or IM daily for 5 days. Repeat after ≥ 1 wk, according to response or toxicity. *Acute lymphocytic leukemia* — **Adults and children:** 3.3 mg/m²/day PO, IM, or IV for 4 to 6 wk or until remission; then 20 to 30 mg/m² PO or IM weekly in 2 divided doses or 2.5 mg/kg IV q 14 days. *Meningeal leukemia* — **Adults and children:** 12 mg/m² or less (max 15 mg) intrathecally q 2 to 5 days until CSF normal, then 1 additional dose.	▪ Use cautiously and at modified dosage in impaired hepatic or renal function, bone marrow suppression, aplasia, leukopenia, thrombocytopenia, or anemia. Also use cautiously in infection, peptic ulceration, or ulcerative colitis and in very young, elderly, or debilitated patients. ▪ Contraindicated in hypersensitivity to drug and during pregnancy or breast-feeding. Also contraindicated in patients with psoriasis or rheumatoid arthritis who also have alcoholism, alcoholic liver, chronic liver disease, immunodeficiency syndromes, or pre-existing blood dyscrasias.

methoxsalen (topical) Oxsoralen *Psoralen derivative* *Pigmenting antipsoriatic* Preg. Risk Category: C	lotion: 1%	*To induce repigmentation in vitiligo; psoriasis* — **Adults and children > 12 yr:** apply lotion to small, well-defined vitiliginous lesions. For optimum effect, apply about 1 to 2 hr before exposure to UV light.	<ul><li>Use cautiously in family history of sunlight allergy, GI diseases, or chronic infection.</li><li>Contraindicated in sensitivity to psoralen compounds, diseases associated with photosensitivity, and in melanoma, invasive squamous cell carcinoma, and aphakia.</li></ul>
methylcellulose Citrucel, Cologel *Adsorbent* *Bulk-forming laxative* Preg. Risk Category: C	powder: 105, 364 mg/g; tab: 500 mg	*Chronic constipation* — **Adults:** max 6 g daily, divided into 0.45 to 3 g/dose. **Children 6 to 12 yr:** Max 3 g daily, divided into 0.45 to 1.5 g/dose.	<ul><li>Contraindicated in abdominal pain, nausea, vomiting, or symptoms of appendicitis or acute surgical abdomen and in intestinal obstruction or ulceration, disabling adhesions, and difficulty swallowing.</li></ul>
methyldopa Aldomet, Apo-Methyldopa†, Dopamet†, Novomedopa† methyldopate hydrochloride Aldomet, Aldomet Ester Injection‡ *Centrally acting antiadrenergic* *Antihypertensive* Preg. Risk Category: B	methyldopa — tab: 125, 250, 500 mg; oral susp: 250 mg/5 ml. methyldopate hydrochloride — inj: 250 mg/5 ml	*Hypertension, hypertensive crisis* — **Adults:** initially, 250 mg PO bid to tid in first 48 hr. Then increase prn q 2 days. Maintenance 500 mg to 2 g daily in 2 to 4 divided doses; max recommended 3 g daily. Or, 250 to 500 mg IV q 6 hr, diluted in D₅W and given over 30 to 60 min; max dose 1 g q 6 hr. **Children:** 10 mg/kg PO qd in 2 to 4 divided doses; or 20 to 40 mg/kg IV qd in 4 divided doses. Dosage increased qd prn. Max daily dosage 65 mg/kg or 3 g.	<ul><li>Use cautiously in history of impaired hepatic function and in breast-feeding patients.</li><li>Contraindicated in hypersensitivity to drug or active hepatic disease (such as acute hepatitis) and active cirrhosis. Also contraindicated if previous methyldopa therapy linked to liver disorder.</li></ul>
methylphenidate hydrochloride PMS-Methylphenidate‡, Ritalin, Ritalin-SR *Piperidine CNS stimulant* *CNS stimulant (analeptic)* Preg. Risk Category: NR Controlled Sub. Sched.: II	tab: 5, 10, 20 mg; tab (sustrelease): 20 mg	*Attention deficit hyperactivity disorder (ADHD)* — **Children ≥ 6 yr:** initial dose, 5 to 10 mg PO daily before breakfast and lunch, with 5- to 10-mg increments weekly prn, up to 2 mg/kg or 60 mg daily. Usual effective dose 20 to 30 mg. *Narcolepsy* — **Adults:** 10 mg PO bid or tid 30 to 45 min before meals. Dosage varies with patient needs; average 40 to 60 mg/day.	<ul><li>Use cautiously in history of drug abuse, hypertension, history of seizures, or EEG abnormalities.</li><li>Contraindicated in hypersensitivity to drug, glaucoma, motor tics, family history of or diagnosis of Tourette syndrome, or history of marked anxiety, tension, or agitation.</li></ul>

DRUG/CLASS/ CATEGORY	DOSAGE FORMS	INDICATIONS/ DOSAGES	KEY PRECAUTIONS
methylprednisolone Medrol **methylprednisolone acetate** depMedalone-40, Depoject-40, Depo-Medrol, Depopred-40, Depo-Predate 40, Duralone-40, Medralone-40, Rep-pred 40 **methylprednisolone sodium succinate** A-methaPred, Solu-Medrol *Glucocorticoid* *Anti-inflammatory/immuno-suppressant* Preg. Risk Category: C	**tab:** 2, 4, 8, 16, 24, 32 mg. **acetate — *inj* (*susp*):** 20, 40, 80 mg/ml. **sodium succinate — *inj*:** 40-, 125-, 500-, 1,000-, 2,000-mg vial	*Multiple sclerosis —* **Adults:** 200 mg PO daily for 1 wk, followed by 80 mg qod for 1 mo. *Severe inflammation or immunosuppression —* **Adults:** 2 to 60 mg PO daily in 4 divided doses; 10 to 80 mg acetate IM daily, or 10 to 250 mg succinate IM or IV up to q 4 hr; or 4 to 40 mg acetate into smaller joints or 20 to 80 mg acetate into larger joints. **Children:** 0.03 to 0.2 mg/kg succinate or 1 to 6.25 mg/m² IM qd or bid. *Shock —* **Adults:** 100 to 250 mg succinate IV at 2- to 6-hr intervals; or 30 mg/kg IV initially, repeated q 4 to 6 hr, prn. Continue therapy for 2 or 3 days or until patient stable.	▪ Use cautiously in GI ulceration or renal disease, hypertension, osteoporosis, diabetes mellitus, hypothyroidism, cirrhosis, diverticulitis, nonspecific ulcerative colitis, recent intestinal anastomoses, thromboembolic disorders, seizures, myasthenia gravis, heart failure, TB, ocular herpes simplex, emotional instability, and psychotic tendencies. ▪ Contraindicated in allergy to any component of formulation, in systemic fungal infections, and in premature infants (acetate and succinate).
methyltestosterone Android, Metandren, Testred *Androgen* *Androgen replacement* Preg. Risk Category: X Controlled Sub. Sched.: II	**tab:** 10, 25 mg; **tab (*buccal*):** 10 mg, **cap:** 10 mg	*Breast cancer in women —* **Adults:** 50 to 200 mg PO daily or 25 to 100 mg buccally daily. *Male hypogonadism —* **Adults:** 10 to 50 mg PO daily or 5 to 25 mg buccally daily. Evaluate semen q 3 to 4 months.	▪ Use cautiously in elderly patients; in cardiac, renal, or hepatic disease; or in healthy males with delayed puberty. ▪ Contraindicated in pregnant and breast-feeding patients or in males with breast cancer or prostate cancer. ▪ Avoid use in women of childbearing age until pregnancy ruled out.
methysergide maleate Deseril; Sansert *Ergot alkaloid* *Vasoconstrictor* Preg. Risk Category: X	**tab:** 1 mg‡, 2 mg	*Prevention of frequent, severe, uncontrollable, or disabling migraine or vascular headaches —* **Adults:** 4 to 8 mg PO daily with meals.	▪ Use cautiously in peptic ulceration, suspected CAD, sensitivity to aspirin or tartrazine. ▪ Evaluate ECG and cardiac status and before giving to patients > 40 yr.

Drug	Forms	Indications & Dosage	Contraindications & Precautions
metipranolol hydrochloride OptiPranolol *Beta-adrenergic blocker* *Antiglaucoma agent* Preg. Risk Category: C	**ophth sol:** 0.3% in 5-, 10-ml dropper bottles	*IOP reduction in ocular conditions, including ocular hypertension and chronic open-angle glaucoma* — **Adults:** 1 drop into affected eye bid. If IOP not at satisfactory level, may institute concomitant therapy to lower IOP.	■ Use cautiously in nonallergic bronchospasm, chronic bronchitis, emphysema, diabetes mellitus (especially in those subject to spontaneous hypoglycemia), hyperthyroidism, or cerebrovascular insufficiency. ■ Contraindicated in hypersensitivity to drug or its components and in bronchial asthma, history of bronchial asthma or severe COPD, sinus bradycardia, 2nd- or 3rd-degree AV block, heart failure, and cardiogenic shock.
metoclopramide hydrochloride Apo-Metoclop†, Clopra, Maxolon, Octamide, Reclomide, Reglan *PABA derivative* *Antiemetic/GI stimulant* Preg. Risk Category: B	**inj:** 5 mg/ml	*Prevention or reduction of nausea and vomiting associated with cancer chemotherapy* — **Adults:** 1 to 2 mg/kg IV 30 min before chemotherapy, then repeated q 2 hr for 2 doses, then q 3 hr for 3 doses.	■ Use cautiously in history of depression, Parkinson's disease, or hypertension. ■ Contraindicated when stimulation of GI motility might be dangerous and in hypersensitivity to drug, pheochromocytoma, or seizure disorders.
metolazone Diulo, Mykrox, Zaroxolyn *Quinazoline derivative (thiazide-like)* *diuretic* *Diuretic/antihypertensive* Preg. Risk Category: B	**tab (ext-release):** 2.5, 5, 10 mg; **tab (prompt-release):** 0.5 mg	*Edema in heart failure or renal disease* — **Adults:** 5 to 20 mg (ext-release) PO daily. *Hypertension* — **Adults:** 2.5 to 5 mg (ext-release) PO daily. Maintenance dosage based on BP. Or 0.5 mg (prompt-release) PO qd in morning, increased to 1 mg PO qd.	■ Use cautiously in impaired renal or hepatic function. ■ Contraindicated in anuria, hepatic coma or precoma, or hypersensitivity to thiazides or other sulfonamide-derived drugs.

(top of first column, continued entry for preceding drug):
■ Contraindicated in severe hypertension or arteriosclerosis, peripheral vascular insufficiency, renal or hepatic disease, CAD, phlebitis or cellulitis of lower limbs, collagen diseases, fibrotic processes, or valvular heart disease; in debilitated patients; and during pregnancy.

†Canadian ‡Australian

DRUG/CLASS/ CATEGORY	DOSAGE FORMS	INDICATIONS/ DOSAGES	KEY PRECAUTIONS
metoprolol succinate Toprol XL **metoprolol tartrate** Apo-Metoprolol†, Lopresor SR†, Lopressor, Minax‡ *Beta-adrenergic blocker* Antihypertensive/adjunctive treatment of acute MI Preg. Risk Category: C	**succinate —** *tab (ext-release):* 50, 100, 200 mg. **tartrate —** *tab:* 50, 100 mg; *tab (ext-release):* 100 mg‡; 200 mg‡; *inj:* 1 mg/ml in 5-ml ampules	*Hypertension —* **Adults:** 100 mg PO in single or divided doses; maint 100 to 450 mg qd in 2 or 3 divided doses. Or, 50 to 100 mg of ext-release tab qd (max 400 mg qd). *Early intervention in acute MI —* **Adults:** three 5-mg (tartrate) IV boluses q 2 min. Then, 15 min after last dose, 25 to 50 mg PO q 6 hr for 48 hr. Maint 100 mg PO bid. *Angina pectoris —* **Adults:** initially, 100 mg PO qd in 2 divided doses. Maint 100 to 400 mg qd.	▪ Use cautiously in heart failure, diabetes, or respiratory or hepatic disease. ▪ Contraindicated in hypersensitivity to drug or other beta blockers and in sinus bradycardia, heart block > first-degree, cardiogenic shock, or overt cardiac failure when used to treat hypertension or angina. When used to treat MI, contraindicated in HR < 45, second- or third-degree heart block, PR interval ≥ 0.24 sec or longer with first-degree heart block, systolic BP < 100, or moderate to severe cardiac failure.
metronidazole Apo-Metronidazole†, Flagyl, Metrozine‡, Neo-Metric†, PMS Metronidazole†, Protostat, Trikacide† **metronidazole hydrochloride** Flagyl IV RTU, Metro IV, Novonidazol *Nitroimidazole* Antibacterial/antiprotozoal/ amebicide Preg. Risk Category: B	*tab:* 200 mg‡; 250, 375, 400 mg‡; 500 mg; *oral susp (benzoyl metronidazole):* 200 mg/5 ml‡; *inj:* 500 mg/100 ml ready to use; *powder for inj:* 500-mg single-dose vials	*Intestinal amebiasis —* **Adults:** 750 mg PO tid for 5 to 10 days. **Children:** 30 to 50 mg/kg daily (in 3 doses) for 10 days. *Trichomoniasis —* **Adults:** 250 mg PO tid for 7 days or 2 g PO in single dose; 4 to 6 wk should elapse between courses of therapy. **Children:** 5 mg/kg dose PO tid for 7 days. *Refractory trichomoniasis —* **Adults:** 250 or 500 mg PO bid for 10 or 7 days, respectively. *Bacterial infections caused by anaerobic microorganisms —* **Adults:** *load* —15 mg/kg IV infused over 1 hr. Maint dose 7.5 mg/kg IV or PO q 6 hr. Give 1st maint dose 6 hr after loading dose. Max 4 g qd. *Prevention of postop infection in contaminated or potentially contaminated colorectal surgery —* **Adults:** 15 mg/kg IV infused over 30 to 60 min 1 hr before surgery. Then 7.5 mg/kg IV infused over 30 to 60 min at 6 and 12 hr after initial dose.	▪ Use cautiously in history of blood dyscrasia or CNS disorder; in retinal or visual field changes, hepatic disease, or alcoholism; or in conjunction with hepatotoxic drugs. ▪ Contraindicated in hypersensitivity to drug or other nitroimidazole derivatives.

metronidazole (topical) MetroGel, MetroGel-Vaginal Nitroimidazole Antiprotozoal/antibacterial Preg. Risk Category: B	*topical gel:* 0.75%; *vag gel:* 0.75%	*Acne rosacea* — **Adults:** apply thin film to affected area bid, morning and evening. Frequency and duration of therapy adjusted after response evaluated. *Bacterial vaginosis* — **Adults:** 1 applicatorful bid, morning and evening, for 5 days.	• Use cautiously in history or evidence of blood dyscrasia. • Use vag gel cautiously in history of CNS diseases. • Contraindicated in hypersensitivity to drug or ingredients (such as parabens) or to other nitromidazole derivatives.
mexiletine hydrochloride Mexitil *Lidocaine analogue, sodium channel antagonist* Ventricular antiarrhythmic Preg. Risk Category: C	*cap:* 50‡, 100, 150, 200, 250 mg; *inj:* 250 mg/10 ml‡	*Refractory life-threatening ventricular arrhythmias, including ventricular tachycardia and PVCs* — **Adults:** 200 mg PO q 8 hr. May increase dose in increments of 50 to 100 mg q 8 hr. Or, loading dose of 400 mg with maintenance dose of 200 mg q 8 hr. Max shouldn't exceed 1,200 mg daily.	• Use cautiously in preexisting first-degree heart block, ventricular pacemaker, preexisting sinus node dysfunction, intraventricular conduction disturbances, hypotension, severe heart failure, or seizure disorder. • Contraindicated in cardiogenic shock or preexisting second- or third-degree AV block in absence of artificial pacemaker.
mezlocillin sodium Mezlin *Extended-spectrum penicillin/acylaminopenicillin* Antibiotic Preg. Risk Category: B	*inj:* 1, 2, 3, 4 g; *pharm bulk pkg:* 20 g	*Systemic infections caused by susceptible strains of gram-pos and especially gram-neg organisms* — **Adults:** 200 to 300 mg/kg daily IV or IM in 4 to 6 divided doses. Usual dose 3 g q 4 hr or 4 g q 6 hr. For very serious infections, up to 24 g daily may be given. **Children ≤ 12 yr:** 200 to 300 mg/kg per day IM or IV in divided doses q 4 to 6 hr.	• Use cautiously in other drug allergies, especially to cephalosporins (possible cross-sensitivity) or in bleeding tendencies, uremia, or hypokalemia. • Contraindicated in hypersensitivity to drug or other penicillins.
miconazole nitrate Micatin, Monistat-Derm Cream and Lotion, Monistat 3 Vaginal Suppository, Monistat 7 Vaginal Cream, Monistat 7 Vaginal Suppository *Imidazole derivative* Antifungal Preg. Risk Category: C	*cream:* 2%; *powder:* 2%; *spray:* 2%; *vag cream:* 2%; *vag supp:* 100, 200 mg	*Tinea pedis, tinea cruris, tinea corporis* — **Adults and children:** apply or spray sparingly bid for 2 to 4 wk. *Vulvovaginal candidiasis* — **Adults:** 1 applicatorful or 100 mg supp (Monistat 7) inserted intravaginally hs for 7 days; repeat course if necessary. Alternatively, 200 mg supp (Monistat 3) intravaginally hs for 3 days.	• Use cautiously in hepatic insufficiency. • Contraindicated in hypersensitivity to drug.

‡Canadian †Australian

DRUG/CLASS/CATEGORY	DOSAGE FORMS	INDICATIONS/DOSAGES	KEY PRECAUTIONS
midazolam hydrochloride Hypnovel‡, Versed *Benzodiazepine* Preoperative sedative/agent for conscious sedation/adjunct for induction of general anesthesia/amnesic agent Preg. Risk Category: D Controlled Sub. Sched.: IV	*inj:* 1, 5 mg/ml	*Preop sedation —* **Adults:** 0.07 mg to 0.08 mg/kg IM 1 hr before surgery. *Conscious sedation before short diagnostic procedures —* **Adults:** 1 to 2 mg by slow IV injection before procedure. *Induction of general anesthesia —* **Adults:** 0.15 to 0.35 mg/kg given over 20 to 30 sec. Additional increments of 25% of initial dose may be needed. Max dose up to 0.6 mg/kg. **Unpremedicated adults ≥ 55 yr:** initially, 0.3 mg/kg. For debilitated patients, initial dose 0.2 to 0.25 mg/kg.	▪ Use cautiously in uncompensated acute illness and in elderly or debilitated patients. ▪ Contraindicated in hypersensitivity to drug, acute angle-closure glaucoma, shock, coma, or acute alcohol intoxication.
milrinone lactate Primacor *Bipyridine phosphodiesterase inhibitor* *Inotropic vasodilator* Preg. Risk Category: C	*inj:* 1 mg/ml	*Short-term treatment of heart failure —* **Adults:** initial loading dose 50 mcg/kg IV, given slowly over 10 min, followed by continuous IV infusion of 0.375 to 0.75 mcg/kg/min. Adjust infusion dose according to clinical and hemodynamic responses.	▪ Use cautiously in atrial flutter or fibrillation. ▪ Contraindicated in hypersensitivity to drug. ▪ Avoid use in severe aortic or pulmonic valvular disease in place of surgical correction of obstruction or during acute phase of MI.
minocycline hydrochloride Apo-Minocline†, Dynacin, Minocin, Minomycin IV‡, Syn-Mynocycline† *Tetracycline* *Antibiotic* Preg. Risk Category: NR	*tab (film-coated):* 50, 100 mg; *cap (pellet-filled):* 50, 100 mg; *oral susp:* 50 mg/5 ml; *inj:* 100 mg	*Infections caused by susceptible gram-neg and gram-pos organisms —* **Adults:** 200 mg IV; then 100 mg IV q 12 hr. Max 400 mg/day. Or, 200 mg PO; then 100 mg PO q 12 hr. Some clinicians use 100 or 200 mg PO, followed by 50 mg qid. **Children > 8 yr:** 4 mg/kg PO or IV, then 2 mg/kg q 12 hr. Given IV in 500- to 1,000-ml sol without calcium over 6 hr. *Gonorrhea in patients allergic to penicillin —* **Adults:** initially, 200 mg PO; then 100 mg q 12 hr for at least 4 days. *Syphilis in patients allergic to penicillin —* **Adults:** 200 mg PO; then 100 mg q 12 hr for 10 to 15 days.	▪ Use cautiously in impaired renal or hepatic function. ▪ Contraindicated in hypersensitivity to drug or other tetracyclines. ▪ Use during last half of pregnancy and in children < 9 yr may cause permanent tooth discoloration, enamel defects, and bone growth retardation.

*Meningococcal carrier state — **Adults:** 100 mg PO q 12 hr for 5 days.*
Uncomplicated urethral, endocervical, or rectal infection caused by C. trachomatis — 100 mg PO bid for at least 7 days.

---

mirtazapine
Remeron
Piperazinoazepine
Tetracyclic antidepressant
Preg. Risk Category: C

tab: 15, 30 mg

Depression — **Adults:** initially, 15 mg PO hs. Maintenance range 15 to 45 mg daily. Dosage adjustments at intervals of at least 1 to 2 wk.

- Use cautiously in CV or cerebrovascular disease, seizure disorders, suicidal ideations, impaired hepatic or renal function, history of mania or hypomania, or predisposition to hypotension.
- Contraindicated in hypersensitivity to drug.
- Safety and efficacy in children not established.

---

misoprostol
Cytotec
Prostaglandin E$_1$ analogue
Antiulcer agent/gastric mucosal protectant
Preg. Risk Category: X

tab: 100, 200 mcg

Prevention of NSAID-induced gastric ulcer in elderly or debilitated patients at high risk for complications from gastric ulcer and in patients with history of NSAID-induced ulcer — **Adults:** 200 mcg PO qid with food; if not tolerated, may decrease to 100 mcg PO qid. Give for duration of NSAID therapy. Give last dose hs.

- Shouldn't be routinely given to women of childbearing age unless at high risk for developing ulcers or complications from NSAID-induced ulcers.
- Contraindicated in pregnant and breast-feeding patients.

**mitomycin
(mitomycin-C)**
Mutamycin
Antineoplastic antibiotic (cell cycle–phase nonspecific)
Antineoplastic
Preg. Risk Category: NR

inj: 5-, 20-, 40-mg vials

Dosage and indications vary. Check treatment protocol.
Disseminated adenocarcinoma of stomach or pancreas — **Adults:** 20 mg/m^2 as IV single dose. Cycle repeated after 6 to 8 wk when WBC and platelet counts return to normal.

- Contraindicated in hypersensitivity to drug and in thrombocytopenia, coagulation disorders, or increased bleeding tendency due to other causes.

DRUG/CLASS/ CATEGORY	DOSAGE FORMS	INDICATIONS/ DOSAGES	KEY PRECAUTIONS
mitotane (o,p'-DDD) Lysodren *Chlorophenothane (DDT) analogue* *Antineoplastic/antiadrenal agent* Preg. Risk Category: C	*tab (scored):* 500 mg	*Inoperable adrenocortical cancer* — **Adults:** initially, 2 to 6 g PO daily in divided doses tid or qid; increase to 9 to 10 g PO daily, in divided doses tid or qid. Adjust dosage until max tolerated dosage achieved (varies from 2 to 16 g/day; usually 8 to 10 g/day).	▪ Use cautiously in hepatic disease. ▪ Contraindicated in hypersensitivity to drug. ▪ Shouldn't be used in shock or trauma.
mitoxantrone hydrochloride Novantrone *Antibiotic antineoplastic* *Antineoplastic* Preg. Risk Category: D	*inj:* 2 mg/ml in 10-, 12.5-, 15-ml vials	*Combination initial therapy for acute nonlymphocytic leukemia* — **Adults:** induction 12 mg/m² IV qd on days 1 to 3, in combination with 100 mg/m² qd of cytarabine on days 1 to 7. Give second induction if response not adequate. Maintenance therapy 12 mg/m² on days 1 and 2 with cytarabine on days 1 to 5. *Combination initial therapy for pain related to advanced hormone-refractory prostate cancer* — **Adults:** 12 to 14 mg/m² IV infusion over 15 to 30 min q 21 days.	▪ Use cautiously in prior exposure to anthracyclines or other cardiotoxic drugs, prior radiation therapy to mediastinal area, and preexisting heart disease. ▪ Contraindicated in hypersensitivity to drug.
moexipril hydrochloride Univasc *ACE inhibitor* *Antihypertensive* Preg. Risk Category: C (D in 2nd and 3rd trimesters)	*tab:* 7.5, 15 mg	*Hypertension* — **Adults:** initially, 7.5 mg (3.75 mg if patient receiving diuretic) PO qd 1 hr before meal. If control inadequate, dose may be increased or divided. Recommended maintenance dosage 7.5 mg to 30 mg daily, in 1 or 2 divided doses 1 hr before meals. Subsequent dosage depends on response.	▪ Use cautiously in impaired renal function, heart failure, or renal artery stenosis and in breast-feeding women. ▪ Contraindicated in hypersensitivity to drug or history of angioedema related to ACE inhibitor use. ▪ Safety in children not established.
molindone hydrochloride Moban *Dihydroindolone* *Antipsychotic* Preg. Risk Category: NR	*tab:* 5, 10, 25, 50, 100 mg; *oral sol:* 20 mg/ml	*Psychotic disorders* — **Adults:** initially, 50 to 75 mg PO daily, increased to 100 to 225 mg/day in 3 or 4 days. Maint dosage as follows: mild severity — 5 to 15 mg PO tid to qid; moderate severity — 10 to 25 mg PO tid or qid; extreme severity — 225 mg/day PO.	▪ Use cautiously when increased physical activity would be harmful and in patients subject to seizures. ▪ Contraindicated in hypersensitivity to drug or in coma or severe CNS depression.

mometasone furoate
Elocon
Synthetic corticosteroid
Anti-inflammatory
Preg. Risk Category: C

cream: 0.1%; *oint:* 0.1%; *lotion:* 0.1%

Inflammation associated with corticosteroid-responsive dermatoses — **Adults:** apply to affected areas qd.

- Use cautiously in young children.
- Contraindicated in hypersensitivity to drug or other corticosteroids.

monoctanoin
Moctanin
Esterified glycerol
Cholelitholytic
Preg. Risk Category: C

infusion: 120-ml bottles

To solubilize cholesterol (radiolucent) gallstones retained in biliary tract after cholecystectomy — **Adults:** given as continuous infusion for 2 to 10 days (to eliminate stones or reduce their size) through catheter inserted directly into common bile duct at rate of 3 to 5 ml/hr and pressure of 10 cm H_2O.

- Contraindicated in impaired hepatic function, biliary tract infection, or history of recent duodenal ulceration or jejunitis, portosystemic shunting, acute pancreatitis, or any active life-threatening problems that would be complicated by perfusion into biliary tract.

moricizine hydrochloride
Ethmozine
Sodium channel blocker
Antiarrhythmic
Preg. Risk Category: B

tab: 200, 250, 300 mg

Life-threatening ventricular arrhythmias — **Adults:** individualized. Therapy should begin in hospital. Most patients respond to 600 to 900 mg PO daily in divided doses q 8 hr. Daily dosage increased q 3 days by 150 mg.

- Use with extreme caution in sick sinus syndrome, CAD, and left ventricular dysfunction. Use cautiously in liver impairment.
- Contraindicated in hypersensitivity to drug; preexisting second- or third-degree AV block or right bundle branch block when associated with left hemiblock (bifascicular block) unless artificial pacemaker present; and cardiogenic shock.
- Drug detected in breast milk.

DRUG/CLASS/CATEGORY	DOSAGE FORMS	INDICATIONS/DOSAGES	KEY PRECAUTIONS
morphine hydrochloride Morphitec†, M.O.S.† **morphine sulfate** Astramorph PF, Duramorph, Epimorph†, Infumorph 200, Morphine H.P.†, MS Contin, Roxanol **morphine tartrate‡** *Opioid* *Narcotic analgesic* Preg. Risk Category: C Controlled Sub. Sched.: II	**hydrochloride** — *tab*: 10†, 20†, 40†, 60 mg†; *tab (ext-release)*: 30†, 60 mg†; *oral sol*: 1, 5, 10, 20, 50 mg/ml; *syrup*: 1†, 5†, 10†, 20†, 50 mg/ml†; *supp*: 10†, 20†, 30 mg†. **sulfate** — *tab*: 15, 30 mg; *tab (ext-release)*: 15, 30, 60, 100, 200 mg; *solu-ble tab*: 10, 15, 30 mg; *oral sol*: 10 mg/5 ml, 20 mg/5 ml, 20 mg/ml (conc); *syrup*: 1, 5 mg/ml; *inj (with preserv)*: 0.5, 1, 2, 3, 4, 5, 8, 10, 15, 25, 50 mg/ml; *inj (without preserv)*: 0.5,	*Severe pain* — **Adults:** 5 to 20 mg SC or IM, or 2.5 to 15 mg IV q 4 hr prn; or 10 to 30 mg PO or 10 to 20 mg PR q 4 hr, prn. When given by continuous IV, loading dose of 15 mg IV may be followed by contin-uous infusion of 0.8 to 10 mg/hour. May also give 15 to 30 mg contr-release tab PO q 8 to 12 hr. As epidur-al inj, 5 mg; then, if adequate pain relief not obtained within 1 hr, additional doses of 1 to 2 mg. Max total epidural dose shouldn't exceed 10 mg/24 hr. **Chil-dren:** 0.1 to 0.2 mg/kg SC or IM q 4 hr. Max single dose 15 mg.	▪ Use with extreme caution in head injury, in-creased ICP, seizures, chronic pulmonary disease, prostatic hyperplasia, severe hepat-ic or renal disease, acute abdominal condi-tions, hypothyroidism, Addison's disease, or urethral stricture and in elderly or debilitated patients. ▪ Contraindicated in hypersensitivity to drug or conditions that preclude IV opioid admin-istration (acute bronchial asthma or upper airway obstruction).

	1, 10, 25 mg/ml; **supp:** 5, 10, 20, 30 mg. **tartrate — inj:** 80 mg/ml‡	
mupirocin Bactroban *Antibiotic* *Topical antibacterial* Preg. Risk Category: B	**oint:** 2%	*Impetigo* — **Adults and children:** apply to affected areas tid for 1 to 2 wk.	▪ Use cautiously in burns or impaired renal function. ▪ Contraindicated in hypersensitivity to drug.
muromonab-CD3 Orthoclone OKT3 *Monoclonal antibody* *Immunosuppressant* Preg. Risk Category: C	**inj:** 1 mg/1 ml in 5-ml ampules	*Acute allograft rejection in renal transplant patients; in steroid-resistant hepatic or cardiac allograft rejection* — **Adults:** 5 mg IV bolus qd for 10 to 14 days.	▪ May potentiate immunosuppressive effects of other immunosuppressant drugs. ▪ Contraindicated in pregnancy and lactation. Also contraindicated in hypersensitivity to drug or any other product of murine (mouse) origin; if antimurine antibody titers ≥ 1:1,000; in fluid overload, as evidenced by chest X-ray or weight gain > 3% within wk before treatment; or in history of seizures or predisposition to seizures.
mycophenolate mofetil CellCept *Mycophenolic acid derivative* *Immunosuppressant* Preg. Risk Category: C	**cap:** 250 mg	*Prophylaxis of organ rejection in patients receiving allogenic renal transplants* — **Adults:** 1 g PO bid within 72 hr after transplantation, together with corticosteroids and cyclosporine.	▪ Use cautiously in GI disorders. ▪ Not recommended for pregnant patients unless benefits outweigh risks to fetus, or in breast-feeding patients. ▪ Contraindicated in hypersensitivity to drug, mycophenolic acid, or any drug component.

†Canadian ‡Australian

n

DRUG/CLASS/CATEGORY	DOSAGE FORMS	INDICATIONS/DOSAGES	KEY PRECAUTIONS
nabumetone Relafen *Nonsteroidal anti-inflammatory* *Antiarthritic* Preg. Risk Category: C	*tab:* 500, 750 mg	*Rheumatoid arthritis or osteoarthritis* — **Adults:** initially, 1,000 mg PO daily as single dose or in divided doses bid. Max 2,000 mg daily.	▪ Use cautiously in renal or hepatic impairment; heart failure, hypertension, or other conditions that may predispose to fluid retention; and in history of peptic ulcer disease. ▪ Contraindicated in hypersensitivity reactions or history of aspirin- or NSAID-induced asthma, urticaria, or other allergic-type reactions. ▪ Use in third trimester of pregnancy and in children not recommended.
nadolol Corgard *Beta-adrenergic blocker* *Antihypertensive/antianginal* Preg. Risk Category: C	*tab:* 20, 40, 80, 120, 160 mg	*Long-standing angina pectoris* — **Adults:** 40 mg PO qd. Increased in 40- to 80-mg increments until optimum response occurs. Usual maint dosage 40 to 80 mg qd. *Hypertension* — **Adults:** 40 mg PO qd. Increased in 40- to 80-mg increments until optimum response occurs. Usual maint dosage 40 to 80 mg qd. Doses of 320 mg may be needed.	▪ Use cautiously in heart failure, diabetes mellitus, chronic bronchitis, emphysema, or renal or hepatic impairment and in patients undergoing major surgery involving general anesthesia. ▪ Contraindicated in bronchial asthma, cardiogenic shock, sinus bradycardia and > first-degree heart block.
nafarelin acetate Synarel *Synthetic decapeptide* *GnRH analogue* Preg. Risk Category: X	*nasal sol:* 200 mcg/spray in metered-dose spray bottle (2 mg/ml)	*Management of endometriosis, pain relief, reduction of endometriotic lesions* — **Adults:** usual daily dose 1 spray (400 mcg) in one nostril in morning and 1 spray in other nostril in evening. If menstruation persists after 2 mo, may increase to 800 mcg daily. Begin treatment on day 2, 3, or 4 of menstrual cycle. Max duration of therapy 6 mo. *Central precocious puberty* — **Children:** 2 sprays (400 mcg) in each nostril in morning and evening. Total daily dosage 9 sprays (1,600 mcg).	▪ Slight loss in bone density occurs after 6 mo. Patients with chronic alcohol or tobacco use, strong family history of osteoporosis, or use of drugs that may reduce bone mass shouldn't receive additional therapy; weigh risks and benefits before initial trial. ▪ Contraindicated in hypersensitivity to GnRH analogues or any component of formulation, in undiagnosed vaginal bleeding, in breast-feeding patients, and during pregnancy.

nafcillin sodium
Nafcil, Nallpen, Unipen
Penicillinase-resistant penicillin
Antibiotic
Preg. Risk Category: B

cap: 250 mg;
oral sol: 250
mg/5 ml (after
reconst); **inj:**
500 mg and 1,
2 g; **IV infu-
sion piggy-
back:** 1, 2 g;
**pharm bulk
pkg:** 10 g

*Systemic infections caused by penicillinase-produc-
ing staphylococci —* **Adults:** 2 to 4 g PO daily in divided doses q 6 hr; or 2 to 12 g IM or IV daily in divided doses q 4 to 6 hr. **Children:** 25 to 50 mg/kg PO
daily in divided doses q 6 hr. **Neonates:** 25 mg/kg IV
bid.

- Use cautiously in other drug allergies, especially to cephalosporins, or in GI distress.
- Contraindicated in hypersensitivity to drug
or other penicillins.

naftifine
Naftin
Synthetic allylamine derivative
Antifungal agent
Preg. Risk Category: B

cream: 1%;
gel: 1%

Tinea corporis, tinea cruris, and tinea pedis —
Adults: apply cream to affected area qd, or apply gel
bid in morning and evening.

- Contraindicated in hypersensitivity to drug.
- Safety and efficacy in children < 12 yr not
established.

naloxone hydrochloride
Narcan
Narcotic (opioid) antagonist
Narcotic antagonist
Preg. Risk Category: B

inj: 0.02, 0.4,
1 mg/ml

*Known or suspected narcotic-induced respiratory de-
pression, including that caused by pentazocine and
propoxyphene —* **Adults:** 0.4 to 2 mg IV, SC, or IM
repeated q 2 to 3 min, prn. If no response after 10 mg
given, reconsider diagnosis of narcotic-induced toxicity. **Children:** 0.01 mg/kg IV, followed by 2nd dose of
0.1 mg/kg IV, if needed. If IV route not available, may
give IM or SC in divided doses. **Neonates:** 0.01
mg/kg IV, IM, or SC. May repeat dose q 2 to 3 min
prn.
Postop narcotic depression — **Adults:** 0.1 to 0.2 mg
IV q 2 to 3 min prn. May repeat dosage within 1 to 2
hr, if needed. **Children:** 0.005 to 0.01 mg IV. Repeat
q 2 to 3 min prn. **Neonates (asphyxia neonatorum):**
0.01 mg/kg IV into umbilical vein. May repeat q 2 to
3 min.

- Use cautiously in cardiac irritability and opi-
ate addiction.
- Contraindicated in hypersensitivity to drug.

DRUG / CLASS / CATEGORY	DOSAGE FORMS	INDICATIONS / DOSAGES	KEY PRECAUTIONS
naltrexone hydrochloride ReVia *Narcotic (opioid) antagonist* *Narcotic detoxification adjunct* Preg. Risk Category: C	**tab:** 50 mg	*Adjunct for maintenance of opioid-free state in detoxified individuals* — **Adults:** 25 mg PO. If no withdrawal signs < 1 hr, give additional 25 mg. When patient on 50 mg q 24 hr, may use flexible maint schedule. *Treatment of alcohol dependence* — **Adults:** 50 mg PO qd.	▪ Use cautiously in mild hepatic disease or history of recent hepatic disease. ▪ Contraindicated in patients receiving opioid analgesics, in opioid dependency, in acute opioid withdrawal, in patients with positive urine screen for opioids, in acute hepatitis or liver failure, or in hypersensitivity to drug.
nandrolone decanoate Androlone-D, Decolone, Hybolin Decanoate **nandrolone phenpropionate** Anabolin IM, Androlone, Durabolin, Nandrobolic *Anabolic steroid* *Erythropoietin/antineoplastic* Preg. Risk Category: X Controlled Sub. Sched.: III	**decanoate** — **inj (in oil):** 50, 100, 200 mg/ml. **phenpropionate** — **inj:** 25 mg/ml, 50 mg/ml (in oil)	*Anemias associated with renal insufficiency (decanoate)* — **Adults:** 100 to 200 mg IM weekly in males; 50 to 100 mg/wk in females. **Children 2 to 13 yr:** 25 to 50 mg decanoate IM q 3 to 4 wk. *Control of metastatic breast cancer* — **Adults:** 50 to 100 mg phenpropionate IM weekly.	▪ Use cautiously in diabetes; cardiac, renal, or hepatic disease; epilepsy; or migraine or other conditions that may be aggravated by fluid retention. ▪ Contraindicated in hypersensitivity to anabolic steroids, in males with breast cancer or prostate cancer, in nephrosis, during nephrotic phase of nephritis, in women with breast cancer and hypercalcemia, during pregnancy, or in breast-feeding patients. ▪ Avoid in women of childbearing age until pregnancy ruled out.
naphazoline hydrochloride Allerest, Clear Eyes, Optazine‡, Vasoclear, Privine *Sympathomimetic* *Decongestant/vasoconstrictor* Preg. Risk Category: C	**ophth sol:** 0.012, 0.02, 0.03, 0.1%; **nasal drops and spray (Privine):** 0.05% sol	*Ocular congestion, irritation, itching* — **Adults:** 1 drop 0.1% sol instilled q 3 to 4 hr, or 1 drop 0.012% to 0.03% sol up to qid. *Nasal congestion (Privine)* — **Adults and children >12 yr:** 2 drops or sprays in each nostril q 3 to 4 hr (drops) or 3 to 6 hr (spray). **Children 6 to 12 yr:** 1 to 2 drops or sprays in each nostril q 3 to 6 hr, prn. Don't use > 3 to 5 days.	▪ Use cautiously in hyperthyroidism, cardiac disease, hypertension, or diabetes mellitus. ▪ Contraindicated in hypersensitivity to any drug ingredient. Ophth sol contraindicated in acute angle-closure glaucoma. 0.1% ophth sol contraindicated in children.

naproxen
EC Naprosyn, Inza-250‡, Naprosyn, Naprosyn SR‡, Novo-Naprox†
naproxen sodium
Aleve, Anaprox, Apo-Napro-Na†, Naprelan, Naprogesic‡, Synflex‡
Nonsteroidal anti-inflammatory
Nonnarcotic analgesic/antipyretic/anti-inflammatory
Preg. Risk Category: B

naproxen —
tab: 250, 375, 500 mg; **tab (delayed-release):** 375, 500 mg; **tab (ext-release):** 750, 1,000 mg; **oral susp:** 125 mg/5 ml; **supp:** 500 mg‡. **sodium — tab (contr-release):** 421.5, 550 mg; **tab (film-coated):** 220, 275, 550 mg.
Note: 275 mg naproxen sodium contains 250 mg naproxen.

Rheumatoid arthritis, osteoarthritis, ankylosing spondylitis, pain, dysmenorrhea, tendinitis, bursitis —
Adults: 250 to 500 mg (naproxen) bid; max 1.5 g/day. Or, 375 to 500 mg delayed-release (EC-Naprosyn) bid; or 750 to 1,000 mg contr-release (Naprelan) bid; or 275 to 550 mg naproxen sodium bid.

Juvenile arthritis — **Children:** 10 mg/kg PO in 2 divided doses.

Acute gout — **Adults:** 750 mg (naproxen) PO, then 250 mg q 8 hr until attack subsides. Or, 825 mg naproxen sodium, then 275 mg q 8 hr until attack subsides; or 1,000 to 1,500 mg/day contr-release (Naprelan) on first day, then 1,000 mg qd.

Mild to moderate pain — **Adults:** 500 mg (naproxen) PO, then 250 mg q 6 to 8 hr, up to 1.25 g/day. Or, 550 mg naproxen sodium, then 275 mg q 6 to 8 hr, up to 1.375 g/day; or 1,000 mg contr-release (Naprelan) qd.

- Use cautiously in elderly patients and in renal disease, CV disease, GI disorders, hepatic disease, or history of peptic ulcer disease.
- Contraindicated in hypersensitivity to drug or in syndrome of asthma, rhinitis, and nasal polyps.
- Avoid in last trimester of pregnancy.

---

nedocromil sodium
Tilade
Pyranoquinoline
Anti-inflammatory respiratory inhalant
Preg. Risk Category: B

inhalation aerosol: 1.75 mg/activation

Maintenance in mild to moderate bronchial asthma — **Adults and children ≥ 12 yr:** 2 inhalations qid at regular intervals.

- Contraindicated in hypersensitivity to formulation or during acute asthmatic attack or acute bronchospasm.

DRUG / CLASS / CATEGORY	DOSAGE FORMS	INDICATIONS / DOSAGES	KEY PRECAUTIONS
nefazodone hydrochloride Serzone *Phenylpiperazine* *Antidepressant* Preg. Risk Category: C	**tab:** 100, 150, 200, 250 mg	*Depression* — **Adults:** initially, 200 mg/day PO in 2 divided doses. Increase in increments of 100 to 200 mg/day at intervals of no less than 1 wk. prn. Usual range 300 to 600 mg/day.	■ Use cautiously in CV or cerebrovascular disease that could be exacerbated by hypotension or conditions that predispose to hypotension and in history of mania. ■ Contraindicated in hypersensitivity to drug or other phenylpiperazine antidepressants, within 14 days of MAO inhibitor therapy, and in coadministration with astemizole.
neomycin sulfate Mycifradin, Neo-fradin, Neosulf†, Neo-Tabs *Aminoglycoside* *Antibiotic* Preg. Risk Category: NR	**tab:** 500 mg; **oral sol:** 125 mg/5 ml	*Infectious diarrhea caused by enteropathogenic* E. coli — **Adults:** 50 mg/kg daily PO in 4 divided doses for 2 to 3 days; max 3 g daily usually adequate. **Children:** 50 to 100 mg/kg daily PO divided q 4 to 6 hr for 2 to 3 days. *Suppression of intestinal bacteria preoperatively* — **Adults:** 1 g PO q 1 hr for 4 doses, then 1 g q 4 hr for balance of 24 hr. Saline cathartic should precede therapy. **Children:** 40 to 100 mg/kg PO divided q 4 to 6 hr. First dose should follow saline cathartic.	■ Use cautiously in impaired renal function, neuromuscular disorders, or ulcerative bowel lesions and in elderly patients. Never give parenterally. ■ Contraindicated in hypersensitivity to other aminoglycosides and in intestinal obstruction.
neomycin sulfate Mycifradin†, Myciguent, Neo-Rx *Aminoglycoside* *Antibiotic* Preg. Risk Category: C	**cream:** 0.5%; **oint:** 0.5%	*Prevention or treatment of superficial bacterial infections* — **Adults and children:** rub into affected area qd to tid.	■ Use cautiously in extensive dermatologic conditions. Don't use on > 20% of body surface. ■ Contraindicated in hypersensitivity to drug.
neostigmine bromide Prostigmin **neostigmine methylsulfate**	**inj:** 0.25, 0.5, 1 mg/ml; **tab:** 15 mg	*Symptomatic control of myasthenia gravis* — **Adults:** 0.5 mg SC or IM. PO dose ranges from 15 to 375 mg/day. Subsequent dosages must be individualized. **Children:** 7.5 to 15 mg PO tid to qid.	■ Use cautiously in bronchial asthma, bradycardia, seizure disorders, recent coronary occlusion, vagotonia, hyperthyroidism, arrhythmias, and peptic ulcer.

Prostigmin
Cholinesterase inhibitor
Muscle stimulant
Preg. Risk Category: C

tab: 200 mg

Diagnosis of myasthenia gravis — **Adults:** 0.022 mg/kg IM 30 min after 0.011 mg/kg atropine sulfate IM. **Children:** 0.025 to 0.04 mg/kg IM after 0.011 mg/kg atropine sulfate SC.
Postop abdominal distention and bladder atony — **Adults:** 0.25 to 0.5 mg IM or SC q 4 to 6 hr for 2 to 3 days.
Antidote for nondepolarizing neuromuscular blocking agents — **Adults:** 0.5 to 2 mg IV slowly. Repeat prn to total of 5 mg. Before antidote dose, give 0.6 to 1.2 mg atropine sulfate IV. **Neonates and infants:** 0.04 mg/kg IV with 0.02 mg/kg of atropine sulfate.

- Contraindicated in hypersensitivity to cholinergics and in peritonitis or mechanical obstruction of intestine or urinary tract.

nevirapine
Viramune
Nonnucleoside reverse transcriptase inhibitor
Antiviral
Preg. Risk Category: C

tab: 200 mg

Adjunctive treatment in patients with HIV-1 infection who have experienced clinical or immunologic deterioration — **Adults:** 200 mg PO daily for first 14 days, then 200 mg PO bid. Used in combination with nucleoside analogue antiretroviral agents.

- Use cautiously in impaired renal and hepatic function.
- Contraindicated in hypersensitivity to drug.
- Drug excreted in breast milk.
- Safety and efficacy in children not established.

niacin (vitamin B₃, nicotinic acid)
Niac, Niacor, Nico-400, Nicobid, Nicolar

niacinamide (nicotinamide)
B-complex vitamin
Vitamin B₃/antilipemic
Preg. Risk Category: C

niacin — **tab:** 25, 50, 100, 250, 500 mg; **elixir:** 50 mg/5 ml; **inj:** 100 mg/ml in 30-ml vials. **niacinamide** — **tab:** 50, 100, 125, 250, 500 mg

Pellagra — **Adults:** 300 to 500 mg PO, SC, IM, or IV daily in divided doses, depending on severity of deficiency. **Children:** up to 300 mg PO daily in divided doses, depending on severity of deficiency.
Hyperlipidemias, especially with hypercholesterolemia (niacin only) — **Adults:** 1 to 2 g PO tid with or after meals, increased at intervals to 6 g daily.

- Use cautiously in gallbladder disease, diabetes mellitus, or CAD and in history of liver disease, peptic ulcer, allergy, or gout.
- Contraindicated in hepatic dysfunction, active peptic ulcers, severe hypotension, arterial hemorrhage, or hypersensitivity to drug.

NIACINAMIDE   **175**

†Canadian   ‡Australian

DRUG / CLASS / CATEGORY	DOSAGE FORMS	INDICATIONS / DOSAGES	KEY PRECAUTIONS
nicardipine Cardene, Cardene IV, Cardene SR *Calcium channel blocker* *Antianginal/antihypertensive* Preg. Risk Category: C	*cap (immed-release):* 20, 30 mg; *cap (sust-release):* 30, 45, 60 mg; *inj:* 2.5 mg/ml	*Chronic stable angina, hypertension* — **Adults:** 20 mg PO tid (immed-release only). Titrate according to patient response q 3 days. Usual range 20 to 40 mg tid. *Short-term management of hypertension* — **Adults:** if unable to take orally, give 5 mg/hr IV infusion, titrated to 2.5 mg/hr q 15 min to max 15 mg/hr.	▪ Use cautiously in hypotension, heart failure, and impaired hepatic or renal function. ▪ Contraindicated in hypersensitivity to drug and in advanced aortic stenosis.
nicotine polacrilex [nicotine-polacrilin resin complex] Nicorette, Nicorette DS *Nicotinic agonist* *Smoking cessation aid* Preg. Risk Category: X	*chew gum:* 2, 4 mg/square	*Relief of nicotine withdrawal symptoms in patients undergoing smoking cessation* — **Adults:** initially, one 2-mg square; highly dependent patients should start with 4-mg squares. Patients should chew 1 piece of gum slowly and intermittently for 30 min whenever urge to smoke occurs. Most patients require 9 to 12 pieces of gum daily during 1st mo. For patients using 4-mg squares, max 20 pieces daily. For patients using 2-mg squares, max 30 pieces daily.	▪ Use cautiously in hyperthyroidism, pheochromocytoma, insulin-dependent diabetes, peptic ulcer disease, history of esophagitis, oral or pharyngeal inflammation, or dental conditions that might be exacerbated by chewing gum. ▪ Contraindicated in nonsmokers, recent MI, life-threatening arrhythmias, severe or worsening angina pectoris, temporomandibular joint disease; and during pregnancy.
nicotine transdermal system Habitrol, Nicoderm, Nicotrol, ProStep *Nicotinic cholinergic agonist* *Smoking cessation aid* Preg. Risk Category: D	*transderm system* (releases nicotine at fixed rate): **Habitrol** — 21, 14, 7 mg/day. **Nicoderm** — 21, 14, 7 mg/day. **Nicotrol** — 15, 10, 5 mg/16 hr. **ProStep** — 22, 11 mg/day	*Relief of nicotine withdrawal symptoms in patients undergoing smoking cessation* — **Adults:** initially, 1 transderm system, delivering largest available nicotine dosage in its dosage series, applied qd to nonhairy body part. For Habitrol, Nicoderm, and ProStep, patch should be kept on 24 hr, then removed and new system applied to alternate skin site. For Nicotrol, patch should be applied on awakening and removed hs. After 4 to 12 wk, dosage tapered to next lowest available nicotine dosage in its dosage series, followed in 2 to 4 wk by lowest nicotine dosage system in series being used. Drug then stopped in 2 to 4 wk.	▪ Use cautiously in hyperthyroidism, pheochromocytoma, hypertension, insulin-dependent diabetes, or peptic ulcer disease. ▪ Contraindicated in hypersensitivity to nicotine or any component of transdermal system. Also contraindicated in nonsmokers and in recent MI, life-threatening arrhythmias, and severe or worsening angina pectoris.

Drug	Forms	Indications & dosages	Nursing considerations
nifedipine Adalat, Adalat CC, Anpine‡, Apo-Nifed†, Nu-Nifed†, Procardia, Procardia XL *Calcium channel blocker* *Antianginal* Preg. Risk Category: C	**tab (ext-release):** 30, 60, 90 mg; **cap:** 10, 20 mg	*Prinzmetal's (variant) angina* — **Adults:** starting dose 10 mg PO tid. Usual effective range 10 to 20 mg tid. Max 180 mg daily. *Hypertension* — **Adults:** 30 or 60 mg PO qd. Titrate over 7 to 14 days. Doses > 90 mg (for Adalat CC) and 120 mg (for Procardia XL) not recommended.	▪ Use cautiously in heart failure or hypotension and in elderly patients. Use ext-release tablets cautiously in severe GI narrowing. ▪ Contraindicated in hypersensitivity to drug.
nimodipine Nimotop *Calcium channel blocker* *Cerebral vasodilator* Preg. Risk Category: C	**cap:** 30 mg	*Improvement of neurologic deficits after subarachnoid hemorrhage from ruptured congenital aneurysm* — **Adults:** 60 mg PO q 4 hr for 21 days. Begin therapy within 96 hr after subarachnoid hemorrhage. In patients with hepatic failure, 30 mg PO q 4 hr for 21 days.	▪ Use cautiously in hepatic failure.
nisoldipine Sular *Calcium channel blocker* *Antihypertensive* Preg. Risk Category: C	**tab (ext-release):** 10, 20, 30, 40 mg	*Hypertension* — **Adults:** initially, 20 mg (10 mg if patient > 65 or has liver dysfunction) PO qd; increased by 10 mg/wk or at longer intervals, as needed. Usual maintenance dosage 20 to 40 mg/day. Dosages > 60 mg/day not recommended.	▪ Use cautiously in heart failure or compromised ventricular function, particularly in patients receiving beta blockers and in those with severe hepatic dysfunction. ▪ Contraindicated in hypersensitivity to dihydropyridine calcium channel blockers. ▪ Avoid use in breast-feeding patients.
nitrofurantoin macrocrystals Macrobid, Macrodantin **nitrofurantoin microcrystals** Furadantin, Macrodantin, Nephronex† *Nitrofuran* *Urinary tract anti-infective* Preg. Risk Category: B	**macrocrystals — cap:** 25, 50, 100 mg. **microcrystals — oral susp:** 25 mg/5 ml	*UTI caused by susceptible organisms* — **Adults and children > 12 yr:** 50 to 100 mg PO qid with meals and hs. **Children 1 mo to 12 yr:** 5 to 7 mg/kg PO daily divided qid. *Long-term suppression therapy* — **Adults:** 50 to 100 mg PO daily hs. **Children:** 1 mg/kg PO daily in single dose hs or divided into 2 doses.	▪ Use cautiously in renal impairment, anemia, diabetes mellitus, electrolyte abnormalities, vitamin B deficiency, debilitating disease, and G6PD deficiency. ▪ Contraindicated in children ≤ 1 mo; in moderate to severe renal impairment, anuria, oliguria, or creatinine clearance < 60 ml/min; and in pregnancy at term.

†Canadian ‡Australian

DRUG / CLASS / CATEGORY	DOSAGE FORMS	INDICATIONS / DOSAGES	KEY PRECAUTIONS
nitrofurazone Furacin *Synthetic antibacterial nitrofuran derivative* *Topical antibacterial* Preg. Risk Category: C	*cream:* 0.2%; *oint:* 0.2% (soluble dressing); *topical sol:* 0.2%	*Adjunctive treatment of 2nd- and 3rd-degree burns; prevention of skin allograft rejection* — **Adults and children:** apply directly to lesion daily or q few days, depending on burn severity. May also apply to dressings used to cover affected area.	▪ Use cautiously in known or suspected renal impairment. Monitor serum creatinine regularly. ▪ Contraindicated in hypersensitivity to drug.
nitroglycerin (glyceryl trinitrate) Anginine‡, Coro-Nitra, Nitro-Bid, Nitrocine, Nitrodisc, Nitro-Dur, Nitrogard, Nitroglyn, Nitrol, Nitrolingual, Nitrostat, Transderm-Nitro, Transiderm-Nitro‡, Tridil *Nitrate* *Antianginal/vasodilator* Preg. Risk Category: C	*tab (buccal):* 1, 2, 3 mg; *tab (SL):* 0.15 mg (¹⁄₄₀₀ gr), 0.3 mg (¹⁄₂₀₀ gr), 0.4 mg (¹⁄₁₅₀ gr), 0.6 mg (¹⁄₁₀₀ gr); *tab (sust-release):* 2.6, 6.5, 9, 13 mg; *cap (sust-release):* 2.5, 6.5, 9, 13 mg; *aerosol (translingual):* 0.4 mg metered spray; *topical:* 2% ointment; *transderm:* 0.1, 0.2, 0.3, 0.4, 0.6, 0.8 mg/hr release rate; *inj:* 0.5, 5 mg/ml	*Prophylaxis against chronic anginal attacks* — **Adults:** 2.5 mg or 2.6 mg sust-release capsule q 8 to 12 hr. Or, use 2% ointment range 1/20 to 59. Or, transderm disc or pad 0.2 to 0.4 mg/hr qd. *Acute angina pectoris, prophylaxis to prevent or minimize anginal attacks before stressful events* — **Adults:** 1 SL tab. Repeat q 5 min, if needed, for 15 min. Or, using Nitrolingual spray, 1 or 2 sprays into mouth. Repeat q 3 to 5 min, prn, to max 3 doses in 15-min period. Or, 1 to 3 mg transmucosally q 3 to 5 hr during waking hours. *Hypertension, heart failure, acute angina pectoris, to produce controlled hypotension during surgery (by IV infusion)* — **Adults:** 5 mcg/min, increased prn by 5 mcg/min q 3 to 5 min until response.	▪ Use cautiously in hypotension or volume depletion. ▪ Contraindicated in hypersensitivity to nitrates and in early MI (SL nitroglycerin), severe anemia, increased ICP, angle-closure glaucoma, orthostatic hypotension, and allergy to adhesives (transdermal). IV nitroglycerin contraindicated in hypersensitivity to IV form, cardiac tamponade, restrictive cardiomyopathy, or constrictive pericarditis.

nitroprusside sodium
Nitropress
Vasodilator
Antihypertensive
Preg. Risk Category: C

inj: 50 mg/vial in 2-ml, 5-ml vials

Hypertensive emergencies — Adults and children: 50-mg vial diluted with 2 to 3 ml of D_5W and then added to 250, 500, or 1,000 ml of D_5W; infuse at 0.3 to 10 mcg/kg/min titrated to BP. Max infusion rate 10 mcg/kg/min.

Acute heart failure — Adults and children: IV infusion titrated to cardiac output and systemic BP. Same dosage range as for hypertensive emergencies.

- Use with extreme caution in increased ICP. Use cautiously in hypothyroidism, hepatic or renal disease, hyponatremia, or low vitamin B_{12} concentration.
- Contraindicated in hypersensitivity to drug, compensatory hypertension, inadequate cerebral circulation, acute heart failure associated with reduced peripheral vascular resistance, congenital optic atrophy, or tobacco-induced amblyopia.

nizatidine
Axid, Tazac‡
Histamine₂-receptor antagonist
Antiulcer agent
Preg. Risk Category: C

cap: 150, 300 mg

Active duodenal ulcer — Adults: 300 mg PO daily hs. Or, 150 mg PO bid.
Maintenance therapy for duodenal ulcer — Adults: 150 mg PO daily hs.
Benign gastric ulcer — Adults: 150 mg PO bid or 300 mg hs for 8 wk.
Gastroesophageal reflux disease — Adults: 150 mg PO bid.

- Use cautiously and in reduced dosages in renal impairment.
- Contraindicated in hypersensitivity to H_2-receptor antagonists.
- Safety and efficacy in children not established.

norepinephrine bitartrate
Levophed
Adrenergic
Vasopressor
Preg. Risk Category: C

inj: 1 mg/ml

To maintain BP in acute hypotensive states — Adults: initially, 8 to 12 mcg/min IV infusion, then adjust to maintain normal BP. Avg maintenance dosage 2 to 4 mcg/min. *Children:* 2 mcg/m²/min IV infusion. Adjust dose per response.

- Use with extreme caution in patients receiving MAO inhibitors or triptyline- or imipramine-type antidepressants. Use cautiously in sulfite sensitivity.
- Contraindicated in mesenteric or peripheral vascular thrombosis, profound hypoxia, hypercapnia, or hypotension resulting from blood volume deficit and during cyclopropane and halothane anesthesia.

NOREPINEPHRINE BITARTRATE 179

†Canadian ‡Australian

DRUG/CLASS/CATEGORY	DOSAGE FORMS	INDICATIONS/DOSAGES	KEY PRECAUTIONS
norethindrone Micronor, Norlutin, Nor-Q.D. **norethindrone acetate** Aygestin, Norlutate *Progestin* *Contraceptive* Preg. Risk Category: X	*tab:* 0.35, 5 mg. **acetate** — *tab:* 5 mg	*Amenorrhea, abnormal uterine bleeding* — **Adults:** 2.5 to 20 mg PO daily on days 5 to 25 of menstrual cycle. *Endometriosis* — **Adults:** 5 to 10 mg PO daily for 14 days; then increase by 2.5 to 5 mg daily q 2 wk up to 15 to 30 mg daily. *Contraception in women* — **Adults:** initially, 0.35 mg norethindrone PO on first day of menstruation; then 0.35 mg daily.	▪ Use cautiously in diabetes mellitus, seizures, migraine, cardiac or renal disease, asthma, and mental depression. ▪ Contraindicated in thromboembolic disorders; cerebral apoplexy, or history of these conditions; hypersensitivity to drug, breast cancer, undiagnosed abnormal vaginal bleeding, severe hepatic disease, or missed abortion and during pregnancy.
norfloxacin Noroxin *Fluoroquinolone* *Broad-spectrum antibiotic* Preg. Risk Category: C	*film-coated* *tab:* 400 mg	*UTI caused by susceptible strains of* E. faecalis, E. coli, *and* K. pneumoniae — **Adults:** for uncomplicated infections, 400 mg PO q 12 hr for 7 to 10 days. For complicated infections, 400 mg PO q 12 hr for 10 to 21 days. *Acute, uncomplicated urethral and cervical gonorrhea* — **Adults:** 800 mg PO as single dose, followed by doxycycline to treat coexisting chlamydial infection.	▪ Use cautiously in conditions that may predispose to seizure disorders such as cerebral arteriosclerosis. Also use cautiously in renal impairment. ▪ Contraindicated in hypersensitivity to fluoroquinolones. ▪ Safety in children < 18 yr not established.
norfloxacin Chibroxin *Fluoroquinolone* *Broad-spectrum antibiotic* Preg. Risk Category: C	*ophth sol:* 0.3% in 5-ml containers	*Conjunctivitis caused by susceptible strains of bacteria* — **Adults and children ≥ 1 yr:** 1 drop in affected eye qid for ≤ 7 days. In severe infections, 1 or 2 drops q 2 hr while awake for initial 1 to 2 days of treatment.	▪ Use with caution in breast-feeding patients. ▪ Contraindicated in history of hypersensitivity to norfloxacin or other fluoroquinolone antibiotics. Shouldn't be injected into eye.
norgestrel Ovrette *Progestin* *Contraceptive* Preg. Risk Category: X	*tab:* 0.075 mg	*Contraception in women* — **Adults:** 0.075 mg PO daily.	▪ Use cautiously in diabetes mellitus, seizures, migraine, cardiac or renal disease, asthma, and mental depression. ▪ Contraindicated in thromboembolic disorders, cerebral apoplexy, or history of these

nortriptyline hydrochloride
Allegron‡, Aventyl, Nortab‡, Pamelor
Tricyclic antidepressant
Antidepressant
Preg. Risk Category: NR

tab: 10 mg†, 25 mg†; *cap*: 10, 25, 50, 75 mg; *oral sol*: 10 mg/5 ml (4% alcohol)

Depression — **Adults:** 25 mg PO tid or qid, gradually increased to max 150 mg daily. Entire dosage may be given hs. Monitor plasma levels when giving doses > 100 mg/day.

- conditions; hypersensitivity to drug; breast cancer, undiagnosed abnormal vaginal bleeding, severe hepatic disease, and missed abortion and during pregnancy.
- Use with extreme caution in glaucoma, suicidal tendency, history of urine retention or seizures, CV disease, or hyperthyroidism and in patients taking thyroid medication.
- Contraindicated during acute recovery phase of MI, in hypersensitivity to drug, or within 14 days of MAO inhibitor therapy.

nystatin
Mycostatin, Nadostine†, Nilstat, Nystat-Rx, Nystex
Polyene macrolide
Antifungal
Preg. Risk Category: NR

tab: 500,000 units; *oral susp*: 100,000 units/ml; 50, 150, 500 million units; 1, 2 billion units; *powder*: 150, 250, 500 million units; 1, 2, 5 billion units; *vag supp (as tab)*: 100,000 units; *cream*: 100,000 units/g; *oint*: 100,000 units/g; *powder*: 100,000 units/g; *vag tab*: 100,000 units

Intestinal candidiasis — **Adults:** 500,000 to 1 million units as oral tab tid.
Oral infections — **Adults and children:** 400,000 to 600,000 units oral susp qid. **Infants:** 200,000 units oral susp qid. **Neonates and premature infants:** 100,000 units oral susp qid.
Vaginal infections — **Adults:** 100,000 units as vaginal tablets high into vagina, daily for 14 days.
Cutaneous and mucocutaneous infections caused by C. albicans — **Adults and children:** apply to affected area up to several times daily.

- Safety in breast-feeding patients not established.
- Contraindicated in hypersensitivity to drug.

DRUG/CLASS/ CATEGORY	DOSAGE FORMS	INDICATIONS/ DOSAGES	KEY PRECAUTIONS
octreotide acetate Sandostatin *Synthetic octapeptide* *Somatotropic hormone* Preg. Risk Category: B	*inj (ampules):* 0.05, 0.1, 0.5 mg; *inj (multidose vials):* 0.2, 1 mg/ml	*Flushing and diarrhea associated with carcinoid tumors* — **Adults:** 100 to 600 mcg daily SC in 2 to 4 divided doses for first 2 wk of therapy, then dosage per response. *Watery diarrhea associated with vasoactive intestinal polypeptide secreting tumors* — **Adults:** 200 to 300 mcg daily SC in 2 to 4 divided doses for first 2 wk of therapy. *Acromegaly* — **Adults:** initially, 50 mcg SC tid, then adjusted according to somatomedin C levels q 2 wk.	▪ Monitor baseline thyroid function tests. ▪ Contraindicated in hypersensitivity to drug or any drug component.
ofloxacin Floxin, Floxin IV **ofloxacin 0.3%** Ocuflox *Fluoroquinolone* *Antibiotic* Preg. Risk Category: C	*tab (film-coated):* 200, 300, 400 mg; *inj:* 20, 40 mg/ml; 4 mg/ml premixed in D₅W; *ophth sol:* 0.3%	*Lower resp tract infections* — **Adults:** 400 mg IV or PO q 12 hr for 10 days. *Cervicitis or urethritis* — **Adults:** 300 mg IV or PO q 12 hr for 7 days. *Acute, uncomplicated gonorrhea* — **Adults:** 400 mg IV or PO as single dose with doxycycline. *Mild to moderate skin infections* — **Adults:** 400 mg IV or PO q 12 hr for 10 days. *Cystitis, UTI* — **Adults:** 200 mg IV or PO q 12 hr for 3 to 7 days. *Prostatitis* — **Adults:** 300 mg IV or PO q 12 hr for 6 wk. *Pelvic inflammatory disease (outpatient)* — **Adults:** 400 mg PO q 12 hr for 14 days. *Conjunctivitis* — **Adults and children > 1 yr:** 1 to 2 drops in conjunctival sac 2 to 4 hr qd, while awake, for 1st 2 days and then qid for up to 5 more days.	▪ Use cautiously in history of seizure disorders or other CNS diseases, such as cerebral arteriosclerosis. ▪ Contraindicated in hypersensitivity to drug or other fluoroquinolones and in breast-feeding patients (ophth). ▪ Safety in children < 18 yr unknown.

olanzapine
Zyprexa
Cholinergic
Antipsychotic
Preg. Risk Category: C

tab: 5, 7.5, 10 mg

Psychotic disorders — **Adults:** initially, 5 to 10 mg PO qd. Dosage adjustments in 5-mg daily increments should occur at intervals of not less than 1 wk. Most patients respond to 10 mg/day. Don't exceed 20 mg/day.

- Use cautiously in heart disease, cerebrovascular disease, conditions that predispose to hypotension, history of seizures or conditions that might lower seizure threshold, and hepatic impairment. Also use cautiously in elderly patients, history of paralytic ileus, and patients at risk for aspiration pneumonia, prostatic hypertrophy, or narrow-angle glaucoma.
- Contraindicated in known hypersensitivity to drug.
- Use in pregnancy only if benefit justifies potential risk to fetus. Women taking drug should not breast-feed.
- Safety and effectiveness in children < 18 yr not established.

olsalazine sodium
Dipentum
Salicylate
Anti-inflammatory
Preg. Risk Category: C

cap: 250 mg

Maintenance of remission of ulcerative colitis in patients intolerant of sulfasalazine — **Adults:** 500 mg PO bid with meals.

- Use cautiously in preexisting renal disease.
- Contraindicated in hypersensitivity to salicylates.

omeprazole
Losec‡, Prilosec
Substituted benzimidazole
Gastric acid suppressant
Preg. Risk Category: C

cap (delayed-release): 10, 20 mg

Severe erosive esophagitis; poorly responsive GERD — **Adults:** 20 mg PO daily for 4 to 8 wk.
Pathologic hypersecretory conditions — **Adults:** initially, 60 mg PO daily; titrate according to response. If daily dosage > 80 mg, give in divided doses.
Duodenal ulcer (short-term treatment) — **Adults:** 20 mg PO daily for 4 to 8 wk.
Short-term treatment of active benign gastric ulcer — **Adults:** 40 mg PO qd for 4 to 8 wk.

- Contraindicated in hypersensitivity to drug or any component.
- Safety in children not established.
- Not known if drug excreted in breast milk. Breast-feeding not recommended.

DRUG / CLASS / CATEGORY	DOSAGE FORMS	INDICATIONS / DOSAGES	KEY PRECAUTIONS
ondansetron hydrochloride Zofran *Serotonin (5-HT₃) receptor antagonist* *Antiemetic* Preg. Risk Category: B	*tab:* 4, 8 mg; *inj:* 2, 4 mg/ml; *premixed inj:* 32 mg/50 ml	*Prevention of nausea and vomiting associated with chemotherapy —* **Adults and children ≥ 12 yr:** 8 mg PO 30 min before chemotherapy. Then 8 mg PO 8 hr after first dose, then 8 mg q 12 hr for 1 to 2 days. Or, single dose of 32 mg by IV infusion over 15 min, given 30 min before chemotherapy; or 3 divided doses of 0.15 mg/kg IV given over 15 min, 4 and 8 hr after first dose (30 min before chemotherapy). **Children 4 to 12 yr:** 4 mg PO 30 min before chemotherapy. Then 4 mg PO 4 and 8 hr after first dose, and 4 mg q 8 hr for 1 to 2 days. Or, 3 doses of 0.15 mg/kg IV, given as for adults. *Prevention of nausea and vomiting associated with radiotherapy —* **Adults:** 8 mg PO tid.	• Use cautiously in liver failure. • Contraindicated in hypersensitivity to drug. • Little information available on use in children ≤ 3 yr. • Unknown if excreted in breast milk. Caution recommended.
opium tincture, camphorated (paregoric) *Opiate* *Antidiarrheal* Preg. Risk Category: NR Controlled Sub. Sched.: II (tincture) or III (camphorated)	*oral sol:* equiv to morphine 10 mg/ml; *camphorated — oral sol:* each 5 ml contains morphine, 2 mg; anise oil, 0.2 ml; benzoic acid 20 mg; camphor, 20 mg; glycerin, 0.2 ml; and ethanol to make 5 ml	*Acute diarrhea — tincture —* **Adults:** 0.6 ml (range 0.3 to 1 ml) PO qid. Max 6 ml daily. *camphorated tincture —* **Adults:** 5 to 10 ml PO qd, bid, tid, or qid until diarrhea subsides. **Children:** 0.25 to 0.5 ml/kg camphorated tincture PO qd, bid, tid, or qid until diarrhea subsides.	• Use cautiously in asthma, prostatic hyperplasia, hepatic disease, and history of opioid dependence. • Contraindicated in acute diarrhea caused by poisoning until toxic material removed from GI tract or in diarrhea caused by organisms that penetrate intestinal mucosa. • Do not confuse opium tincture with opium tincture, camphorated.

oxacillin sodium
Bactocill, Prostaphlin
Penicillinase-resistant penicillin
Antibiotic
Preg. Risk Category: B

cap: 250, 500 mg; **oral sol:** 250 mg/5 ml (after reconstitution); **inj:** 250, 500 mg and 1, 2, 4 g; **IV infusion:** 1, 2, 4 g; **pharm bulk pkg:** 4, 10 g

Infections caused by penicillinase-producing staphylococci — **Adults and children > 40 kg:** 500 mg to 1 g PO q 4 to 6 hr; or 2 to 12 g IM or IV qd in divided doses q 4 to 6 hr. **Children ≤ 40 kg:** 50 to 100 mg/kg PO qd in divided doses q 6 hr; or 50 to 200 mg/kg IM or IV qd in divided doses q 4 to 6 hr.

- Use cautiously in other drug allergies, especially to cephalosporins, and in neonates and infants.
- Contraindicated in hypersensitivity to drug or other penicillins.

oxazepam
Alepam‡, Serax, Zapex†
Benzodiazepine
Antianxiety agent/sedative-hypnotic
Preg. Risk Category: NR
Controlled Sub. Sched.: IV

tab: 10, 15, 30 mg; **cap:** 10, 15, 30 mg

Alcohol withdrawal, severe anxiety — **Adults:** 15 to 30 mg PO tid or qid.
Mild to moderate anxiety — **Adults:** 10 to 15 mg PO tid or qid. **Elderly patients:** initially 10 mg tid, increased to 15 mg tid to qid prn.

- Avoid during pregnancy, especially first trimester.
- Contraindicated in psychosis or hypersensitivity to drug.

oxiconazole nitrate
Oxistat
Ergosterol synthesis inhibitor
Antifungal
Preg. Risk Category: B

cream: 1%; **lotion:** 1%

Tinea pedis, tinea cruris, and tinea corporis caused by T. rubrum or T. mentagrophytes — **Adults:** apply to affected area qd or bid. Treat tinea cruris and tinea corporis for 2 wk and tinea pedis for 1 mo to minimize risk of recurrence.

- Use cautiously in breast-feeding patients.
- Contraindicated in hypersensitivity to drug.

oxtriphylline (choline salt of theophyllinate)
Choledyl
Xanthine derivative
Bronchodilator
Preg. Risk Category: C

tab: 100, 200 mg; **tab (ext-release):** 400, 600 mg; **tab (delayed-release)** 200 mg; **elixir:** 100 mg/ 5 ml; **syrup:** 50 mg/5 ml

Acute bronchial asthma and reversible bronchospasm associated with chronic bronchitis and emphysema — **Adults and children > 12 yr:** 200 mg PO q 6 hr; or 400 to 600 mg sust-release tab q 12 hr. **Children 2 to 12 yr:** 4 mg/kg PO q 6 hr. Increase as needed to maintain therapeutic theophylline levels (usually 10 to 20 mcg/ml, but some patients may respond to lower levels).

- Use cautiously in young children, elderly patients, and peptic ulcer, COPD, cardiac failure, cor pulmonale, renal or hepatic impairment, glaucoma, severe hypoxemia, hypertension, compromised cardiac or circulatory function, angina, acute MI, sulfite sensitivity, hyperthyroidism, or diabetes mellitus.
- Contraindicated in hypersensitivity to xanthines and in preexisting arrhythmias, especially tachyarrhythmias.

†Canadian ‡Australian

OXTRIPHYLLINE **185**

DRUG/CLASS / CATEGORY	DOSAGE FORMS	INDICATIONS / DOSAGES	KEY PRECAUTIONS
oxybutynin chloride Ditropan *Synthetic tertiary amine* *Antispasmodic* Preg. Risk Category: B	*tab:* 5 mg; *syrup:* 5 mg/5 ml	*Antispasmodic for uninhibited or reflex neurogenic bladder* — **Adults:** 5 mg PO bid to tid, to max 5 mg qid. **Children > 5 yr:** 5 mg PO bid, to max 5 mg tid.	▪ Use cautiously in elderly patients and in autonomic neuropathy, reflux esophagitis, and hepatic or renal disease. ▪ Contraindicated in hypersensitivity to drug, myasthenia gravis, GI obstruction, untreated narrow-angle glaucoma, adynamic ileus, megacolon, severe colitis, ulcerative colitis when megacolon present, or obstructive uropathy; in elderly or debilitated patients with intestinal atony; and in hemorrhaging patients with unstable CV status.
oxycodone hydrochloride Endone‡, Roxicodone, Roxicodone Intensol, Supeudol† **oxycodone pectinate** Proladone‡ *Opioid* *Analgesic* Preg. Risk Category: C Controlled Sub. Sched.: II	*cap:* 5 mg; *tab:* 5 mg; *tab (con-tr-release):* 10, 20, 40 mg; *oral sol:* 5 mg/5 ml, 20 mg/ml (con-centrate); *supp:* 10, 20 mg. **pectinate —** *supp:* 30 mg‡	*Moderate to severe pain* — **Adults:** 5 mg PO q 6 hr, prn. Or, 1 to 3 supp rectally daily, prn.	▪ Use with extreme caution in head injury, increased ICP, seizures, asthma, COPD, prostatic hyperplasia, severe hepatic or renal disease, acute abdominal conditions, urethral stricture, hypothyroidism, Addison's disease, and arrhythmias. Also use with extreme caution in elderly or debilitated patients. ▪ Contraindicated in hypersensitivity to drug.
oxymetazoline hydrochloride Afrin, Allerest 12-Hr Nasal *Sympathomimetic* *Decongestant/vasoconstrictor* Preg. Risk Category: NR	*nasal sol:* 0.025%, 0.05%	*Nasal congestion* — **Adults and children ≥ 6 yr:** 2 to 3 drops or sprays of 0.05% sol in each nostril bid. **Children 2 to 6 yr:** 2 to 3 drops of 0.025% sol in each nostril bid. Don't use > 3 to 5 days.	▪ Use cautiously in hyperthyroidism, cardiac disease, hypertension, or diabetes mellitus. ▪ Contraindicated in hypersensitivity to drug.

oxymetazoline hydrochloride
OcuClear, Visine L.R.
Sympathomimetic
Decongestant/vasoconstrictor
Preg. Risk Category: C

ophth sol: 0.025%

Relief of eye redness due to minor eye irritations — **Adults and children ≥ 6 yr:** 1 to 2 drops in conjunctival sac 2 to 4 times daily (spaced ≥ 6 hr apart).

- Use cautiously in hyperthyroidism, cardiac disease, hypertension, eye disease, infection, or injury.
- Contraindicated in hypersensitivity to any component of drug and in angle-closure glaucoma.

oxymorphone hydrochloride
Numorphan, Numorphan H.P.
Opioid
Analgesic
Preg. Risk Category: C
Controlled Sub. Sched.: II

inj: 1, 1.5 mg/ml; **supp:** 5 mg

Moderate to severe pain — **Adults:** 1 to 1.5 mg IM or SC q 4 to 6 hr, prn; or 0.5 mg IV q 4 to 6 hr, prn; or 5 mg rectally q 4 to 6 hr, prn.
Analgesia during labor — **Adults:** 0.5 to 1 mg IM.

- Use with extreme caution in head injury, increased ICP, seizures, asthma, COPD, acute abdominal conditions, prostatic hyperplasia, severe hepatic or renal disease, urethral stricture, respiratory depression, hypothyroidism, Addison's disease, and arrhythmias. Also use with extreme caution in elderly or debilitated patients.
- Contraindicated in hypersensitivity to drug.

oxytetracycline hydrochloride
Terramycin, Uri-Tet
Tetracycline
Antibiotic
Preg. Risk Category: D

cap: 250 mg; **inj:** 50 mg/ml, 125 mg/ml (with lidocaine 2%)

Infections caused by susceptible gram-neg and gram-pos organisms — **Adults:** 250 mg PO q 6 hr; 250 mg IM q 24 hr; or 300 mg IM divided q 8 to 12 hr. **Children > 8 yr:** 25 to 50 mg/kg PO daily, in divided doses q 6 hr; 15 to 25 mg/kg IM daily, in divided doses q 8 to 12 hr.
Syphilis in patients allergic to penicillin — **Adults:** 30 to 40 g total dosage PO, divided equally over 10 to 15 days.
Gonorrhea in patients allergic to penicillin — **Adults:** initially, 1.5 g PO, then 0.5 g qid, for total of 9 g.

- Use cautiously in impaired renal or hepatic function.
- Use during last half of pregnancy and in children < 9 yr may cause permanent tooth discoloration, enamel defects, and bone growth retardation.
- Contraindicated in hypersensitivity to drug or other tetracyclines.

oxytocin, synthetic injection
Oxytocin, Pitocin, Syntocinon
Exogenous hormone
Oxytocic

inj: 10 units/ml ampule, vial, or tubex

Induction or stimulation of labor — **Adults:** initially, 1-ml (10 units) ampule in 1,000 ml D₅W inj or 0.9% NaCl sol IV infused at 1 to 2 milliunits/min. Rate increased in increments of not > 1 to 2 milliunits/min at 15- to 30-min intervals.

- Use with extreme caution during 1st and 2nd stages of labor and, if at all, in history of cervical or uterine surgery (including cesarean section), grand multiparity, uterine

(continued)

DRUG/CLASS/ CATEGORY	DOSAGE FORMS	INDICATIONS/ DOSAGES	KEY PRECAUTIONS
oxytocin, synthetic injection *(continued)* Preg. Risk Category: NR		*Reduction of postpartum bleeding after placenta expulsion* — **Adults:** 10 to 40 units added to 1,000 ml D₅W or 0.9% NaCl sol infused at rate necessary to control bleeding, usually 20 to 40 milliunits/min. Also, 1 ml (10 units) can be given IM after placenta delivery. *Incomplete or inevitable abortion* — **Adults:** 10 units IV in 500 ml 0.9% NaCl sol or dextrose 5% in 0.9% NaCl sol. Infuse at 10 to 20 milliunits (20 to 40 drops)/min.	sepsis, traumatic delivery, or overdistended uterus and in invasive cervical cancer. ▪ Contraindicated in cephalopelvic disproportion or when delivery requires conversion, as in transverse lie; fetal distress when delivery not imminent, prematurity, and other obstetric emergencies; severe toxemia, hypertonic uterine patterns, total placenta previa, or vasoprevia; and hypersensitivity.
oxytocin, synthetic nasal solution Syntocinon *Exogenous hormone* *Lactation stimulant* Preg. Risk Category: X	**nasal sol:** 40 units/ml	*Promotion of initial milk ejection* — **Adults:** 1 spray into one or both nostrils 2 or 3 min before breast-feeding.	▪ Contraindicated in hypersensitivity to drug and during pregnancy.
p			
paclitaxel Taxol *Novel antimicrotuble* *Antineoplastic* Preg. Risk Category: D	**inj:** 30 mg/5 ml, 100 mg/17 ml	*Metastatic ovarian cancer after failure of 1st-line or subsequent chemotherapy* — **Adults:** 135 or 175 mg/m² IV over 3 hr q 3 wk. *Breast cancer after failure of combination chemotherapy for metastatic disease or relapse within 6 mo of adjuvant chemotherapy* — **Adults:** 175 mg/m² IV over 3 hr q 3 wk.	▪ Use cautiously in hepatic impairment. ▪ Contraindicated in hypersensitivity to drug or to polyoxyethylated castor oil and in baseline neutrophil count <1,500/mm³.

pamidronate disodium Aredia *Bisphosphonate/pyrophosphate analogue* *Antihypercalcemic* Preg. Risk Category: C	*inj:* 30-, 60-, 90-mg vials	*Moderate to severe hypercalcemia associated with cancer (with or without bone metastases)* — **Patients with CCa levels 12 to 13.5 mg/dl:** 60 to 90 mg by IV infusion over 4 hr for 60-mg dose and over 24 hr for 90-mg dose. **Patients with CCa levels > 13.5 mg/dl:** 90 mg by IV infusion over 24 hr. Min of 7 days before retreatment. *Moderate to severe Paget's disease* — **Adults:** 30 mg IV as 4-hr infusion qd on 3 consecutive days for total dose of 90 mg. Repeat as needed. *Osteolytic bone lesions of multiple myeloma in combination with standard antineoplastic therapy* — **Adults:** 90 mg IV infusion over 4 hr q 4 wk.	• Use with extreme caution in renal impairment and weigh risks against benefits. • Contraindicated in hypersensitivity to drug or to other biphosphonates such as etidronate.
pancreatin Bioglan Panazyme†, Dizymes Tablets, 4X Pancreatin 600 mg, Hi-Vegi-Lip Tablets, Pancrezyme 4X Tablets *Pancreatic enzyme* *Digestant* Preg. Risk Category: C	*tab (reg or enteric-coated):* 250 to 7,200 mg pancreatin, plus varying amt of lipase, protease, and amylase. Consult reference or pkg insert for specifics.	*Exocrine pancreatic secretion insufficiency; digestive aid in diseases associated with deficiency of pancreatic enzymes, such as cystic fibrosis* — **Adults and children:** 1 to 2 tab PO with meals.	• Use with caution in pregnant or breast-feeding patients. • Contraindicated in hypersensitivity to drug or to pork protein or enzymes, in acute pancreatitis, or in acute exacerbation of chronic pancreatitis.
pancrelipase Cotazym Capsules, Creon 5 Capsules, Creon 10 Capsules, Ilozyme tab, Ku-Zyme HP Capsules, Pancrease Capsules, Pancrease MT 16, Pancrelipase Capsules, Protilase Capsules, Ultrase	*cap (enteric-coated, delayed-release), tab, powder, enteric-coated microtabs:*	*Exocrine pancreatic secretion insufficiency, cystic fibrosis, steatorrhea and other disorders of fat metabolism secondary to insufficient pancreatic enzymes* — **Adults and children ≥ 12 yr:** dosage titrated to patient response. Usual initial dosage 4,000 to 48,000 units lipase with each meal. **Children 7 to 12 yr:** 4,000 to 12,000 units (more, if needed) lipase with	• Should be used only after confirmed diagnosis of exocrine pancreatic insufficiency. Not effective in GI disorders unrelated to enzyme deficiency. • Contraindicated in severe hypersensitivity to pork or in acute pancreatitis or acute exacerbations of chronic pancreatic diseases. *(continued)*

PANCRELIPASE **189**

DRUG/CLASS/CATEGORY	DOSAGE FORMS	INDICATIONS/DOSAGES	KEY PRECAUTIONS
pancrelipase *(continued)* MT 12, Viokase Powder, Zymase Capsules *Pancreatic enzyme Digestant* Preg. Risk Category: C	contain varying amt of lipase, protease, and amylase	each meal or snack. **Children 1 to 6 yr:** 4,000 to 8,000 units lipase with each meal and 4,000 units lipase with each snack. **Children 6 mo to 1 yr:** 2,000 units lipase with each meal. **Children < 6 mo:** dosage not established.	
pancuronium bromide Pavulon *Nondepolarizing neuromuscular blocker Skeletal muscle relaxant* Preg. Risk Category: C	*inj:* 1, 2 mg/ml	*Adjunct to anesthesia to induce skeletal muscle relaxation; to facilitate intubation; to lessen muscle contractions in pharmacologically or electrically induced seizures; to assist with mechanical ventilation —* Dosage depends on anesthetic used, individual needs, and response. Dosages listed are representative only. **Adults and children ≥ 1 mo:** initially, 0.04 to 0.1 mg/kg IV; then 0.01 mg/kg q 30 to 60 min.	▪ Use cautiously in elderly or debilitated patients; in renal, hepatic, or pulmonary impairment; in respiratory depression, myasthenia gravis, myasthenic syndrome of lung cancer or bronchogenic carcinoma, dehydration, thyroid disorders, collagen diseases, porphyria, electrolyte disturbances, hyperthermia, and toxemic states. ▪ Use large doses cautiously in patients undergoing cesarean section. ▪ Contraindicated in hypersensitivity to bromides or preexisting tachycardia and when even minor increase in HR undesirable.
paromomycin sulfate Humatin *Aminoglycoside Antibacterial amebicide* Preg. Risk Category: C	*cap:* 250 mg	*Intestinal amebiasis, acute and chronic —* **Adults and children:** 25 to 35 mg/kg daily PO in 3 doses with meals for 5 to 10 days. *Tapeworms (fish, beef, pork, dog) —* **Adults:** 1 g PO q 15 min for 4 doses. **Children:** 11 mg/kg PO q 15 min for 4 doses.	▪ Use cautiously in ulcerative bowel lesions. Poorly absorbed orally, but will accumulate in patients with renal impairment or ulcerative lesions. ▪ Contraindicated in hypersensitivity to drug, impaired renal function, or intestinal obstruction.

paroxetine hydrochloride
Paxil
Selective serotonin reuptake inhibitor
Antidepressant
Preg. Risk Category: B

tab: 20, 30 mg

Depression — **Adults:** initially, 20 mg PO qd, in morning. If no response, may increase in 10-mg/day increments to max 50 mg qd. **Elderly or debilitated patients, patients with severe hepatic or renal disease:** initially, 10 mg PO qd, in morning. If no response, may increase in 10-mg/day increments to max 40 mg qd.
Panic disorder — **Adults:** initially, 10 mg/day. May increase in 10-mg/wk increments. Max dosage ≤ 60 mg/day.

- Use cautiously in history of seizure disorders or mania, in severe, concomitant systemic illness, and in high risk for volume depletion.
- Contraindicated in hypersensitivity to drug, in patients taking MAO inhibitors, or within 14 days of MAO inhibitor therapy.

---

pemoline
Cylert, Cylert Chewable
Oxazolidinedione derivative/CNS stimulant
Analeptic
Preg. Risk Category: B
Controlled Sub. Sched.: IV

tab: 18.75, 37.5, 75 mg;
tab (chew): 37.5 mg

Attention deficit hyperactivity disorder (ADHD) — **Children ≥ 6 yr:** initially, 37.5 mg PO in morning with daily dosage raised by 18.75 mg weekly, prn. Effective dosage range 56.25 to 75 mg daily; max 112.5 mg daily.

- Use cautiously in impaired renal function.
- Contraindicated in hepatic dysfunction and hypersensitivity or idiosyncrasy to drug.

---

penbutolol sulfate
Levatol, Lobeta‡
Beta-adrenergic blocker
Antihypertensive
Preg. Risk Category: C

tab: 20 mg

Mild to moderate hypertension — **Adults:** 20 mg PO qd. Usually given with other antihypertensives, such as thiazide diuretics.

- Use cautiously in diabetes mellitus, in heart failure controlled by drug therapy, and in history of bronchospastic disease.
- Contraindicated in hypersensitivity to drug or other beta blockers and in sinus bradycardia, cardiogenic shock, overt cardiac failure, > first-degree heart block, or bronchial asthma.

---

penicillin G benzathine (benzylpenicillin benzathine)
Bicillin L-A, Permapen
Natural penicillin
Antibiotic
Preg. Risk Category: B

inj: 300,000, 600,000 units/ml

Congenital syphilis — **Children < 2 yr:** 50,000 units/kg IM once.
Group A strep upper resp infections — **Adults:** 1.2 million units IM once. **Children > 27 kg:** 900,000 units IM once. **Children < 27 kg:** 300,000 to 600,000 units IM once.

- Use cautiously in other drug allergies, especially to cephalosporins.
- Contraindicated in hypersensitivity to drug or other penicillins.

(continued)

†Canadian ‡Australian

PENICILLIN G BENZATHINE 191

DRUG / CLASS / CATEGORY	DOSAGE FORMS	INDICATIONS / DOSAGES	KEY PRECAUTIONS
penicillin G benzathine *(continued)*		*Prophylaxis of poststreptococcal rheumatic fever* — **Adults and children:** 1.2 million units IM q mo or 600,000 units twice monthly. *Syphilis* — **Adults:** 2.4 million units IM once (< 1-yr duration), or q wk for 3 wk (> 1-yr duration).	
penicillin G potassium (benzylpenicillin potassium) Megacillin†, Pfizerpen *Natural penicillin* *Antibiotic* Preg. Risk Category: B	**tab:** 500,000 units†; **oral susp:** 250,000†, 500,000 units†; **inj:** 1 million, 5 million, 10 million, 20 million units	*Moderate to severe systemic infection* — **Adults and children ≥ 12 yr:** individualized; 1.6 to 3.2 million units PO qd in divided doses q 6 hr; 1.2 to 24 million units IM or IV qd in divided doses q 4 hr. **Children < 12 yr:** 25,000 to 100,000 units/kg PO qd in divided doses q 6 hr; or 25,000 to 400,000 units/kg IM or IV qd in divided doses q 4 hr.	▪ Use cautiously in other drug allergies, especially to cephalosporins. ▪ Contraindicated in hypersensitivity to drug or other penicillins.
penicillin G procaine (benzylpenicillin procaine) Ayercillin†, Crysticillin 300 A.S., Wycillin *Natural penicillin* *Antibiotic* Preg. Risk Category: B	**inj:** 300,000, 500,000, 600,000 units/ml	*Moderate to severe systemic infection* — **Adults:** 600,000 to 1.2 million units IM qd in single dose. **Children > 1 mo:** 25,000 to 50,000 units/kg IM qd in single dose. *Uncomplicated gonorrhea* — **Adults and children > 12 yr:** 1 g probenecid PO; after 30 min, 4.8 million units IM, divided between 2 sites. *Pneumococcal pneumonia* — **Adults and children > 12 yr:** 600,000 to 1.2 million units IM qd for 7 to 10 days.	▪ Use cautiously in other drug allergies, especially to cephalosporins. Some formulations contain sulfites, which may cause allergic reactions in sensitive persons. ▪ Contraindicated in hypersensitivity to drug or other penicillins.
penicillin G sodium (benzylpenicillin sodium) Crystapen†	**inj:** 5 million-units vial	*Moderate to severe systemic infection* — **Adults and children ≥ 12 yr:** 1.2 to 24 million units daily IM or IV	▪ Use cautiously in other drug allergies, especially to cephalosporins.

Drug		Indications & dosages	Nursing considerations
Natural penicillin *Antibiotic* Preg. Risk Category: B		in divided doses q 4 to 6 hr. **Children < 12 yr:** 25,000 to 400,000 units/kg daily IM or IV in divided doses q 4 to 6 hr.	▪ Contraindicated in hypersensitivity to drug or other penicillins and in patients on sodium-restricted diets.
penicillin V (phenoxyethylpenicillin) penicillin V potassium (phenoxyethylpenicillin potassium) Abbocillin VK‡, Pen Vee K *Natural penicillin* *Antibiotic* Preg. Risk Category: B	*tab:* 250, 500 mg; *oral susp:* 125, 250 mg/5 ml (after reconst). **potassium — tab:** 125, 250, 500 mg; *tab (film-coated):* 250, 500 mg; *cap:* 250 mg‡; *oral susp:* 125, 250 mg/5 ml (after reconst)	*Mild to moderate systemic infections* — **Adults and children ≥ 12 yr:** 250 to 500 mg (400,000 to 800,000 units) PO q 6 hr. **Children < 12 yr:** 15 to 62.5 mg/kg (25,000 to 100,000 units/kg) PO qd, in divided doses q 6 to 8 hr. *Endocarditis prophylaxis for dental surgery* — **Adults:** 2 g PO 30 to 60 min before procedure; then 1 g 6 hr after. **Children < 30 kg:** ½ adult dose.	▪ Use cautiously in other drug allergies, especially to cephalosporins. ▪ Contraindicated in hypersensitivity to drug or other penicillins.
pentamidine isethionate NebuPent, Pentacarinat *Diamidine derivative* *Antiprotozoal* Preg. Risk Category: C	*inj:* 300-mg vial; *aerosol:* 300-mg vial	*Pneumocystis carinii pneumonia* — **Adults and children:** 3 to 4 mg/kg IV or IM qd for 14 to 21 days. *Prevention of P. carinii pneumonia in high-risk individuals* — **Adults:** 300 mg by inhalation q 4 wk.	▪ Use cautiously in hypertension, hypotension, hypoglycemia, hypocalcemia, leukopenia, thrombocytopenia, anemia, or hepatic or renal dysfunction. ▪ Contraindicated in history of anaphylactic reaction to drug.
pentazocine hydrochloride Fortral‡, Talwin † **pentazocine hydrochloride and naloxone hydrochloride** Talwin-Nx	*tab:* 25 mg‡, 50 mg‡. **hydrochloride and naloxone — tab:** 50 mg hydrochloride and	*Moderate to severe pain* — **Adults:** 50 to 100 mg PO q 3 to 4 hr, prn. Max oral dosage 600 mg/day. Or, 30 mg IM, IV, or SC q 3 to 4 hr, prn. Max parenteral dosage 360 mg/day. Single doses > 30 mg IV or 60 mg IM or SC not recommended.	▪ Use cautiously in hepatic or renal disease, acute MI, head injury, increased ICP, and respiratory depression. ▪ Contraindicated in hypersensitivity to drug or any component.

(continued)

DRUG/CLASS/CATEGORY	DOSAGE FORMS	INDICATIONS/DOSAGES	KEY PRECAUTIONS
pentazocine *(continued)* **pentazocine lactate** Fortral‡, Talwin *Narcotic agonist-antagonist/opioid partial agonist Analgesic/adjunct to anesthesia* Preg. Risk Category: C Controlled Sub. Sched.: IV	500 mcg naloxone. **lactate** — *inj:* 30 mg/ml	*Labor* — **Adults:** 30 mg IM or 20 mg IV q 2 to 3 hr with regular contractions.	▪ Not recommended for children < 12 yr.
pentobarbital (pentobarbitone) Nembutal **pentobarbital sodium** Carbrital‡, Nembutal Sodium, Nova Rectal† *Barbiturate Anticonvulsant/sedative-hypnotic* Preg. Risk Category: D (suppositories C) Controlled Sub. Sched.: II (suppositories III)	*elixir:* 18.2 mg/5 ml. **sodium** — *cap:* 50, 100 mg; *inj:* 50 mg/ml; *supp:* 30, 60, 120, 200 mg	*Sedation* — **Adults:** 20 to 40 mg PO bid, tid, or qid. **Children:** 2 to 6 mg/kg daily PO in 3 divided doses. Max 100 mg daily. *Insomnia* — **Adults:** 100 to 200 mg PO hs or 150 to 200 mg deep IM; 100 mg initially IV, then additional doses up to 500 mg; 120 or 200 mg PR. **Children:** 2 to 6 mg/kg or 125 mg/m² IM. Max 100 mg. For child 2 mo to 1 yr, 30 mg PR; 1 yr to 4 yr, 30 or 60 mg; 5 to 11 yr, 60 mg; 12 to 14 yr, 60 or 120 mg. *Preop sedation* — **Adults:** 150 to 200 mg IM. **Children:** 5 mg/kg PO or IM ≥ 10 yr; 5 mg/kg IM or rectally if < 10 yr.	▪ Use cautiously in acute or chronic pain, mental depression, suicidal tendencies, history of drug abuse, or hepatic impairment and in elderly or debilitated patients. ▪ Contraindicated in hypersensitivity to barbiturates, or porphyria.
pentostatin (2'-deoxyco-formycin) Nipent *Antimetabolite (adenosine deaminase inhibitor) Antineoplastic* Preg. Risk Category: D	*powder for inj:* 10 mg-vial	*Alpha-interferon-refractory hairy-cell leukemia* — **Adults:** 4 mg/m² IV every other wk.	▪ Use cautiously and only under supervision of doctor qualified and experienced in use of chemotherapeutic agents. Adverse reactions common. ▪ Contraindicated in hypersensitivity to drug.

pentoxifylline Trental *Xanthine derivative* *Hemorrheologic* Preg. Risk Category: C	**tab (ext-release):** 400 mg	*Intermittent claudication caused by chronic occlusive vascular disease* — **Adults:** 400 mg PO tid with meals. May decrease to 400 mg bid if adverse GI and CNS effects occur.	▪ Contraindicated in intolerance to methylxanthines (such as caffeine, theophylline, and theobromine) and in recent cerebral or retinal hemorrhage.
pergolide mesylate Permax *Dopaminergic agonist* *Antiparkinson agent* Preg. Risk Category: B	**tab:** 0.05, 0.25, 1 mg	*Adjunctive treatment with carbidopa-levodopa in Parkinson's disease* — **Adults:** initially, 0.05 mg PO every day for first 2 days, then increase to 0.1 to 0.15 mg every third day over 12 days. Subsequent dosage increased by 0.25 mg every third day, if needed, until optimum clinical response seen. Usually given in divided doses tid.	▪ Use cautiously in predisposition to arrhythmias. ▪ Contraindicated in hypersensitivity to drug or ergot alkaloids.
permethrin Elimite, Nix *Synthetic pyrethroid* *Scabicide/pediculicide* Preg. Risk Category: B	**topical liq (cream-rinse):** 1%; **cream:** 5%	*Infestation with Pediculus humanus capitis (head lice) and its nits* — **Adults and children:** use after hair washed with shampoo, rinsed with water, and towel-dried. Apply 25 to 50 ml liquid to saturate hair and scalp. Allow to remain on hair for 10 min before rinsing off with water. *Treatment of Sarcoptes scabiei* — **Adults and children:** thoroughly massage into skin from head to soles. Infants should be treated on hairline, neck, scalp, temple, and forehead. Cream should be removed after 8 to 14 hr by washing.	▪ Contraindicated in hypersensitivity to pyrethrins or chrysanthemums.
perphenazine Apo-Perphenazine†, PMS Perphenazine†, Trilafon, Trilafon Concentrate *Phenothiazine (piperazine derivative)* *Antipsychotic/antiemetic* Preg. Risk Category: NR	**tab:** 2, 4, 8, 16 mg; **oral conc:** 16 mg/5 ml; **syrup:** 2 mg/5 ml‡; **inj:** 5 mg/ml	*Psychosis in nonhospitalized patients* — **Adults:** 4 to 8 mg PO tid, reduced soon to minimum effective dosage. **Children > 12 yr:** lowest adult dose. *Psychosis in hospitalized patients* — **Adults:** initially, 8 to 16 mg PO bid, tid, or qid, increased to 64 mg daily, prn. Or, 5 to 10 mg IM q 6 hr, prn. Max 30 mg. **Children > 12 yr:** lowest adult dose.	▪ Use cautiously with other CNS depressants or anticholinergics and in elderly or debilitated patients, alcohol withdrawal, depression, suicidal tendency, severe adverse reactions to other phenothiazines, impaired renal function, and respiratory disorders.

(continued)

†Canadian ‡Australian

PERPHENAZINE 195

DRUG/CLASS/ CATEGORY	DOSAGE FORMS	INDICATIONS/ DOSAGES	KEY PRECAUTIONS
perphenazine (continued)		*Severe nausea and vomiting* — **Adults:** 8 to 16 mg PO daily in divided doses to max 24 mg. Or, 5 to 10 mg IM, prn. May give IV, diluted to 0.5 mg/ml with 0.9% NaCl solution. Max 5 mg.	▪ Contraindicated in hypersensitivity to drug; in coma, CNS depression, blood dyscrasia, bone marrow depression, liver damage, or subcortical damage; and in patients receiving large doses of CNS depressants.
phenobarbital (phenobarbitone) Ancalix†, Barbita, Solfoton phenobarbital sodium (phenobarbitone sodium) Luminal Sodium Barbiturate Anticonvulsant/sedative-hypnotic Preg. Risk Category: D Controlled Sub. Sched.: IV	*tab:* 15, 16, 30, 32, 60, 65, 100 mg; *cap:* 16 mg; *elixir:* 15, 20 mg/5 ml; *inj:* 30, 60, 65, 130 mg/ml	*All forms of epilepsy, febrile seizures* — **Adults:** 60 to 200 mg PO daily in divided doses tid or as single dose hs. **Children:** 3 to 6 mg/kg PO daily, usually divided q 12 hr. Can give qd, usually hs. *Status epilepticus* — **Adults:** 200 to 600 mg IV. **Children:** 100 to 400 mg IV. Max 50 mg/min. *Sedation* — **Adults:** 30 to 120 mg PO daily in 2 or 3 divided doses. **Children:** 3 to 5 mg/kg PO daily in divided doses tid. *Insomnia* — **Adults:** 100 to 200 mg PO or IM hs. *Preop sedation* — **Adults:** 100 to 200 mg IM 60 to 90 min before surgery. **Children:** 16 to 100 mg IM or 1 to 3 mg/kg IV, IM, or PO 60 to 90 min before surgery.	▪ Use cautiously in acute or chronic pain, depression, suicidal tendencies, history of drug abuse, BP alterations, CV disease, shock, or uremia and in elderly or debilitated patients. ▪ Contraindicated in barbiturate hypersensitivity, history of manifest or latent porphyria, hepatic dysfunction, respiratory disease with dyspnea or obstruction, and nephritis.
phensuximide Milontin *Succinimide derivative* Anticonvulsant Preg. Risk Category: NR	*cap:* 500 mg	*Absence seizures* — **Adults and children:** 500 mg to 1 g PO bid or tid.	▪ Use with extreme caution in hepatic or renal disease. ▪ Contraindicated in hypersensitivity to succinimide derivatives.

phentermine hydrochloride
Fastin, Obe-Mar, Panshape M, Phentercot, Phentride
Amphetamine congener
Short-term adjunctive anorexigenic/indirect acting sympathomimetic amine
Preg. Risk Category: X

tab: 8, 30, 37.5 mg; *cap:* 15, 18.75, 37.5 mg; *cap (resin complex,* *sust-rel):* 15, 30 mg

Short-term adjunct in exogenous obesity — **Adults:** 8 mg PO tid ½ hr before meals. Or, 15 to 30 mg (resin complex) or 15 to 37.5 mg (hydrochloride) PO daily as single dose in morning.

- Use cautiously in mild hypertension.
- Contraindicated in hyperthyroidism, moderate to severe hypertension, advanced arteriosclerosis, symptomatic CV disease, glaucoma, or hypersensitivity or idiosyncrasy to sympathomimetic amines; within 14 days of MAO inhibitor therapy; and in agitated patients.

---

phentolamine mesylate
Regitine, Rogitine†
Alpha-adrenergic blocker
Antihypertensive agent for pheochromocytoma/cutaneous vasodilator
Preg. Risk Category: C

inj: 5 mg/ml in 1-ml vials

To aid pheochromocytoma diagnosis; to control or prevent hypertension before or during pheochromocytomectomy — **Adults:** IV diagnostic dose 2.5 mg. Before tumor removal, 5 mg IM or IV. During surgery, may give 5 mg IV. **Children:** IV diagnostic dose 1 mg. Before tumor removal, 1 mg IV or IM. During surgery, may give 1 mg IV.
Dermal necrosis and sloughing after IV extravasation of norepinephrine — **Adults and children:** infiltrate with 5 to 10 mg in 10 ml 0.9% NaCl solution, or half through infiltrated IV and other half around site. Must be done within 12 hr.

- Use cautiously in gastritis or peptic ulcer.
- Contraindicated in angina, CAD, MI or history of MI, or hypersensitivity to drug.

---

phenylephrine hydrochloride
Neo-Synephrine
Adrenergic
Vasoconstrictor
Preg. Risk Category: C

inj: 10 mg/ml

Mild to moderate hypotension — **Adults:** 2 to 5 mg SC or IM; repeated in 1 to 2 hr prn. Initial dose ≤ 5 mg. Alternatively, 0.1 to 0.5 mg by slow IV; repeat 10 to 15 min. **Children:** 0.1 mg/kg IM or SC; repeated in 1 to 2 hr prn.
Severe hypotension and shock — **Adults:** 10 mg in 250 to 500 ml D₅W or 0.9% NaCl. Start IV infusion at 100 to 180 mcg/min; decrease to maintenance infusion of 40 to 60 mcg/min when BP stabilizes.

- Use with extreme caution in heart disease, hyperthyroidism, severe atherosclerosis, bradycardia, partial heart block, myocardial disease, or sulfite sensitivity and in elderly patients.
- Contraindicated in hypersensitivity to drug and in severe hypertension or ventricular tachycardia.

DRUG / CLASS / CATEGORY	DOSAGE FORMS	INDICATIONS / DOSAGES	KEY PRECAUTIONS
phenylephrine hydrochloride AK-Dilate, AK-Nefrin Ophthalmic, Isopto Frin, Mydfrin, Neo-Synephrine *Adrenergic Vasoconstrictor* Preg. Risk Category: C	*ophth sol:* 0.12, 2.5, 10%	*Mydriasis without cycloplegia* — **Adults and children:** 1 drop of 2.5% or 10% sol before exam. May repeat in 1 hr. *Mydriasis and vasoconstriction* — **Adults and adolescents:** 1 drop 2.5% or 10% sol before exam. **Children:** 1 drop 2.5% sol before exam. *Chronic mydriasis* — **Adults and adolescents:** 1 drop 2.5% or 10% sol bid or tid. **Children:** 1 drop 2.5% sol bid or tid.	▪ Use cautiously in marked hypertension, cardiac disorders, advanced arteriosclerotic changes, type 1 diabetes, hyperthyroidism, children with low body weight, and elderly patients. ▪ Contraindicated in angle-closure glaucoma, hypersensitivity to drug, and patients who wear soft contact lenses.
phenylephrine hydrochloride Alconefrin 12, Alconefrin 25, Neo-Synephrine, Sinex *Adrenergic Vasoconstrictor* Preg. Risk Category: NR	*nasal jelly:* 0.5%; *nasal sol:* 0.125, 0.16, 0.2, 0.25, 0.5, 1%	*Nasal congestion* — **Adults and children ≥ 12 yr:** 1 to 2 sprays in nostril or small amount of jelly to nasal mucosa q 4 hr. Don't use > 3 to 5 days. **Children 6 to 12 yr:** 1 to 2 sprays of 0.25% sol in nostril q 4 hr. **Children < 6 yr:** 2 to 3 drops of 0.125% sol q 4 hr.	▪ Use cautiously in hyperthyroidism, marked hypertension, type 1 diabetes, cardiac disease, advanced arteriosclerotic changes, children with low body weight, and elderly patients. ▪ Contraindicated in hypersensitivity to drug.
phenytoin (diphenylhydantoin) Dilantin, Dilantin Infatabs **phenytoin sodium** Dilantin, Phenytex **phenytoin sodium (extended)** Dilantin Kapseals *Hydantoin derivative Anticonvulsant* Preg. Risk Category: NR	*tab (chew):* 50 mg; *oral susp:* 30, 125 mg/5 ml. **sodium** — *cap:* 30 mg (27.6-mg base), 100 mg (92-mg base); *inj:* 50 mg/ml (46-mg base).	*Control of tonic-clonic and complex partial seizures* — **Adults:** 100 mg PO tid, increased in increments of 100 mg PO q 2 to 4 wk until desired response obtained. **Children:** 5 mg/kg or 250 mg/m² PO divided bid or tid. Max 300 mg daily. *For patients requiring loading dose* — **Adults:** initially, 1 g PO daily divided into 3 doses given at 2-hr intervals. Or, 10 to 15 mg/kg IV at rate not > 50 mg/min. Start normal maintenance dosage 24 hr later. **Children:** 5 mg/kg/day PO in 2 or 3 equally divided doses with later dosage individualized to max 300 mg daily.	▪ Use cautiously in hepatic dysfunction, hypotension, myocardial insufficiency, diabetes, and respiratory depression; in elderly or debilitated patients; and in patients receiving other hydantoin derivatives. ▪ Contraindicated in hydantoin hypersensitivity, sinus bradycardia, SA block, second- or third-degree AV block, or Adams-Stokes syndrome.

Drug	Forms	Indications & dosages	Contraindications & precautions
sodium (extended) —	cap: 30 mg (27.6-mg base), 100 mg base), 100 mg (92-mg base)	Status epilepticus — Adults: loading dose 10 to 15 mg/kg IV at rate not > 50 mg/min, then maintenance doses of 100 mg PO or IV q 6 to 8 hr. Children: loading dose 15 to 20 mg/kg IV, at rate not > 1 to 3 mg/kg/min, then individualized maintenance dosages.	
physostigmine sulfate Eserine Sulfate *Cholinesterase inhibitor* *Antimuscarinic antidote/ antiglaucoma agent* Preg. Risk Category: C	ophth oint: 0.25%	Open-angle glaucoma — Adults and children: apply thin strip of oint qd to tid.	■ Contraindicated in intolerance to physostigmine, active uveitis, and corneal injury.
phytonadione (vitamin K₁) AquaMEPHYTON, Konakion, Mephyton *Vitamin K* *Blood coagulation modifier* Preg. Risk Category: C	tab: 5 mg; inj (aqueous colloid sol): 2, 10 mg/ml; inj (aqueous dispers): 2, 10 mg/ml	Hypoprothrombinemia secondary to vitamin K malabsorption, drug therapy, or excessive vitamin A dosage — Adults: 2.5 to 10 mg PO, SC, or IM; repeat and increase up to 50 mg PO, IM, or SC. Children: 5 to 10 mg PO, IM, or SC. Infants: 2 mg PO, IM, or SC. Hypoprothrombinemia secondary to effect of oral anticoagulants — Adults: 2.5 to 10 mg PO, SC, or IM based on PT and INR. In emergency, 10 to 50 mg slow IV, rate ≤ 1 mg/min, repeated q 4 hr, prn.	■ Use cautiously in breast-feeding patients. ■ Contraindicated in hypersensitivity to drug. ■ Severe reactions, including deaths, have occurred during and after IV injection. Use IV route only if other routes not feasible and serious risk is considered justified.
pilocarpine Ocusert Pilo **pilocarpine hydrochloride** Adsorbocarpine, Isopto Carpine, Miocarpine†, Pilocar, Pilopt‡ **pilocarpine nitrate** Pilagan, P.V.	ext-release insert: 20, 40 mcg/hr for 7 days. hydrochloride: ophth sol: 0.25, 0.5, 1, 2, 3, 4, 5, 6, 8, 10%; ophth gel: 4%.	Primary open-angle glaucoma — Adults and children: 1 drop instilled up to qid, or 1-cm ribbon of 4% gel (Pilopine HS) applied hs. Or, 1 Ocusert Pilo system (20 or 40 mcg/hr) applied q 7 days. Emergency treatment of acute-angle-closure glaucoma — Adults and children: 1 drop 2% sol instilled q 5 to 10 min for 3 to 6 doses, followed by 1 drop q 1 to 3 hr until pressure controlled.	■ Use cautiously in acute cardiac failure, bronchial asthma, peptic ulcer, hyperthyroidism, GI spasm, urinary tract obstruction, and Parkinson's disease. ■ Contraindicated in hypersensitivity to drug and when cholinergic effects such as constriction undesirable (for example, in acute

PILOCARPINE NITRATE 199

†Canadian ‡Australian

DRUG / CLASS / CATEGORY	DOSAGE FORMS	INDICATIONS / DOSAGES	KEY PRECAUTIONS
pilocarpine (continued) *Cholinergic agonist* *Miotic* Preg. Risk Category: C	**nitrate — oph-th sol:** 1, 2, 4%	*Mydriasis caused by mydriatic or cycloplegic agents —* **Adults and children:** 1 drop 1% sol.	iritis, some forms of secondary glaucoma, pupillary block glaucoma, and acute inflammatory disease of anterior chamber).
pilocarpine hydrochloride Salagen *Cholinergic agonist* *Anti-xerostomia agent* Preg. Risk Category: C	**tab:** 5 mg	*Treatment of xerostomia from salivary gland hypofunction caused by radiotherapy for cancer of head and neck —* **Adults:** 5 mg PO tid; may increase to 10 mg PO tid, as needed.	■ Use cautiously in CV disease, controlled asthma, chronic bronchitis, COPD, cholelithiasis, biliary tract disease, nephrolithiasis, and cognitive or psychiatric disturbances. ■ Contraindicated in uncontrolled asthma, hypersensitivity to pilocarpine, and when miosis undesirable, such as in acute iritis and narrow-angle glaucoma. ■ Don't use in breast-feeding patients.
pimozide Orap *Diphenylbutylpiperidine* *Antipsychotic* Preg. Risk Category: C	**tab:** 2 mg, 4 mg†, 10 mg†	*Suppression of motor and phonic tics in Tourette syndrome refractory to first-line therapy —* **Adults and children > 12 yr:** initially, 1 to 2 mg PO daily in divided doses, then increased qod, prn. Maintenance dose < 0.2 mg/kg/day or 10 mg/day, whichever less. Max 10 mg daily.	■ Use cautiously in hepatic or renal dysfunction, glaucoma, prostatic hyperplasia, seizure disorder, or EEG abnormalities. ■ Contraindicated in hypersensitivity to drug, in simple tics or tics other than those associated with Tourette syndrome, concurrent drug therapy known to cause motor and phonic tics, congenital long-QT syndrome or history of arrhythmias, severe toxic CNS depression, or coma.

pindolol
Apo-Pindol‡, Barbloc‡, Visken
Beta-adrenergic blocker
Antihypertensive
Preg. Risk Category: B

tab: 5, 10, 15 mg‡

Hypertension — **Adults:** initially, 5 mg PO bid. Increase as needed or tolerated to max 60 mg daily.

- Use cautiously in heart failure, nonallergic bronchospastic disease, diabetes, hyperthyroidism, and impaired renal or hepatic function.
- Contraindicated in hypersensitivity to drug, bronchial asthma, severe bradycardia, first-degree heart block, cardiogenic shock, or overt cardiac failure.

---

piperacillin sodium
Pipracil, Pipril‡
Extended-spectrum penicillin/
acylaminopenicillin
Antibiotic
Preg. Risk Category: B

inj: 2, 3, 4 g;
pharm bulk pkg: 40 g

Systemic infections caused by susceptible strains of gram-pos and especially gram-neg organisms —
Adults and children > 12 yr: 100 to 300 mg/kg IV or IM daily in divided doses q 4 to 6 hr, max 24 g daily.
Prophylaxis of surgical infections — **Adults:** 2 g IV 30 to 60 min before surgery.

- Use cautiously in other drug allergies, especially to cephalosporins, and in bleeding tendencies, uremia, or hypokalemia.
- Contraindicated in hypersensitivity to drug or other penicillins.

---

piperacillin sodium and tazobactam sodium
Zosyn
Extended-spectrum penicillin/
beta-lactamase inhibitor
Antibiotic
Preg. Risk Category: B

powder for inj: 2 g piper and 0.25 g tazo/ vial, 3-g piper and 0.375 g tazo/vial, 4 g piper and 0.5 g tazo/vial;
pharm bulk: 40.5 g

Appendicitis, skin and skin-structure infections, post-partum endometritis or PID, moderately severe community-acquired pneumonia — **Adults:** 3.375 g piperacillin and 0.375 g tazobactam IV q 6 hr.
In renal impairment — **Adults:** if creatinine clearance 20 to 40 ml/min, 2 g piperacillin and 0.25 g tazobactam IV q 6 hr; if < 20 ml/min, 2 g piperacillin and 0.25 g tazobactam IV q 8 hr.
Moderate to severe nosocomial pneumonia — **Adults:** initially, 3.375 g IV over 30 min q 4 hr. Give with aminoglycoside.

- Use cautiously in other drug allergies, especially to cephalosporins, and in bleeding tendencies, uremia, or hypokalemia.
- Contraindicated in hypersensitivity to drug or other penicillins.

---

pirbuterol
Maxair, Maxair Autohaler
Beta-adrenergic agonist
Bronchodilator
Preg. Risk Category: C

inhaler: 0.2 mg/metered dose

Prevention and reversal of bronchospasm, asthma — **Adults and children ≥ 12 yr:** 1 or 2 inhalations (0.2 to 0.4 mg) repeated q 4 to 6 hr. Max 12 inhalations daily.

- Use cautiously in CV disorders, hyperthyroidism, diabetes, and seizure disorders or in unusual responsiveness to sympathomimetic amines.
- Contraindicated in hypersensitivity to drug.

DRUG/CLASS/CATEGORY	DOSAGE FORMS	INDICATIONS/DOSAGES	KEY PRECAUTIONS
piroxicam Apo-Piroxicam†, Feldene, Novo-Pirocam *Nonsteroidal anti-inflammatory* *Nonnarcotic analgesic/ antipyretic/anti-inflammatory* Preg. Risk Category: NR	*cap:* 10, 20 mg	*Osteoarthritis and rheumatoid arthritis* — **Adults:** 20 mg PO daily. If desired, may divide dosage bid.	▪ Use cautiously in elderly patients and in GI disorders, history of renal or peptic ulcer disease, cardiac disease, hypertension, or conditions predisposing to fluid retention. ▪ Contraindicated in hypersensitivity to drug or in history of bronchospasm or angioedema precipitated by aspirin or NSAIDs. Also contraindicated during pregnancy or breast-feeding.
plasma protein fraction Plasmanate, Plasma-Plex, Plasmatein, Protenate *Blood derivative* *Plasma volume expander* Preg. Risk Category: C	*inj:* 5% sol in 50-, 250-, 500-ml vials	*Shock* — **Adults:** varies with patient condition and response; usual dose 250 to 500 ml IV (12.5 to 25 g protein), usually no faster than 10 ml/min. **Children:** 6.6 to 33 ml/kg (0.33 to 1.65 g/kg of protein) IV, 5 to 10 ml/min. *Hypoproteinemia* — **Adults:** 1,000 to 1,500 ml IV daily. Max infusion rate 8 ml/min.	▪ Use cautiously in hepatic or renal failure, low cardiac reserve, and restricted sodium intake. ▪ Contraindicated in severe anemia or heart failure and in patients undergoing cardiac bypass.
plicamycin (mithramycin) Mithracin *Antibiotic antineoplastic (cell cycle–phase nonspecific)* *Antineoplastic/hypocalcemic* Preg. Risk Category: X	*inj:* 2.5-mg vials	Dosage and indications vary. *Hypercalcemia and hypercalciuria associated with advanced malignant disease* — **Adults:** 25 mcg/kg/day IV for 3 to 4 days. Repeat dosage at weekly intervals until desired response seen. *Testicular cancer* — **Adults:** 25 to 30 mcg/kg/day IV for 8 to 10 days or until toxicity occurs. Course of therapy > 10 days not recommended.	▪ Use with extreme caution in significant renal or hepatic impairment. ▪ Contraindicated in thrombocytopenia, bone marrow suppression, coagulation and bleeding disorders, and women who are or may become pregnant.

polyethylene glycol and electrolyte solution
Colovage, GoLYTELY
Polyethylene glycol 3350 nonabsorbable solution
Bowel evacuant
Preg. Risk Category: C

oral sol: contains drug components in varying combinations and amt. Consult reference or pkg insert for specifics.

Bowel preparation before GI exam — **Adults:** 240 ml PO q 10 min until 4 L consumed or until watery stool clear. Typically, give 4 hr before exam, allowing 3 hr for drinking and 1 hr for bowel evacuation.

- Contraindicated in GI obstruction or perforation, gastric retention, toxic colitis, or megacolon.
- Various preparations may contain sodium and potassium.

polymyxin B sulfate
Aerosporin
Polymyxin antibiotic
Antibiotic
Preg. Risk Category: B

powder for inj: 500,000-unit vials

Meningitis caused by sensitive organisms — **Adults and children > 2 yr:** 50,000 units intrathecally qd for 3 to 4 days, then 50,000 units qod for ≥ 2 wk after CSF tests negative and CSF glucose level normal. **Children < 2 yr:** 20,000 units intrathecally qd for 3 to 4 days, then 25,000 units qod for ≥ 2 wk after CSF tests negative and CSF glucose level normal.

- Use cautiously in impaired renal function or myasthenia gravis.
- Contraindicated in hypersensitivity to drug.

polymyxin B sulfate
Aerosporin
Polymyxin antibiotic
Ophthalmic antibiotic
Preg. Risk Category: C

ophth sterile powder for sol: 500,000-unit vials to be recons to 20 to 50 ml

Used alone or with other agents to treat superficial eye infections involving conjunctiva and cornea resulting from infection with Pseudomonas or other gram-neg organism — **Adults and children:** 1 to 3 drops of 0.1% to 0.25% (10,000 to 25,000 units/ml) q hr. Increase interval per response or up to 10,000 units injected subconjunctivally qd.

- Contraindicated in hypersensitivity to drug.

polysaccharide iron complex
Hytinic, Niferex, Niferex-150, Nu-Iron, Nu-Iron-150
Oral iron supplement
Hematinic
Preg. Risk Category: NR

cap: 150 mg; ***sol:*** 100 mg/5 ml; ***tab (film-coated):*** 50 mg

Treatment of uncomplicated iron deficiency anemia — **Adults:** 50 to 100 mg of elemental iron PO tid. **Children:** 4 to 6 mg/kg/day of elemental iron PO in 3 divided doses.

- Contraindicated in hypersensitivity to any component of drug, hemochromatosis, and hemosiderosis.
- Lethal dose between 200 and 250 mg/kg; deaths have occurred at lower doses. Symptoms may follow ingestion of 20 to 60 mg/kg.

POLYSACCHARIDE IRON COMPLEX 203

†Canadian ‡Australian

DRUG/CLASS/ CATEGORY	DOSAGE FORMS	INDICATIONS/ DOSAGES	KEY PRECAUTIONS
potassium acetate Potassium supplement Therapeutic agent for electrolyte balance Preg. Risk Category: C	**inj:** 2 mEq/ml in 20-ml, 30-ml vials; 4 mEq/ml in 50-ml vials	Treatment of hypokalemia — **Adults:** no more than 20 mEq hourly in conc of < 40 mEq/L. Total 24-hr dosage shouldn't exceed 150 mEq (3 mEq/kg in children). Potassium replacement should be done with ECG monitoring and frequent serum potassium determinations. Use IV route only for life-threatening hypokalemia or when oral replacement not feasible. Prevention of hypokalemia — **Adults:** dosage individualized to patient's needs, not to exceed 150 mEq/day. Administer as additive to IV infusions. Usual dose 20 mEq/L infused at rate not to exceed 20 mEq/hr. **Children:** individualized dosage not to exceed 3 mEq/kg/day. Administer as additive to IV infusions.	▪ Use cautiously in cardiac disease or renal impairment. ▪ Contraindicated in severe renal impairment with oliguria, anuria, or azotemia; untreated Addison's disease; and acute dehydration; heat cramps; hyperkalemia; hyperkalemic form of familial periodic paralysis; and conditions associated with extensive tissue breakdown.
potassium bicarbonate K-Gen ET, K-Ide, Klor-Con/EF, K-Lyte Potassium supplement Therapeutic agent for electrolyte balance Preg. Risk Category: NR	**efferv tab:** 6.5, 25 mEq	Hypokalemia — **Adults:** 25 to 50 mEq dissolved in half to full glass of water (120 to 240 ml) qd to qid.	▪ Use cautiously in cardiac disease and renal impairment. ▪ Contraindicated in severe renal impairment with oliguria, anuria, or azotemia; in untreated Addison's disease; and in acute dehydration, heat cramps, hyperkalemia, hyperkalemic form of familial periodic paralysis, and other conditions associated with extensive tissue breakdown.
potassium chloride K+10, Kaochlor 10%, K-Dur, K-Lyte/Cl, K-Tab, Slow-K Potassium supplement Therapeutic agent for electrolyte balance Preg. Risk Category: C	**tab (contr-release):** 6.7 mEq, 8 mEq, 10 mEq, 20 mEq; **tab (film-coated):** 2.5 mEq, 8 mEq, 10 mEq;	Hypokalemia — **Adults:** 40 to 100 mEq PO daily in 3 or 4 divided doses or 10 to 20 mEq for prevention. **Children:** 3 mEq/kg daily. Max daily dosage 40 mEq/m². If potassium < 2 mEq/ml, max infusion rate 40 mEq/hr; max infusion conc 80 mEq/L; and max 24-hr dose 400 mEq. If potassium > 2 mEq/ml, max	▪ Use cautiously in cardiac disease and renal impairment. ▪ Contraindicated in severe renal impairment with oliguria, anuria, or azotemia; untreated Addison's disease; acute dehydration; heat cramps; hyperkalemia; hyperkalemic form

of familial periodic paralysis; and other conditions associated with extensive tissue breakdown.

Drug	Forms	Indications & Dosage	Nursing considerations
		infusion rate 10 mEq/hr; max infusion conc 40 mEq/L; and max 24-hr dose 200 mEq.	
	cap (contr-release): 8 mEq, 10 mEq; *oral liq:* range from 5 to 20% (10 to 40 mEq/15 ml); *powder for oral use:* 15-, 20-, 25-mEq pkt; *inj:* 20- 40-mEq amp; 30-mEq amp; 30- or 40-mEq; *syringes:* 10-, 20-, 30-, 40-, 60-, 100-, 200-, 400-, or 1,000- mEq vials		
potassium gluconate Glu-K, Kaon Liquid *Therapeutic agent for electrolyte balance* Preg. Risk Category: C	*tab:* 500 mg (2 mEq K+); 1,170 mg (5 mEq K+); *elixir:* 4.68 g (20 mEq K+)/15 ml	*Hypokalemia* — **Adults:** 40 to 100 mEq PO daily in 3 or 4 divided doses for treatment; 10 to 20 mEq daily for prevention. Further dosage adjustments based on serum potassium levels.	■ Use cautiously in cardiac disease and renal impairment. ■ Contraindicated in severe renal impairment with oliguria, anuria, or azotemia; untreated Addison's disease; acute dehydration; heat cramps; hyperkalemia; hyperkalemic form of familial periodic paralysis; and other conditions associated with extensive tissue breakdown.
potassium iodide Iostat, Pima, Thyro-Block **potassium iodide, saturated solution (SSKI), strong iodine solution**	*tab:* 130 mg; *tab (enteric-coated):* 300 mg; oral sol: 500 mg/15 ml;	*Preparation for thyroidectomy* — **Adults and children:** strong iodine sol (USP), 0.1-0.3 ml PO tid, or SSKI, 1 to 5 drops in water PO tid after meals for 10 to 14 days before surgery.	■ Use cautiously in hypocomplementemic vasculitis, goiter, or autoimmune thyroid disease.

(continued)

POTASSIUM IODIDE 205

†Canadian ‡Australian

DRUG/CLASS/ CATEGORY	DOSAGE FORMS	INDICATIONS/ DOSAGES	KEY PRECAUTIONS
potassium iodide *(continued)* Electrolyte *Antihyperthyroid agent* Preg. Risk Category: D	**syrup:** 325 mg/5 ml. **SSKI — oral sol:** 1 g/ml. **strong iodine sol — oral sol:** iodine 50 mg/ml and pot. iodide 100 mg/ml	*Thyrotoxic crisis* — **Adults and children:** 500 mg PO q 4 hr (SSKI) or 1 ml strong iodine sol tid. *Radiation protectant for thyroid gland* — **Adults and children ≥ 1 yr:** 130 mg PO daily for 7 to 14 days after radiation exposure. **Children < 1 yr:** 65 mg PO daily for 7 to 14 days after exposure.	▪ Contraindicated in TB, acute bronchitis, iodide hypersensitivity, or hyperkalemia. Some formulations contain sulfites, which may induce allergic reactions in hypersensitive patients.
pralidoxime chloride (pyridine-2-aldoxime methochloride; 2-PAM) Protopam Chloride *Quaternary ammonium oxime* Antidote Preg. Risk Category: C	**inj:** 1 g/20 ml in 20-ml vial without diluent or syringe; 1 g/20 ml in 20-ml vial with diluent, syringe, needle, and alcohol swab (emergency kit); 600 mg/2 ml autoinjector, parenteral	*Antidote for organophosphate poisoning* — **Adults:** 1 to 2 g in 100 ml NaCl sol by IV infusion over 15 to 30 min. If pulmonary edema present, give by slow IV push over 5 min. Repeat in 1 hr if muscle weakness persists. May give additional doses cautiously. May use IM or SC inj if IV not feasible. **Children:** 20 to 40 mg/kg IV, administered as for adults. *Cholinergic crisis in myasthenia gravis* — **Adults:** 1 to 2 g IV, followed by 250 mg IV q 5 min as needed.	▪ Use with extreme caution in myasthenia gravis. ▪ Contraindicated in hypersensitivity to pralidoxime.
pravastatin sodium (eptastatin) Pravachol *HMG-CoA reductase inhibitor* Antilipemic Preg. Risk Category: X	**tab:** 10, 20, 40 mg	*Reduction of LDL and total cholesterol levels in primary hypercholesterolemia (types IIa and IIb)* — **Adults:** 10 or 20 mg PO daily hs. Adjust q 4 wk per response; max 40 mg qd. Most elderly patients respond to ≤ 20 mg qd.	▪ Use cautiously in patients who consume large quantities of alcohol or in history of liver disease. ▪ Contraindicated in hypersensitivity to drug; in patients with active liver disease or conditions that cause unexplained, persistent

Drug	Indications/dosage	Preparations	Nursing considerations
			serum transaminase elevations; in pregnant and breast-feeding patients; and in women of childbearing age unless no risk of pregnancy. ■ Use cautiously in patients receiving other antihypertensives.
prazosin hydrochloride Minipress *Alpha-adrenergic blocker* *Antihypertensive* Preg. Risk Category: C	*Mild to moderate hypertension* — **Adults:** PO test dose 1 mg hs. Initial dose 1 mg PO bid or tid. Increase slowly. Max 20 mg qd. Maint. 6 to 15 mg qd in 3 divided doses.	*cap:* 1, 2, 5 mg	
prednisolone Cortalone, Delta-Cortef **prednisolone sodium phosphate** Hydeltrasol, Key-Pred-SP **prednisolone tebutate** Hydeltra-TBA, Nor-Pred TBA *Glucocorticoid* *Anti-inflammatory/immuno-suppressant* Preg. Risk Category: C	*Severe inflammation or immunosuppression* — **Adults:** 2.5 to 15 mg PO bid, tid, or qid; 2 to 30 mg IM (phosphate) or IV (phosphate) q 12 hr; or 2 to 30 mg (phosphate) into joints (depending on joint size); lesions, or soft tissue; or 4 to 40 mg (tebutate) into joints (depending on joint size) and lesions prn.	*tab:* 5 mg, *syrup:* 15 mg/5 ml. **sodium phosphate** — *oral sol:* 5 mg/5 ml; *inj:* 20 mg/ml. *tebutate* — *inj (susp):* 20 mg/ml	■ Use with extreme caution in recent MI, GI ulcer, renal disease, hypertension, osteoporosis, diabetes mellitus, hypothyroidism, cirrhosis, diverticulitis, nonspecific ulcerative colitis, recent intestinal anastomoses, thromboembolic disorders, seizures, myasthenia gravis, heart failure, TB, ocular herpes simplex, emotional instability, or psychotic tendencies. ■ Contraindicated in hypersensitivity to drug or any ingredient and in systemic fungal infections.
prednisolone acetate (suspension) Pred-Forte **prednisolone sodium phosphate** AK-Pred, Inflamase Forte *Corticosteroid* *Ophthalmic anti-inflammatory* Preg. Risk Category: C	*Inflammation* — **Adults and children:** 1 to 2 drops instilled into eye. In severe conditions, may use hourly, tapering to discontinuation as inflammation subsides. In mild conditions, may use bid to qid.	*acetate* — *ophth susp:* 0.12, 0.125, 1%. **sodium phosphate** — *ophth susp:* 0.125, 1%	■ Use cautiously in corneal abrasions that may be contaminated (especially with herpes). ■ Contraindicated in acute, untreated, purulent ocular infections; acute, superficial herpes simplex (dendritic keratitis); vaccinia, varicella, or other viral or fungal eye diseases; and ocular TB.

DRUG/CLASS/ CATEGORY	DOSAGE FORMS	INDICATIONS/ DOSAGES	KEY PRECAUTIONS
prednisone Apo-Prednisone†, Liquid Pred, Meticorten, Panasol, Prednicen-M, Prednisone Intensol, Winpred† *Adrenocorticoid* *Anti-inflammatory/immuno-suppressant* Preg. Risk Category: C	**tab:** 1, 2.5, 5, 10, 20, 25, 50 mg; **oral sol:** 5 mg/ml, 5 mg/ml (conc); **syrup:** 5 mg/5 ml	*Severe inflammation or immunosuppression —* **Adults:** 5 to 60 mg PO daily in 2 to 4 divided doses. Give maintenance dosage qd or qod. Dosage individualized. **Children:** 0.14 to 2 mg/kg or 4 to 60 mg/m² daily PO in 4 divided doses.	▪ Use cautiously in GI ulcer, renal disease, hypertension, osteoporosis, diabetes mellitus, hypothyroidism, cirrhosis, diverticulitis, nonspecific ulcerative colitis, recent intestinal anastomoses, thromboembolic disorders, seizures, myasthenia gravis, heart failure, TB, ocular herpes simplex, emotional instability, and psychotic tendencies. ▪ Contraindicated in hypersensitivity to drug or in systemic fungal infections.
primaquine phosphate *8-aminoquinoline* *Antimalarial* Preg. Risk Category: C	**tab:** 15 mg (base)	*Radical cure of relapsing P. vivax malaria, eliminating symptoms and infection completely; prevention of relapse —* **Adults:** 15 mg (base) PO daily for 14 days. (26.3-mg tab provides 15 mg of base.) **Children:** 0.5 mg/kg/day (0.3 mg base/kg/day; max 15 mg base/dose) PO for 14 days.	▪ Use cautiously in previous idiosyncratic reaction (manifested by hemolytic anemia, methemoglobinemia, or leukopenia); in family or personal history of favism; and in erythrocytic G6PD deficiency or NADH methemoglobin reductase deficiency. ▪ Contraindicated in systemic diseases in which agranulocytosis may develop and in patients taking bone marrow suppressants or potentially hemolytic drugs.
primidone Apo-Primidone†, Mysoline, PMS Primidone†, Sertan† *Barbiturate analogue* *Anticonvulsant* Preg. Risk Category: NR	**tab:** 50, 250 mg; **oral susp:** 250 mg/5 ml	*Tonic-clonic, complex partial, and simple partial seizures —* **Adults and children ≥ 8 yr:** initially, 100 to 125 mg PO hs on days 1 to 3; 100 to 125 mg PO bid on days 4 to 6; 100 to 125 mg PO tid on days 7 to 9; followed by dose of 250 mg PO tid. Dose increased to 250 mg qid, prn. Max 2 g qd in divided doses. **Children < 8 yr:** 50 mg PO hs for 3 days, then 50 mg PO bid for days 4 to 6, 100 mg PO bid for days 7 to 9, followed by dose of 125 to 250 mg PO tid.	▪ Contraindicated in phenobarbital hypersensitivity or porphyria.

probenecid Benemid, Benn, Benuryl† Probalan, Robenecid *Sulfonamide derivative* *Uricosuric* Preg. Risk Category: NR	**tab:** 500 mg	*Gonorrhea* — **Adults:** 3.5 g ampicillin PO with 1 g probenecid PO given together; or 1 g probenecid PO 30 min before dose of 4.8 million units of aqueous penicillin G procaine IM, injected at 2 different sites. *Hyperuricemia of gout, gouty arthritis* — **Adults:** 250 mg PO bid for 1st wk, then 500 mg bid, to max 2 g daily.	• Use cautiously in peptic ulcer and renal impairment. • Contraindicated in hypersensitivity to drug, uric acid kidney stones, blood dyscrasias, acute gout attack, and children < 2 yr.
procainamide hydrochloride Procainamide Durules‡, Procan SR, Promine, Pronestyl *Procaine derivative* *Ventricular antiarrhythmic/ supraventricular antiarrhythmic* Preg. Risk Category: C	**tab:** 250, 375, 500 mg; **tab (sust- release):** 250, 500, 750, 1,000 mg; **cap:** 250, 375, 500 mg; **inj:** 100, 500 mg/ml	*Life-threatening ventricular arrhythmias* — **Adults:** 100 mg slow IV push q 5 min, no faster than 25 to 50 mg/min until arrhythmias disappear, adverse reactions develop, or 1 g given. Usual effective dose 500 to 600 mg. When arrhythmias disappear, give continuous infusion of 1 to 6 mg/min. If arrhythmias recur, repeat bolus and increase infusion rate. Or, 0.5 to 1 g IM q 4 to 8 hr until oral therapy begins. Oral: 50 mg/kg qd in divided doses q 3 hr.	• Use with extreme caution when treating patients with ventricular tachycardia during coronary occlusion, heart failure, or other conduction disturbances, such as bundle-branch heart block, sinus bradycardia, or digitalis glycoside intoxication, or with hepatic or renal insufficiency, blood dyscrasias, or bone marrow suppression. • Contraindicated in hypersensitivity to procaine and related drugs; in complete, second-, or third-degree heart block in absence of artificial pacemaker; and in myasthenia gravis or systemic lupus erythematosus. Also contraindicated in atypical ventricular tachycardia (torsade de pointes).
procarbazine hydrochloride Matulane, Natulan† *Antibiotic antineoplastic (cell cycle-phase specific, S phase)* *Antineoplastic* Preg. Risk Category: D	**cap:** 50 mg	*Adjunct treatment of Hodgkin's disease* — **Adults:** 2 to 4 mg/kg PO qd for 1st wk. Then 4 to 6 mg/kg/day until WBC count < 4,000/mm³ or platelet count < 100,000/mm³. After bone marrow recovers, resume maint of 1 to 2 mg/kg/day. For MOPP regimen, 100 mg/m²/day PO for 14 days. **Children:** 50 mg/m² PO daily for 1st wk; then 100 mg/m² until response or toxicity occurs. Maintenance dosage 50 mg/m² PO daily after bone marrow recovery.	• Use cautiously in impaired hepatic or renal function. • Contraindicated in hypersensitivity to drug and inadequate bone marrow reserve (as shown by bone marrow aspiration).

DRUG/CLASS/ CATEGORY	DOSAGE FORMS	INDICATIONS/ DOSAGES	KEY PRECAUTIONS
prochlorperazine Compazine, PMS Prochlorperazine†, Prorazin†, Stemetil† **prochlorperazine edisylate** Compa-Z, Compazine, Cotranzine, Ultrazine-10 **prochlorperazine maleate** Anti-Naus‡, Compazine, PMS Prochlorperazine†, Prorazin†, Stemetil† *Phenothiazine (piperazine derivative) Antipsychotic/antiemetic/antianxiety agent* Preg. Risk Category: NR	*tab:* 5, 10 mg; *inj:* 5 mg/ml; *supp:* 2.5, 5, 25 mg. **edisylate** — *syrup:* 5 mg/5 ml; *inj:* 5 mg/ml. **maleate** — *tab:* 5, 10, 25 mg; *cap (sustrelease):* 10, 15, 30 mg	*Preop nausea control* — **Adults:** 5 to 10 mg IM 1 to 2 hr before anesthesia; repeat once in 30 min, prn. Or, 5 to 10 mg IV 15 to 30 min before anesthesia; repeat once prn. *Severe nausea and vomiting* — **Adults:** 5 to 10 mg PO, tid or qid; 25 mg PR, bid; or 5 to 10 mg IM repeated q 3 to 4 hr, prn. Max IM dosage 40 mg daily. Or, 2.5 to 10 mg IV at max rate 5 mg/min. **Children 9 to 13 kg:** 2.5 mg PO or PR qd or bid. Max 7.5 mg daily. Or give 0.132 mg/kg by IM injection. **Children 14 to 17 kg:** 2.5 mg PO or PR, bid or tid. Max 10 mg daily. Or give 0.132 mg/kg by deep IM injection. Control usually obtained with one dose. **Children 18 to 39 kg:** 2.5 mg PO or PR, tid; or 5 mg PO or PR, bid. Max 15 mg daily. Or give 0.132 mg/kg by deep IM injection. Control usually obtained with one dose. *To manage symptoms of psychotic disorders* — **Adults:** 5 to 10 mg PO, tid or qid. **Children 2 to 12 yr:** 2.5 mg PO or PR, bid or tid. Max 10 mg on day 1. Increase dosage gradually to recommended max (if necessary). In children 2 to 5 yr, max 25 mg daily. In children 6 to 10 yr, max 25 mg daily. *Nonpsychotic anxiety* — **Adults:** 5 to 10 mg by deep IM injection q 3 to 4 hr, not to exceed 20 mg daily or for > 12 wk; or 5 to 10 mg PO, tid or qid. Or, 15 mg ext-release cap qd or 10 mg ext-release cap q 12 hr.	• Use cautiously in impaired CV function, glaucoma, or seizure disorders; in patients exposed to extreme heat; and in children with acute illness. • Contraindicated in hypersensitivity to phenothiazines and in CNS depression including coma; during pediatric surgery; when using spinal or epidural anesthetics, adrenergic blockers, or ethanol; and in children < 2 yr.
progesterone Gesterol 50, Progestilin† *Progestin*	*inj (in oil):* 50 mg/ml	*Amenorrhea* — **Adults:** 5 to 10 mg IM daily for 6 to 8 days, beginning 8 to 10 days before anticipated start of menstruation.	• Use cautiously in diabetes mellitus, seizures, migraine, cardiac or renal disease, asthma, and mental depression.

Progestin/contraceptive
Preg. Risk Category: X

Dysfunctional uterine bleeding — **Adults:** 5 to 10 mg IM daily for 6 doses.

- Contraindicated in thromboembolic disorders; cerebral apoplexy, or history of those conditions; hypersensitivity; breast cancer; undiagnosed abnormal vaginal bleeding; severe hepatic disease; or missed abortion.

promazine hydrochloride
Primazine, Prozine-50, Sparine
Aliphatic phenothiazine
Antipsychotic/antiemetic
Preg. Risk Category: NR

tab: 25, 50, 100 mg; **inj:** 25, 50 mg/ml

Psychosis — **Adults:** 10 to 200 mg PO or IM q 4 to 6 hr, up to 1 g daily, prn. For acutely agitated patients, initial dose 50 to 150 mg IM; repeat within 30 min, if necessary, to total of 300 mg. **Children > 12 yr:** 10 to 25 mg PO or IM q 4 to 6 hr.

- Use cautiously in elderly or debilitated patients; in hepatic or renal disease or severe CV disease; in exposure to extreme heat or cold (including antipyretic therapy) or to organophosphate insecticides; or in respiratory disorders, hypocalcemia, seizure disorder, severe reactions to insulin or electroconvulsive therapy, glaucoma, or prostatic hyperplasia.
- Contraindicated in hypersensitivity to drug or in coma, CNS depression, bone marrow suppression, or subcortical damage.

promethazine hydrochloride
Anergan 25, Histantil†, Pentazine, Phenazine 25, Phencen-50, Phenergan, Phenoject-50, PMS-Promethazine†, Promethegan, Prothazine†, V-Gan-25
promethazine theoclate
Avomine‡
Phenothiazine derivative
Antiemetic/antivertigo agent/antihistamine/sedative/analgesic adjunct
Preg. Risk Category: C

tab: 12.5, 25, 50 mg; **syrup:** 5‡, 6.25, 10‡, 25 mg/5 ml; **inj:** 25, 50 mg/ml; **supp:** 12.5, 25, 50 mg.
theoclate — **tab:** 25 mg‡

Motion sickness — **Adults:** 25 mg PO bid. **Children:** 12.5 to 25 mg PO, IM, or PR bid.
Nausea — **Adults:** 12.5 to 25 mg PO, IM, or PR q 4 to 6 hr, prn. **Children:** 12.5 to 25 mg IM or PR q 4 to 6 hr, prn.
Rhinitis, allergy symptoms — **Adults:** 12.5 mg PO qid; or 25 mg PO hs. **Children:** 6.25 to 12.5 mg PO tid or 25 mg PO or PR hs.
Sedation — **Adults:** 25 to 50 mg PO or IM hs or prn. **Children:** 12.5 to 25 mg PO, IM, or PR hs.
Routine preop or postop sedation or adjunct to analgesics — **Adults:** 25 to 50 mg IM, IV, or PO. **Children:** 12.5 to 25 mg IM, IV, or PO.

- Use cautiously in pulmonary, hepatic, CV disease, or asthma.
- Contraindicated in hypersensitivity to drug; in intestinal obstruction, prostatic hyperplasia, bladder-neck obstruction, seizure disorders, coma, CNS depression, and stenosing peptic ulcerations; in newborns and premature neonates; in breast-feeding patients; and in acutely ill or dehydrated children.

†Canadian ‡Australian

DRUG / CLASS / CATEGORY	DOSAGE FORMS	INDICATIONS / DOSAGES	KEY PRECAUTIONS
propafenone hydrochloride Rythmol *Sodium channel antagonist* *Antiarrhythmic (class 1C)* Preg. Risk Category: C	***tab:*** 150, 225, 300 mg	*Suppression of life-threatening ventricular arrhythmias, such as SVT* — **Adults:** initially, 150 mg PO q 8 hr. May increase dosage at 3- to 4-day intervals to 225 mg q 8 hr; if necessary, increase to 300 mg q 8 hr. Max 900 mg daily.	▪ Use cautiously in heart failure, in patients taking other cardiac depressant drugs, and in hepatic or renal failure. ▪ Contraindicated in hypersensitivity to drug and in severe or uncontrolled heart failure; cardiogenic shock; SA, AV, or intraventricular disorders of impulse conduction in absence of pacemaker; bradycardia; marked hypotension; bronchospastic disorders; and electrolyte imbalance.
propantheline bromide Panthelinе‡, Pro-Banthine *Anticholinergic* *Antimuscarinic/GI antispasmodic* Preg. Risk Category: C	***tab:*** 7.5, 15 mg	*Adjunctive treatment of peptic ulceration* — **Adults:** 15 mg PO tid before meals and 30 mg hs. **Elderly patients:** 7.5 mg PO tid before meals.	▪ Use cautiously in autonomic neuropathy, hyperthyroidism, CAD, arrhythmias, heart failure, hypertension, hiatal hernia associated with reflux esophagitis, hepatic or renal disease, and ulcerative colitis. Also use cautiously in hot or humid environments. ▪ Contraindicated in angle-closure glaucoma, obstructive uropathy, obstructive disease of GI tract, severe ulcerative colitis, myasthenia gravis, hypersensitivity to anticholinergics, paralytic ileus, intestinal atony, unstable CV status in acute hemorrhage, or toxic megacolon.

propoxyphene hydrochloride

Darvon, Dolene, Novopropoxyn†, 642†

cap: 32, 65 mg. **napsylate — *tab:*** 100 mg; *oral susp:* 10 mg/ml

Mild to moderate pain — **Adults:** 65 mg (hydrochloride) PO q 4 hr, prn. Max 390 mg/day.

■ Use cautiously in hepatic or renal disease, emotional instability, or history of drug or alcohol abuse.
■ Contraindicated in hypersensitivity to drug.

propoxyphene napsylate

Darvon-N, Doloxene‡

Narcotic analgesic

Opioid analgesic

Preg. Risk Category: C

Controlled Sub. Sched.: IV

Mild to moderate pain — **Adults:** 100 mg (napsylate) PO q 4 hr, prn. Max 600 mg/day.

propranolol hydrochloride

Betachron E-R, Deralin‡, Detensol†, Inderal, Inderal LA, Novopranol†

Beta-adrenergic blocker

Antihypertensive/antianginal/antiarrhythmic/adjunct for MI therapy

Preg. Risk Category: C

tab: 10, 20, 40, 60, 80, 90 mg; *cap (ext-rel):* 60, 80, 120, 160 mg; *oral sol:* 4, 8 mg/ml, 80 mg/ml (conc); *inj:* 1 mg/ml

Angina pectoris — **Adults:** total daily dose, 80 to 320 mg PO bid, tid, or qid; or one 80-mg ext-rel cap qd. Increase dosage at 7- to 10-day intervals.

Mortality reduction after MI — **Adults:** 180 to 240 mg PO tid or qid 5 to 21 days after MI.

Supraventricular and ventricular arrhythmias; tachyarrhythmias due to excessive catecholamine action during anesthesia, hyperthyroidism, or pheochromocytoma — **Adults:** 0.5 to 3 mg by slow IV push (≤ 1 mg/min). After 3 mg, give next dose in 2 min; other doses > q 4 hr. Maint: 10 to 30 mg PO tid or qid.

Hypertension — **Adults:** 80 mg PO qd in 2 to 4 divided doses or ext-rel qd. Increased at 3- to 7-day intervals to max 640 mg qd. Maint: 160 to 480 mg qd.

Essential tremor — **Adults:** 40 mg PO bid. Maint: 120 to 320 mg qd in 3 divided doses.

Hypertrophic subaortic stenosis — **Adults:** 20 to 40 mg PO tid or qid, or 80 to 160 mg ext-rel capsules once daily.

Adjunct therapy in pheochromocytoma — **Adults:** 60 mg PO qd in divided doses with an alpha-adrenergic blocker 3 days before surgery.

■ Use cautiously in coronary insufficiency, pulmonary disease, diabetes, hypoglycemia, hyperthyroidism, impaired hepatic function.
■ Contraindicated in hypersensitivity, overt heart failure, sinus bradycardia, second- or third-degree AV block, bronchial asthma, cardiogenic shock, and Raynaud's syndrome.

PROPRANOLOL HYDROCHLORIDE   213

†Canadian   ‡Australian

DRUG / CLASS / CATEGORY	DOSAGE FORMS	INDICATIONS / DOSAGES	KEY PRECAUTIONS
propylthiouracil (PTU) Propyl-Thyracil *Thyroid hormone antagonist* *Antihyperthyroid agent* Preg. Risk Category: D	**tab:** 50, 100 mgt	*Hyperthyroidism —* **Adults:** 100 to 150 mg PO tid; up to 1,200 mg qd. Maint.: 100 to 150 mg qd in divided doses tid. **Children > 10 yr:** 150 to 300 mg PO qd in divided doses tid. **Children 6 to 10 yr:** 50 to 150 mg PO qd in divided doses tid. *Thyrotoxic crisis —* **Adults and children:** 200 mg PO q 4 to 6 hr on first day, once symptoms controlled, reduce dosage gradually to usual maintenance level.	▪ Use cautiously in pregnant patients (may require less drug as pregnancy progresses). ▪ Contraindicated in hypersensitivity to drug and in breast-feeding patients.
protamine sulfate *Antidote* *Heparin antagonist* Preg. Risk Category: C	**inj:** 10 mg/ml	*Heparin overdose —* **Adults:** dosage based on blood coagulation studies, usually 1 mg for each 90 to 115 units heparin. Give by slow IV inj over 10 min. Max 50 mg.	▪ Use cautiously after cardiac surgery. ▪ Contraindicated in hypersensitivity to drug.
protriptyline hydrochloride Triptil†, Vivactil *Tricyclic antidepressant* *Antidepressant* Preg. Risk Category: NR	**tab:** 5, 10 mg	*Depression —* **Adults:** 15 to 40 mg PO daily in divided doses, increasing gradually to max 60 mg daily. **Elderly and adolescent patients:** initially, 5 mg tid, increasing dosage gradually. In elderly patients receiving > 20 mg/day, monitor CV status closely.	▪ Use cautiously in elderly patients; in history of seizures or urine retention; in suicidal tendencies, increased intraocular pressure, CV disorders, or hyperthyroidism; and in patients receiving thyroid medications. ▪ Contraindicated during acute recovery phase of MI, in hypersensitivity to drug, and within 14 days of MAO inhibitor therapy.
pseudoephedrine hydrochloride Children's Sudafed, Drixoral, Efidac/24, PediaCare Infant's Decongestant, Pseudofrin†, Sudafed	**tab:** 30, 60 mg; **tab (ext-release):** 120, 240 mg; **cap:** 60 mg; **cap (ext-release):** 120 mg; **oral**	*Nasal and eustachian tube decongestion —* **Adults:** 60 mg PO q 4 hr. Max 240 mg daily. Or, 120 mg extrelease tab PO q 12 hr or 240 mg ext-release qd. **Children > 12 yr:** 120 mg PO q 12 hr, or 240 mg PO qd. **Children 6 to 12 yr:** 30 mg PO reg-release form q 4 to 6 hr. Max 120 mg daily. **Children 2 to 6 yr:** 15 mg PO reg-release form q 4 to 6 hr. Max 60 mg/day.	▪ Use cautiously in hypertension, cardiac disease, diabetes, glaucoma, hyperthyroidism, and prostatic hyperplasia. ▪ Contraindicated in severe hypertension or severe CAD, in patients receiving MAO inhibitors, and in breast-feeding patients. Ext-

pseudoephedrine sulfate

Afrin, Drixoral
Adrenergic
Decongestant
Preg. Risk Category: C

sol: 15 mg,
30 mg/5 ml;
7.5 mg/0.8 ml;
syrup: 30 mg/
5 ml. **sulfate
— tab (ext-
release):** 120
mg (60 mg
immed-
release, 60 mg
delayed-
release)

Children 1 to 2 yr.: 7 drops (0.2 ml)/kg q 4 to 6 hr, up to 4 doses/day. **Children 3 to 12 mo:** 3 drops/kg q 4 to 6 hr, up to 4 doses/day.

release preparations contraindicated in children < 12 yr.

psyllium

Fiberall, Maalox Daily Fiber Therapy, Metamucil, Mylanta Natural Fiber Supplement, Pro-Lax
Absorbent
Bulk laxative
Preg. Risk Category: NR

chew pieces:
1.7 g/piece;
efferv powder:
3.4, 3.7 g/
packet; *gran-
ules:* 2.5, 4.03
g/tsp; *powder:*
3.3, 3.4, 3.5,
4.94 g/tsp;
wafers: 3.4
g/wafer

Constipation; bowel management — **Adults:** 1 to 2 tsp (rounded) PO in full glass of liquid qd, bid, or tid, followed by second glass of liquid; or 1 packet dissolved in water qd, bid, or tid. **Children > 6 yr:** 1 tsp (level) PO in half glass of liquid hs.

- Contraindicated in hypersensitivity to drug, abdominal pain, nausea, vomiting, or other symptoms of appendicitis, and in intestinal obstruction or ulceration, disabling adhesions, or difficulty swallowing.

DRUG/CLASS/ CATEGORY	DOSAGE FORMS	INDICATIONS/ DOSAGES	KEY PRECAUTIONS
pyrantel pamoate Antiminth, Combantrin†, Reese's Pinworm Medicine *Pyrimidine derivative* *Anthelmintic* Preg. Risk Category: C	**tab:** 125 mg†; **oral susp:** 50 mg/ml	*Roundworm and pinworm* — **Adults and children > 2 yr:** 11 mg/kg PO as single dose. Max 1 g. For pinworm, repeat dosage in 2 wk.	▪ Use cautiously in severe malnutrition or anemia or in hepatic dysfunction. ▪ Contraindicated in hypersensitivity to drug.
pyrazinamide Pyrazinamide†, Tebrazid† *Synthetic pyrazine analogue* *Antituberculosis agent* Preg. Risk Category: C	**tab:** 500 mg	*Adjunctive treatment of TB* — **Adults:** 15 to 30 mg/kg PO qd. Max 2 g daily. Or, if patient noncompliant, 50 to 70 mg/kg PO twice weekly.	▪ Use cautiously in diabetes mellitus, renal failure, or gout. ▪ Contraindicated in hypersensitivity to drug, severe hepatic disease, or acute gout.
pyrethrins A-200 Pyrinate, Barc, Blue Gel, Pyrinyl, RID *Synthetic pyrethrin* *Topical pediculicide* Preg. Risk Category: C	**pyrethrins with piperonyl butoxide** — **shampoo:** pyrethrins 0.17, 0.3%; **top gel:** pyrethrins 0.18, 0.3, 0.33%; **top sol:** pyrethrins 0.18, 0.3%; with deodorized kerosene pyrethrins 0.2%	*Infestations of head, body, and pubic (crab) lice and their eggs* — **Adults and children:** apply to hair, scalp, or other infested areas until entirely wet. Allow to remain for 10 min but no longer. Wash thoroughly with warm water and soap or shampoo. Remove dead lice and eggs with fine-tooth comb. Repeat treatment, if necessary, in 7 to 10 days to kill newly hatched lice. Don't exceed 2 applications within 24 hr.	▪ Use cautiously in infants and small children. ▪ Contraindicated in hypersensitivity to drug, ragweed, or chrysanthemums.

pyridoxine hydrochloride (vitamin B₆)

Beesix, Hexa-Betalin, Nestrex, Rodex

Water-soluble vitamin
Nutritional supplement
Preg. Risk Category: A

tab: 10, 25, 50, 100, 200, 250, 500 mg; **cap (timed-release):** 100 mg; **cap:** 500 mg; **tab (timed-release):** 100 mg; **inj:** 100 mg/ml

Dietary vitamin B₆ deficiency — **Adults:** 10 to 20 mg PO, IM, or IV daily for 3 wk, then 2 to 5 mg daily as supplement to proper diet.

Seizures related to vitamin B₆ deficiency or dependency — **Adults and children:** 100 mg IM or IV in single dose.

- Use cautiously in breast-feeding patients.
- Contraindicated in hypersensitivity to pyridoxine.

pyrimethamine

Daraprim

pyrimethamine with sulfadoxine

Fansidar

Aminopyrimidine derivative (folic acid antagonist)
Antimalarial
Preg. Risk Category: C

tab: 25 mg.
sulfadoxine — **tab:** pyrimethamine 25 mg, sulfadoxine 500 mg

Malaria prophylaxis and transmission control (pyrimethamine) — **Adults and children ≥ 10 yr:** 25 mg PO/wk; **4 to 10 yr:** 12.5 mg PO/wk; **< 4 yr:** 6.25 mg PO/wk. Continue 6 to 10 wk after leaving endemic areas.

Acute attacks of malaria (Fansidar) — **Adults and children ≥ 14 yr:** 2 to 3 tab as single dose; **9 to 14 yr:** 2 tab/wk; **4 to 8 yr:** 1 tab/wk; **< 4 yr:** ½ tab/wk.

Malaria prophylaxis (Fansidar) — **Adults and children ≥ 14 yr:** 1 tab/wk; **9 to 14 yr:** ¾ tab/wk; **4 to 8 yr:** ½ tab/wk; **< 4 yr:** ¼ tab/wk.

Acute attacks of malaria (pyrimethamine) — **Adults and children ≥ 15 yr:** 25 mg PO qd for 2 days. **Children < 15 yr:** 12.5 mg PO qd for 2 days.

Toxoplasmosis (pyrimethamine) — **Adults:** 100 mg PO, then 25 mg PO qd for 4 to 5 wk; **Children:** 1 mg/kg PO (< 100 mg) in 2 equally divided doses for 2 to 4 days, then 0.5 mg/kg qd for 4 wk.

- Contraindicated in hypersensitivity to drug and in megaloblastic anemia caused by folic acid deficiency. Fansidar contraindicated in porphyria.
- Repeated Fansidar use contraindicated in severe renal insufficiency, marked liver parenchymal damage or blood dyscrasias, known hypersensitivity to pyrimethamine or sulfonamides, or documented megaloblastic anemia due to folate deficiency; in infants < 2 mo; in pregnancy at term; and during breast-feeding.
- Use cautiously in impaired hepatic or renal function, severe allergy or bronchial asthma, G6PD deficiency, or seizure disorders (smaller doses may be needed) and after chloroquine treatment.

q

DRUG/CLASS/ CATEGORY	DOSAGE FORMS	INDICATIONS/ DOSAGES	KEY PRECAUTIONS
quazepam Doral *Benzodiazepine* *Hypnotic* Preg. Risk Category: X Controlled Sub. Sched.: IV	*tab:* 7.5, 15 mg	*Insomnia* — **Adults:** 15 mg PO hs. Some patients may respond to lower dosages. Lower dosage in elderly after 2 days.	▪ Use cautiously in hepatic, renal, or respiratory disease; depression; and elderly patients. ▪ Contraindicated in hypersensitivity to drug or other benzodiazepines, pregnant patients, and suspected or established sleep apnea.
quinapril hydrochloride Accupril, Asig‡ *ACE inhibitor* *Antihypertensive* Preg. Risk Category: C (D in 2nd and 3rd trimesters)	*tab:* 5, 10, 20, 40 mg	*Hypertension* — **Adults:** initially, 10 mg PO daily or 5 mg daily if patient takes diuretic. Adjust based on response at 2-wk intervals. *Heart failure* — **Adults:** 5 to 10 mg PO bid. Increase at weekly intervals.	▪ Use cautiously in impaired renal function. ▪ Contraindicated in hypersensitivity to ACE inhibitors or history of angioedema related to ACE inhibitor therapy.
quinidine gluconate Quinaglute, Dura-Tabs, Quinalan, Quinate **quinidine sulfate** Apo-Quinidine†, Cin-Quin, Quinidex Extentabs *Cinchona alkaloid* *Antitachyarrhythmic* Preg. Risk Category: C	gluconate — *tab (ext-release):* 324, 325†, 330 mg; *inj:* 80 mg/ml. sulfate — *tab:* 200, 300 mg; *tab (ext-release):* 300 mg; *cap:* 200, 300 mg; *inj:* 200 mg/ml	*Atrial flutter or fib* — **Adults:** 200 mg PO q 2 to 3 hr for 5 to 8 doses, then increase qd. Max 3 to 4 g qd. *PSVT* — **Adults:** 400 to 600 mg IM or PO q 2 to 3 hr. *PACs, PVCs, PAT, PVT, maint after cardioversion of atrial fib* — **Adults:** test dose 200 mg PO or IM. Then 200 to 400 mg (sulf. or equiv. base) PO q 4 to 6 hr; or 600 mg (gluc.) IM, then 400 mg q 2 hr prn; or 800 mg (gluc.) in 40 ml D₅W IV infusion at 16 mg/min. **Children:** test dose 2 mg/kg PO, then 30 mg/kg/24 hr PO or 900 mg/m²/24 hr PO in 5 divided doses.	▪ Use cautiously in impaired renal or hepatic function, asthma, muscle weakness, or infection accompanied by fever. ▪ Contraindicated in idiosyncrasy or hypersensitivity to quinidine or related cinchona derivatives, intraventricular conduction defects, cardiac glycoside toxicity when AV conduction grossly impaired, abnormal rhythms due to escape mechanisms, and history of drug-induced torsade de pointes or QT syndrome.

r

rabies immune globulin, human	*inj:* 150 IU/ml in 2-, 10-ml vials	*Rabies exposure — Adults and children:* 20 IU/kg IM at time of 1st dose of rabies vaccine. Half of dose used to infiltrate wound area; remainder given IM in different site.	• Use cautiously in history of systemic allergic reactions to human immunoglobulin preparations, known hypersensitivity to thimerosal, and immunoglobulin A deficiency.
Hyperab, Imogam Rabies			
Immune serum			
Rabies prophylaxis agent			
Preg. Risk Category: C			
radioactive iodine (sodium iodide) 131I	All radioactivity concentrations determined at time of calibration. **Iodotope Therapeutic — cap:** radioactivity range 1 to 50 mCi/cap. ***oral sol:*** radioactivity conc 7.05 mCi/ml; in vials containing approx 7, 14, 28, 70, 106 mCi. **Sodium Iodide 131I Therapeutic — cap:** radioactivity range 0.8 to 100 mCi/cap. ***oral sol:*** radioactivity range 3.5 to 150 mCi/vial	*Hyperthyroidism — Adults:* usual dosage 4 to 10 mCi PO based on est weight of thyroid gland and thyroid uptake. May repeat treatment in 6 wk based on serum thyroxine level.	• Use cautiously in women of childbearing age.
Iodotope Therapeutic, Sodium Iodide 131I Therapeutic		*Thyroid cancer — Adults:* initially, 50 mCi PO with subsequent doses of 100 to 150 mCi. Dosage based on est malignant thyroid tissue and metastatic tissue as determined by total body scan. Treatment repeated according to clinical status.	• Contraindicated in pregnant patients, except to treat thyroid cancer, and in breast-feeding patients.
Thyroid hormone antagonist			
Antihyperthyroid agent			
Preg. Risk Category: X			

DRUG/CLASS/CATEGORY	DOSAGE FORMS	INDICATIONS/DOSAGES	KEY PRECAUTIONS
ramipril Altace, Ramace†, Tritace‡ *ACE inhibitor* *Antihypertensive* Preg. Risk Category: C (D in 2nd and 3rd trimesters)	*caps:* 1.25, 2.5, 5, 10 mg	*Hypertension —* **Adults:** initially, 2.5 mg PO qd for patient not taking diuretic; 1.25 mg PO qd for patient taking diuretic. Increase prn based on response. Maint. 2.5 to 20 mg qd as single or divided doses. *Heart failure —* **Adults:** 2.5 mg PO bid. If hypotension, decrease to 1.25 mg PO bid. May increase slowly to max 5 mg PO bid prn.	• Use cautiously in impaired renal function. • Contraindicated in hypersensitivity to ACE inhibitors or in history of angioedema related to ACE inhibitor therapy.
ranitidine hydrochloride Apo-Ranitidine†, Zantac, Zantac-C†, Zantac 75 *Histamine₂-receptor antagonist* *Antiulcer agent* Preg. Risk Category: B	*tab:* 75, 150, 300 mg; *dispers tab:* 150 mg‡; *efferv tab:* 150 mg; *efferv granules:* 150 mg; *syrup:* 15 mg/ml; *inj:* 25 mg/ml; *infusion:* 0.5 mg/ml in 100-ml containers	*Duodenal and gastric ulcer (short-term treatment); pathologic hypersecretory conditions, such as Zollinger-Ellison syndrome —* **Adults:** 150 mg PO bid or 300 mg qd hs. Or, 50 mg IV or IM q 6 to 8 hr. Patients with Zollinger-Ellison syndrome may need up to 6 g PO qd. *Maintenance therapy for duodenal or gastric ulcer —* **Adults:** 150 mg PO hs. *GERD —* **Adults:** 150 mg PO bid.	• Use cautiously in impaired renal or hepatic function. • Contraindicated in hypersensitivity to drug or in history of acute porphyria.
reserpine Novoreserpine†, Sandril, Serpalan, Serpasil *Rauwolfia alkaloid/peripherally acting ant-adrenergic agent* *Antihypertensive/antipsychotic* Preg. Risk Category: C	*tab:* 0.1, 0.25 mg	*Mild to moderate essential hypertension —* **Adults:** initially, 0.5 mg PO daily for 1 to 2 wk, then maintenance dose of 0.1 to 0.25 mg PO daily. **Children:** 5 to 20 mcg/kg PO daily.	• Use cautiously in history of peptic ulcer, ulcerative colitis, or gallstones. • Contraindicated in hypersensitivity to drug, mental depression, history of suicidal tendency, ulcerative colitis, or peptic ulcer disease and in patients receiving electroconvulsive therapy or MAO inhibitors.

respiratory syncytial virus immune globulin intravenous, human (RSV-IGIV)
RespiGam
Immunoglobulin G
Immune serum
Preg. Risk Category: C

Inj: 50 mg ± 10 mg/ml in 50-ml single-use vial

Prevention of serious lower respiratory tract infections caused by RSV in children with bronchopulmonary dysplasia (BPD) or premature birth — **Premature infants and children < 2 yr:** single infusion monthly. Give 1.5 ml/kg/hr IV for 15 min; then may increase to 3 ml/kg/hr for 15 min to max 6 ml/kg/hr until infusion ends. Max total per monthly infusion 750 mg/kg.

- Contraindicated in history of severe hypersensitivity to drug or other human immunoglobulin and in selective IgA deficiency.
- Children with fluid overload shouldn't receive drug.

---

reteplase, recombinant
Retavase
Tissue plasminogen activator
Thrombolytic
Preg. Risk Category: C

Inj: 10.8 units (18.8 mg)/vial. Supplied in kit with components for reconstitution for 2 single-use vials.

Management of acute MI — **Adults:** double-bolus of 10 + 10 U. Give each bolus IV over 2 min. If no complications after 1st bolus, give 2nd bolus 30 min after start of 1st.

- Use cautiously in recent major surgery (within 10 days), obstetric delivery, organ biopsy, trauma, previous puncture of noncompressible vessels, cerebrovascular disease, recent GI or GU bleeding, hypertension (systolic pressure of ≥ 180 or diastolic pressure of ≥ 110), conditions that may lead to left heart thrombus (including mitral stenosis), acute pericarditis or subacute bacterial endocarditis, hemostatic defects, diabetic hemorrhagic retinopathy, septic thrombophlebitis, and any other condition in which bleeding would be hard to manage and in patients ≥ 75 yr. Also use cautiously in breast-feeding patients.
- Contraindicated in active internal bleeding, known bleeding diathesis, history of CVA, recent intracranial or intraspinal surgery or trauma, severe uncontrolled hypertension, intracranial neoplasm, arteriovenous malformation, or aneurysm.

DRUG / CLASS / CATEGORY	DOSAGE FORMS	INDICATIONS / DOSAGES	KEY PRECAUTIONS
Rho(D) immune globulin, human Gamulin Rh, HypRho-D, MICRhoGAM, Mini-Gamulin Rh, RhoGAM **Rho(D) immune globulin intravenous, human** WinRho SD *Immune serum* *Anti-Rho(D)-positive prophylaxis agent* Preg. Risk Category: C	*inj:* 300 mcg/ vial (standard dose); 50 mcg/ vial (micro-dose). **Rho(D) immune globulin IV, human** — *inj:* 120, 300 mcg	*Rh exposure* — **Adults (after abortion, miscarriage, ectopic pregnancy, or postpartum):** transfusion unit or blood bank determines fetal packed RBC volume entering patient's blood; then give 1 vial IM if fetal packed RBC volume < 15 ml. More than 1 vial IM may be required if large fetomaternal hemorrhage occurs; must give within 72 hr after delivery or miscarriage. *After postabortion or miscarriage to prevent Rh antibody formation* — **Adults:** consult transfusion unit or blood bank. 1 microdose vial will suppress immune reaction to 2.5 ml Rho(D)-positive RBCs. Ideally, should give within 3 hr, but may give up to 72 hr after abortion or miscarriage. *Transfusion accidents* — **Adults:** 600 mcg IV (IV form) q 8 hr or 1,200 mcg IM q 12 hr until total dose administered. Total dose depends on volume of packed RBCs or whole blood infused.	• Use extreme caution in IgA deficiency. Because of risk of developing IgA antibodies and subsequent anaphylaxis, weigh potential benefits of treatment against potential for hypersensitivity reactions. • Contraindicated in Rho(D)-positive or Du-positive patients and those previously immunized to Rho(D) blood factor. Also contraindicated in anaphylactic or severe systemic reactions to human globulin.
ribavirin Virazole *Synthetic nucleoside* *Antiviral agent* Preg. Risk Category: X	*powder to be reconst for inhalation:* 6 g in 100-ml glass vial	*Hospitalized infants and young children infected by respiratory syncytial virus (RSV)* — **Infants and young children:** sol in conc of 20 mg/ml delivered via Viratek Small Particle Aerosol Generator (SPAG-2) and mechanical ventilation or via O₂ mask, hood, or tent at flow rate of 12.5 L/min mist. Treat for 12 to 18 hr/day for 3 to 7 days, with flow rate of 12.5 L/min of mist.	• Contraindicated in hypersensitivity to drug and in women who are or may become pregnant during treatment.
riboflavin (vitamin B₂) *Water-soluble vitamin* *Vitamin B complex vitamin* Preg. Risk Category: NR	*tab:* 10, 25, 50, 100 mg; *tab (sugar-free):* 50, 100 mg	*Riboflavin deficiency or adjunct to thiamine treatment for polyneuritis or cheilosis secondary to pellagra* — **Adults and children ≥ 12 yr:** 5 to 30 mg PO daily, depending on severity. **Children < 12 yr:** 3 to 10 mg PO daily, depending on severity.	• No known contraindications.

rifabutin
Mycobutin
Semisynthetic ansamycin
Antibiotic
Preg. Risk Category: B

cap: 150 mg

Prevention of disseminated Mycobacterium avium complex in advanced HIV infection — **Adults:** 300 mg PO daily as single dose or divided bid, with food.

- Use cautiously in preexisting neutropenia and thrombocytopenia.
- Contraindicated in hypersensitivity to drug or other rifamycin derivatives (such as rifampin) and in active TB.

---

rifampin (rifampicin)
Rifadin, Rifadin IV, Rimactane, Rimycin‡, Rofact†
Semisynthetic rifamycin B derivative (macrocyclic antibiotic)
Antituberculosis agent
Preg. Risk Category: C

cap: 150, 300 mg; **inj:** 600 mg

Pulmonary TB — **Adults:** 600 mg/day PO or IV in single dose 1 hr before or 2 hr after meals. **Children > 5 yr:** 10 to 20 mg/kg PO or IV daily in single dose 1 hr before or 2 hr after meals. Max 600 mg/day. Give with other antituberculars.
Meningococcal carriers — **Adults:** 600 mg PO or IV bid for 2 days, or 600 mg/day PO or IV for 4 days. **Children 1 mo to 12 yr:** 10 mg/kg PO or IV bid for 2 days, ≤ 600 mg/day, or 10 to 20 mg/kg/day for 4 days. **Neonates:** 5 mg/kg PO or IV bid for 2 days.
Prophylaxis of H. influenzae type b — **Adults and children:** 20 mg/kg/day PO for 4 days; max 600 mg/day.

- Use cautiously in hepatic disease.
- Contraindicated in hypersensitivity to drug.

---

riluzole
Rilutek
Benzothiazole
Neuroprotector
Preg. Risk Category: C

tab: 50 mg

Amyotrophic lateral sclerosis — **Adults:** 50 mg PO q 12 hr, on empty stomach.

- Use cautiously in hepatic or renal dysfunction, elderly patients, and females and Japanese patients.
- Contraindicated of history of severe hypersensitivity to riluzole or drug component.

---

rimantadine hydrochloride
Flumadine
Adamantane
Antiviral
Preg. Risk Category: C

tab (film-coated): 100 mg; **syrup:** 50 mg/5 ml

Influenza A (preventative) — **Adults and children ≥ 10 yr:** 100 mg PO bid. **Children < 10 yr:** 5 mg/kg (max 150 mg) PO daily. **Elderly, severe hepatic or renal dysfunction, or adverse effects at normal dosage:** 100 mg PO daily.
Influenza A — **Adults:** 100 mg PO bid, within 24 to 48 hr of symptom onset and for 48 hr after symptoms disappear.

- Use cautiously during pregnancy, in impaired renal or hepatic function or seizure disorders (especially epilepsy) and in elderly patients.
- Contraindicated in hypersensitivity to drug or amantadine.
- In pregnant patients, consider whether risks of illness outweigh benefits of drug.

RIMANTADINE HYDROCHLORIDE   223

†Canadian ‡Australian

DRUG/CLASS/ CATEGORY	DOSAGE FORMS	INDICATIONS/ DOSAGES	KEY PRECAUTIONS
rimexolone Vexol 1% Ophthalmic Suspension *Ophthalmic steroid* *Ophthalmic anti-inflammatory agent* Preg. Risk Category: C	*ophth susp:* 1%	*Postop inflammation after ocular surgery* — **Adults:** 1 to 2 drops in conjunctival sac qid 24 hr after surgery and for 2 wk. *Anterior uveitis* — **Adults:** 1 to 2 drops in conjunctival sac q hr during waking hours for wk 1, 1 drop q 2 hr during waking hours of wk 2; then taper until uveitis resolved.	▪ Contraindicated in hypersensitivity to any drug component, epithelial herpes simplex keratitis, vaccinia, varicella, and most other viral diseases of cornea and conjunctiva; mycobacterial eye infection; and fungal disease of eye or acute purulent untreated infections masked or enhanced by steroids. ▪ Safety and efficacy in children not established.
Ringer's injection *Electrolyte solution* *Electrolyte and fluid replenishment* Preg. Risk Category: NR	*inj:* 250, 500, 1,000 ml	*Fluid and electrolyte replacement* — **Adults and children:** dosage highly individualized; usually 1.5 to 3 L (2% to 6% body weight), infused IV over 18 to 24 hr.	▪ Use cautiously in heart failure, circulatory insufficiency, renal dysfunction, hypoproteinemia, and pulmonary edema. ▪ Contraindicated in renal failure except as emergency volume expander.
Ringer's injection, lactated (Hartmann's solution, Ringer's lactate solution) *Electrolyte-carbohydrate solution* *Electrolyte and fluid replenishment* Preg. Risk Category: NR	*inj:* 150, 250, 500, 1,000 ml	*Fluid and electrolyte replacement* — **Adults and children:** dosage highly individualized; usually 1.5 to 3 L (2% to 6% body weight) infused IV over 18 to 24 hr.	▪ Use cautiously in heart failure, circulatory insufficiency, renal dysfunction, hypoproteinemia, and pulmonary edema. ▪ Contraindicated in renal failure except as emergency volume expander.
risperidone Risperdal *Benzisoxazole derivative* *Antipsychotic* Preg. Risk Category: C	*tab:* 1, 2, 3, 4 mg	*Psychosis* — **Adults:** initially, 1 mg PO bid, increased in 1-mg increments bid on days 2 and 3 to 3 mg bid. Wait ≥ 1 wk before adjusting dosage. Safety of > 16 mg/day not known. **Elderly or debilitated, hypotension, or severe renal or hepatic impairment:** 0.5 mg PO bid. Increase by 0.5-mg increments bid on days 2 and 3 to 1.5 mg PO bid. Wait ≥ 1 wk before increasing.	▪ Use cautiously in prolonged QT interval, CV disease, cerebrovascular disease, dehydration, hypovolemia, history of seizures or exposure to extreme heat, or conditions that could affect metabolism or hemodynamic responses. ▪ Contraindicated in hypersensitivity to drug and in breast-feeding patients.

ritodrine hydrochloride Yutopar *Beta-receptor agonist* *Adjunctive agent in suppression of preterm labor* Preg. Risk Category: B	*inj:* 10, 15 mg/ml; *inj for IV infusion:* 0.3 mg/ml (150 mg in 500 ml D$_5$W)	*Preterm labor —* **Adults:** dilute 150 mg in 500 ml fluid, yielding final conc of 0.3 mg/ml. Usual initial dose 0.05 mg/min IV, gradually increased by 0.05 mg/min q 10 min until desired result obtained or until maternal HR reaches 130. Effective dosage usually ranges from 0.15 to 0.35 mg/min. *Note:* Continue IV infusion for 24 hr after contractions stop. May treat recurrence of preterm labor with repeated infusion of ritodrine.	▪ Use cautiously in sulfite sensitivity. ▪ Contraindicated in pregnant women before 20th wk of pregnancy and in women with antepartum hemorrhage, eclampsia, severe preeclampsia, intrauterine fetal death, chorioamnionitis, maternal cardiac disease, pulmonary hypertension, maternal hyperthyroidism, or uncontrolled maternal diabetes mellitus. Also contraindicated in hypersensitivity to drug or in preexisting maternal conditions that would be seriously affected by known pharmacologic properties of drug.
ritonavir Norvir *HIV protease inhibitor* *Antiviral* Preg. Risk Category: B	*cap:* 100 mg; *oral sol:* 80 mg/ml	*Treatment of HIV infection with nucleoside analogues or as monotherapy when antiretroviral therapy needed —* **Adults:** 600 mg PO bid before meals. If nausea occurs, adjust dosage: 300 mg bid for 1 day, 400 mg bid for 2 days, 500 mg bid for 1 day, and 600 mg bid thereafter.	▪ Use cautiously in hepatic insufficiency. ▪ Contraindicated in hypersensitivity to any drug component.
rocuronium bromide Zemuron *Nondepolarizing neuromuscular blocker* *Skeletal muscle relaxant* Preg. Risk Category: B	*inj:* 10 mg/ml	*Adjunct to general anesthesia to facilitate endotracheal intubation and to provide skeletal muscle relaxation during surgery or mechanical ventilation —* dosage depends on anesthetic used, individual needs, and response. Dosages listed are representative and must be adjusted. **Adults:** initially, 0.6 mg/kg IV bolus. In most patients, tracheal intubation may be performed within 2 min; muscle paralysis should last about 31 min. Maint dosage of 0.1 mg/kg should provide additional 12 min of muscle relaxation; 0.15 mg/kg adds 17 min; 0.2 mg/kg adds 24 min.	▪ Use cautiously in hepatic disease, severe obesity, bronchogenic carcinoma, electrolyte disturbances, neuromuscular disease, or CV disease, advanced age, or edematous states. ▪ Contraindicated in hypersensitivity to bromides.

†Canadian ‡Australian

S

DRUG/CLASS / CATEGORY	DOSAGE FORMS	INDICATIONS / DOSAGES	KEY PRECAUTIONS
salmeterol xinafoate Serevent *Selective beta₂-adrenergic stimulating agonist* *Bronchodilator* Preg. Risk Category: C	*inhalation aerosol:* 25 mcg/activation	*Long-term maintenance for asthma; prevention of bronchospasm for nocturnal asthma or reversible obstructive airway disease* — **Adults and children > 12 yr:** 2 inhalations bid. *Prevention of exercise-induced bronchospasm* — **Adults and children ≥ 12 yr:** 2 inhalations 30 to 60 min before exercise.	• Use cautiously in coronary insufficiency, arrhythmias, hypertension, other CV disorders, thyrotoxicosis, or seizure disorders and in patients unusually responsive to sympathomimetics. • Contraindicated in hypersensitivity to drug or any component.
salsalate (disalicylic acid, salicylsalicylic acid) Amigesic, Argesic-SA, Arthra-G, Disalcid, Mono-Gesic, Salflex, Salgesic, Salsitab *Salicylate* *Nonnarcotic analgesic/antipyretic/ anti-inflammatory* Preg. Risk Category: C	*tab:* 500, 750 mg; *cap:* 500 mg	*Arthritis* — **Adults:** 3 g PO daily in divided doses bid or tid.	• Use cautiously in renal insufficiency, severely impaired hepatic function, bleeding disorders, peptic ulcer disease, hypoprothrombinemia, vitamin K deficiency, thrombocytopenia, or thrombotic thrombocytopenic purpura. • Not recommended in chickenpox or influenza or flulike symptoms; Reye's syndrome may develop. • Contraindicated in salsalate hypersensitivity.
saquinavir mesylate Invirase *Protease inhibitor* *Antiviral agent* Preg. Risk Category: B	*cap:* 200 mg	*Adjunct treatment of advanced HIV infection in selected patients* — **Adults:** 600 mg PO tid within 2 hr after full meal and with nucleoside analogue.	• Contraindicated in hypersensitivity to drug or to any component in capsule. • Safety in pregnant or breast-feeding women and in children < 16 yr not established.

Drug	Forms	Indications & Dosages	Contraindications & Cautions
sargramostim (granulocyte-macrophage colony-stimulating factor, GM-CSF) Leukine *Biologic response modifier Colony-stimulating factor* Preg. Risk Category: C	*powder for inj:* 250, 500 mcg	*Acceleration of hematopoietic reconstitution after autologous bone marrow transplantation (BMT)* — **Adults:** 250 mcg/m²/day for 21 days given as 2-hr IV infusion starting 2 to 4 hr after BMT. *BMT failure or engraftment delay* — **Adults:** 250 mcg/m²/day for 14 days as 2-hr IV infusion. May repeat dose after 7 days of no therapy.	■ Use cautiously in preexisting cardiac disease or fluid retention, hypoxia, pulmonary infiltrates, heart failure, or impaired renal or hepatic function. ■ Contraindicated in excessive leukemic myeloid blasts in bone marrow or peripheral blood and in hypersensitivity to drug or any component or to yeast-derived products.
scopolamine (hyoscine) Isopto Hyoscine, Scōp†, Transderm-Scōp, Transderm-V† **scopolamine butylbromide (hyoscine butylbromide)** Buscopan†‡ **scopolamine hydrobromide (hyoscine hydrobromide)** *Anticholinergic Antimuscarinic* Preg. Risk Category: C	*patch:* 1.5 mg. **butylbromide** — **tab:** 10 mg†; **cap:** 0.25 mg. **hydrobromide — inj:** 0.3, 0.4, 0.5, 0.6, 1 mg/ml in 1-ml vials and amp; 0.86 mg/ml in 0.5-ml amp	*Spastic states* — **Adults:** 10 to 20 mg PO tid or qid. Or, 10 to 20 mg (butylbromide) SC, IM, or IV tid or qid. *Delirium, preanesthetic sedation and obstetric amnesia with analgesics* — **Adults:** 0.3 to 0.65 mg IM, SC, or IV. **Children:** 0.006 mg/kg IM, SC, IV; max 0.3 mg. *Prevention of motion sickness* — **Adults:** 1 Transderm-Scōp or Transderm-V patch applied to skin behind ear several hr before antiemetic required. Or, 300 to 600 mcg (hydrobromide) SC, IM, or IV. **Children:** 6 mcg/kg or 200 mcg/m² (hydrobromide) SC, IM, or IV.	■ Use cautiously in autonomic neuropathy, hyperthyroidism, CAD, heart failure, hypertension, hiatal hernia associated with reflux esophagitis, hepatic or renal disease, ulcerative colitis, children < 6 yr, and patients in hot or humid environments. ■ Contraindicated in angle-closure glaucoma, obstructive uropathy, obstructive disease of the GI tract, asthma, chronic pulmonary disease, myasthenia gravis, paralytic ileus, intestinal atony, unstable cardiovascular status in acute hemorrhage, or toxic megacolon.
scopolamine hydrobromide Isopto Hyoscine *Antimuscarinic/cycloplegic mydriatic* Preg. Risk Category: NR	*ophth sol:* 0.25%	*Cycloplegic refraction* — **Adults:** 1 to 2 drops 0.25% sol 1 hr before refraction. **Children:** 1 drop 0.25% sol bid for 2 days before refraction. *Iritis, uveitis* — **Adults:** 1 to 2 drops 0.25% sol daily to qid. **Children:** 1 drop qd to qid.	■ Use with extreme caution (if at all) in infants and small children. ■ Use cautiously in cardiac disease and in elderly patients. ■ Contraindicated in shallow anterior chamber and angle-closure glaucoma, hypersensitivity to drug, adhesions (synechia) between iris and lens, and in children with history of severe systemic reaction to atropine. ■ Avoid in breast-feeding patients.

†Canadian ‡Australian

DRUG/CLASS/ CATEGORY	DOSAGE FORMS	INDICATIONS/ DOSAGES	KEY PRECAUTIONS
secobarbital sodium Novosecobarb†, Seconal Sodium *Barbiturate* *Sedative-hypnotic/anticonvulsant* Preg. Risk Category: D Controlled Sub. Sched.: II	**cap:** 50, 100 mg; **inj:** 50 mg/ml	*Preop sedation* — **Adults:** 200 to 300 mg PO 1 to 2 hr before surgery or 1 mg/kg IM 15 min before procedure. **Children:** 2 to 6 mg/kg PO. Max single dose 100 mg. *Insomnia* — **Adults:** 100 to 200 mg PO or IM. *Status epilepticus*— **Adults:** 250 to 350 mg IM or IV. **Children:** 15 to 20 mg/kg IV over 15 min.	▪ Use cautiously in acute or chronic pain, depression, suicidal tendencies, history of drug abuse, or impaired hepatic or renal function. ▪ Contraindicated in respiratory disease with dyspnea or obstruction, hypersensitivity to barbiturates, or porphyria.
selegiline hydrochloride Eldepryl *MAO inhibitor* *Antiparkinsonian agent* Preg. Risk Category: C	**tab:** 5 mg	*Adjunctive treatment with carbidopa-levodopa in managing Parkinson's disease* — **Adults:** 10 mg/day PO (5 mg at breakfast and 5 mg at lunch). After 2 or 3 days, slowly decrease carbidopa-levodopa dosage.	▪ Contraindicated in hypersensitivity to drug and in patients receiving meperidine or other opioids.
senna Fletcher's Castoria, Senexon, Senokot *Anthraquinone derivative* *Stimulant laxative* Preg. Risk Category: C	**tab:** 187, 217, 600 mg; **granules:** 326 mg/ tsp, 1.65 g/ ½ tsp; **supp:** 652 mg; **syrup:** 218 mg/5 ml	*Acute constipation; preparation for bowel or rectal exam* — **Adults:** dosage for Senokot 1 to 8 tab PO; ½ to 4 tsp of granules added to liquid PO; 1 to 2 supp PR hs; or 1 to 4 tsp syrup PO hs.	▪ Contraindicated in ulcerative bowel lesions; nausea, vomiting, abdominal pain, or other symptoms of appendicitis or acute surgical abdomen; fecal impaction; or intestinal obstruction or perforation
sertraline hydrochloride Zoloft *Serotonin uptake inhibitor* *Antidepressant* Preg. Risk Category: B	**tab:** 50, 100 mg	*Depression* — **Adults:** 50 mg/day PO; adjust dosage as tolerated and needed (clinical trials used 50 to 200 mg/day). Adjust dosage at ≥ 1-wk intervals. *Obsessive-compulsive disorder* — **Adults:** 50 mg/day PO. If no response, may increase to max 200 mg/day. Adjust dosage at ≥ 1-wk intervals.	▪ Use cautiously in patients at risk for suicide and in seizure disorders, major affective disorders, or conditions that affect metabolism or hemodynamic responses. ▪ Contraindicated in patients taking MAO inhibitors or within 14 days of discontinuing MAO inhibitor therapy.

silver nitrate 1% *Heavy metal (silver compound)* *Ophthalmic antiseptic* Preg. Risk Category: NR	***ophth sol:** 1%*	■ No known contraindications.
	Prevention of gonorrheal ophthalmia neonatorum — **Neonates:** clean eyelids thoroughly; instill 2 drops 1% sol into lower conjunctival sac of each eye at angle of nasal bridge and eyes, preferably immediately after delivery but no later than 1 hr after delivery.	
silver sulfadiazine Flamazinet, Flint SSD, Silvadene, Thermazene *Synthetic anti-infective* *Topical antibacterial* Preg. Risk Category: B	***cream:** 1%*	■ Use with caution in hypersensitivity to sulfonamides. ■ Contraindicated in premature and full-term neonates < 2 mo, in hypersensitivity to drug, in G6PD deficiency, and in pregnant women at or near term.
	Prevention and treatment of wound infection in 2nd- and 3rd-degree burns — **Adults:** apply 1/16" thickness to clean, debrided burn daily or bid.	
simethicone Gas-X, Mylanta, Mylicon *Dispersant* *Antiflatulent* Preg. Risk Category: NR	***tab:** 40, 60, 80, 95, 125 mg;* ***cap:** 125 mg;* ***drops:** 40 mg/0.6 ml*	■ Not recommended for treatment of infant colic; limited information on safety in infants and children. ■ Contraindicated in hypersensitivity to drug.
	Flatulence, functional gastric bloating — **Adults and children > 12 yr:** 40 to 160 mg before meals and hs. **Children 2 to 12 yr:** 40 mg (drops) PO qid. **Children < 2 yr:** 20 mg (drops) PO qid, up to 240 mg/day.	
simvastatin (syvinolin) Lipex‡, Zocor *HMG-CoA reductase inhibitor* *Antilipemic* Preg. Risk Category: X	***tab:** 5, 10, 20, 40 mg*	■ Use cautiously in history of liver disease or in patients who consume excessive alcohol. ■ Contraindicated in hypersensitivity to drug and in active liver disease or conditions that cause unexplained, persistent serum transaminase elevations; in pregnant and breast-feeding patients; and in women of childbearing age unless no risk of pregnancy exists.
	Reduction of LDL and total cholesterol levels in primary hypercholesterolemia (types IIa and IIb) — **Adults:** initially, 5 to 10 mg/day PO in pm. Adjust dosage q 4 wk based on tolerance and response; max 40 mg/day.	

DRUG/CLASS/ CATEGORY	DOSAGE FORMS	INDICATIONS/ DOSAGES	KEY PRECAUTIONS
sodium bicarbonate Bell/ans, Citrocarbonate, Soda Mint *Alkalizing agent* *Systemic and urinary alkalinizer* Preg. Risk Category: C	***tab:*** 325, 520, 650 mg; ***inj:*** 4% (2.4 mEq/5 ml), 4.2% (5 mEq/10 ml), 5% (297.5 mEq/500 ml), 7.5% (8.92 mEq/10 ml and 44.6 mEq/50 ml), 8.4% (10 mEq/10 ml and 50 mEq/50 ml)	*Cardiac arrest* — **Adults and children:** 1 mEq/kg IV of 7.5% or 8.4% sol, followed by 0.5 mEq/kg IV q 10 min, based on ABGs. If ABG results unavailable, use 0.5 mEq/kg IV q 10 min until spontaneous circulation returns. **Infants < 2 yr:** ≤ 8 mEq/kg/day IV of 4.2% sol. *Metabolic acidosis* — **Adults and children:** usually, 2 to 5 mEq/kg IV over 4 to 8 hr. *Systemic or urinary alkalinization* — **Adults:** initially, 4 g PO, then 1 to 2 g q 4 hr. **Children:** 84 to 840 mg/kg/day PO.	■ Use with extreme caution in heart failure or other edematous or sodium-retaining conditions or renal insufficiency. ■ Contraindicated in metabolic or respiratory alkalosis, in chloride loss due to vomiting or continuous GI suction, in patients receiving diuretics that produce hypochloremic alkalosis, and in hypocalcemia in which alkalosis may produce tetany, hypertension, seizures, or heart failure. Orally administered form contraindicated in acute ingestion of strong mineral acids.
sodium chloride *Electrolyte* *Sodium and chloride replacement* Preg. Risk Category: C	***tab:*** 650 mg; ***tab (slow-release):*** 600 mg; ***inj:*** 0.45, 0.9, 3, 5, 14.6, 23.4% NaCl sol	*Hyponatremia caused by electrolyte loss or in severe salt depletion* — **Adults:** dosage individualized. Use 3% or 5% sol only with frequent electrolyte determination and give only slow IV. With 0.45% sol: 3% to 8% of body weight, according to deficiencies, over 18 to 24 hr; with 0.9% sol: 2% to 6% of body weight, according to deficiencies, over 18 to 24 hr. *Heat cramp caused by excessive perspiration* — **Adults:** 1 g PO with water.	■ Use cautiously in heart failure, circulatory insufficiency, renal dysfunction, and hypoproteinemia and in elderly or postop patients. ■ Contraindicated when sodium and chloride administration detrimental. 3% and 5% NaCl injections contraindicated in increased, normal, or only slightly decreased serum electrolyte levels.

sodium chloride, hypertonic
Adsorbonac Ophthalmic Solution, Muro-128 Ointment, Sodium Chloride Ointment 5%
Hypertonic (hyperosmolar) solution
Hypertonicity agent
Preg. Risk Category: NR

ophth oint: 5%; **ophth sol:** 2%, 5%

Temporary relief of corneal edema — **Adults and children:** 1 to 2 drops q 3 to 4 hr, or oint applied q 3 to 4 hr.

- Contraindicated in hypersensitivity to drug or any component.

sodium fluoride
Fluoritab, Flura-Drops, Luride, Pedi-Dentf, Pharmaflur
sodium fluoride, topical
ACT, Fluorigard, Fluorinse, Listermint with Fluoride, PreviDent, Stop, Thera-Flur
Trace mineral
Dental caries prophylactic
Preg. Risk Category: NR

tab: 1 mg; **tab (chew):** 0.5, 1 mg; **drops:** 0.125, 0.25 mg/drop and 0.2, 0.5 mg/ml; **lozenges:** 1 mg. **topical — gel:** 0.1%, 0.5%, 1.23%; **gel drops:** 0.5%; **drops:** 0.01%, **rinse:** 0.02%, 0.09%

Prevention of dental caries — **Adults and children > 6 yr:** 5 to 10 ml of rinse or thin ribbon of gel applied to teeth with toothbrush or mouth trays for ≥ 1 min hs. **Children < 2 yr:** 0.25 mg PO (tab or drops) daily. **Children 2 to 3 yr:** 0.5 mg PO (tab or drops) daily. **Children 3 to 13 yr:** 1 mg PO (tab or lozenge) daily.

- Contraindicated in hypersensitivity to fluoride or when intake from drinking water > 0.7 ppm.

sodium lactate
Alkalinizing agent
Systemic alkalizer
Preg. Risk Category: NR

inj: 1/6 molar sol (167 mEq/L); **inj:** 5 mEq/ml

Alkalinize urine — **Adults:** 30 ml of 1/6 molar sol/kg body weight IV, given in divided doses over 24 hr.
Metabolic acidosis — **Adults:** 1/6 molar inj (167 mEq lactate/L IV); dosage depends on degree of bicarbonate deficit.

- Use with extreme caution in metabolic or respiratory alkalosis, severe hepatic or renal disease, shock, hypoxia, or beriberi.
- Contraindicated in hypernatremia, lactic acidosis, or conditions in which sodium administration detrimental.

SODIUM LACTATE   **231**

DRUG/CLASS/ CATEGORY	DOSAGE FORMS	INDICATIONS/ DOSAGES	KEY PRECAUTIONS
sodium phosphates (sodium phosphate and sodium biphosphate) Fleet Phospho-Soda, Fleet Enema *Acid salt* *Saline laxative* Preg. Risk Category: C	*liq:* 2.4 g/5 ml sodium phosphate and 900 mg sodium biphosphate/5 ml; *enema:* ready-to-use squeeze bottle (66.5, 133 ml)	*Constipation* — **Adults:** 20 ml sol mixed with 120 ml cold water PO, or as enema, 120 ml PR. **Children:** 5 to 10 ml sol mixed with 120 ml cold water PO; or as enema, 60 ml PR.	▪ Use cautiously in patients with large hemorrhoids or anal excoriations. ▪ Contraindicated in abdominal pain, nausea, vomiting, or other symptoms of appendicitis or acute surgical abdomen; intestinal obstruction or perforation; edema; heart failure; megacolon; or impaired renal function and in patients on sodium-restricted diets.
sodium polystyrene sulfonate Kayexalate, Resonium A, SPS *Cation-exchange resin* *Potassium-removing resin* Preg. Risk Category: C	*powder:* 1-lb jar (3.5 g/tsp); *susp:* 15 g/60 ml	*Hyperkalemia* — **Adults:** 15 g PO daily to qid in water or sorbitol (3 to 4 ml/g of resin). Or, mix powder with appropriate medium (aqueous suspension or diet appropriate for renal failure) and instill through NG tube. Or, 30 to 50 g/100 ml of sorbitol q 6 hr as warm emulsion deep into sigmoid colon (20 cm). **Children:** 1 g/kg of body weight/dose PO or PR prn. PO route preferred (drug should be in intestine ≥ 30 min).	▪ Use cautiously in severe heart failure, severe hypertension, or marked edema. ▪ Contraindicated in hypokalemia or hypersensitivity to drug.
somatrem Protropin **somatropin** Humatrope, Nutropin *Anterior pituitary hormone* *Human growth hormone* Preg. Risk Category: C	**somatrem**— *inj lyophil powder:* 5 mg (about 15 IU)/ vial, 10 mg (about 30 IU)/ vial; *inj:* 2-mg vial (about 6-IU Humatrope) vial†, 5-mg vial† (about 15-IU	*Long-term treatment of children with growth failure from lack of adequate endogenous growth hormone (GH) secretion* —**Children (prepuberty):** somatrem: highly individualized; up to 0.1 mg/kg IM or SC 3 times weekly. Humatrope: up to 0.06 mg/kg SC or IM 3 times weekly. Nutropin: 0.30 mg/kg SC weekly in daily divided doses. *Growth failure in children associated with chronic renal insufficiency up to time of renal transplantation (Nutropin only)* — **Children:** 0.35 mg/kg SC weekly in daily divided doses.	▪ Use cautiously in hypothyroidism and when GH deficiency results from intracranial lesion. ▪ Contraindicated in epiphyseal closure or active underlying intracranial lesion. Somatrem is contraindicated in hypersensitivity to benzyl alcohol.

sotalol
Betapace, Sotacor†‡
Beta-adrenergic blocker
Antiarrhythmic
Preg. Risk Category: B

Humatrope)
vial, 10-mg
(about 30-IU
Nutropin) vial

Long-term treatment of short stature associated with Turner's syndrome (Nutropin) — **Children:** up to 0.375 mg/kg/wk (approx 1.125 IU/kg/wk) SC divided into equal doses given 3 to 7 times per wk.

tab: 80, 120, 160, 240 mg

Documented, life-threatening ventricular arrhythmias — **Adults:** initially, 80 mg PO bid. Increase q 2 to 3 days as needed and tolerated; most respond to 160 to 320 mg/day.

- Use cautiously in impaired renal function or diabetes mellitus.
- Contraindicated in hypersensitivity to drug, severe sinus node dysfunction, sinus bradycardia, second- and third-degree AV block in absence of artificial pacemaker, congenital or acquired long-QT syndrome, cardiogenic shock, uncontrolled heart failure, and bronchial asthma.

sparfloxacin
Zagam
Fluoroquinolone
Anti-infective
Preg. Risk Category: C

tab: 200 mg

Community-acquired pneumonia and acute bacterial exacerbation of chronic bronchitis caused by susceptible organisms — **Adults > 18 yr:** 400 mg PO on day 1 as loading dose, then 200 mg/day for total 10 days.

- Use cautiously in renal impairment and in history of seizure disorder or other CNS disease, such as cerebral arteriosclerosis. Discontinue if patient experiences symptoms of excessive CNS stimulation (restlessness, tremor, confusion, hallucinations).
- Contraindicated in history of hypersensitivity or photosensitivity reactions to drug and in patients who can't stay out of sun. Avoid concomitant use with drugs known to prolong QT interval or cause torsade de pointes.
- Not recommended for patients with cardiac conditions that predispose to arrhythmias.
- Safety and efficacy in pregnant and breast-feeding women and in children < 18 yr not established.

DRUG/CLASS / CATEGORY	DOSAGE FORMS	INDICATIONS / DOSAGES	KEY PRECAUTIONS
spironolactone Aldactone, Novospirotont *Potassium-sparing diuretic* *Antihypertensive/diuretic/treatment of diuretic-induced hypokalemia* Preg. Risk Category: NR	**tab:** 25, 50, 100 mg	*Edema* — **Adults:** 25 to 200 mg PO daily or in divided doses. **Children:** 3.3 mg/kg PO daily or in divided doses. *Hypertension* — **Adults:** 50 to 100 mg PO daily or in divided doses. *Diuretic-induced hypokalemia* — **Adults:** 25 to 100 mg PO daily.	▪ Use cautiously in fluid or electrolyte imbalance, impaired renal function, and hepatic disease. ▪ Contraindicated in known hypersensitivity to drug, anuria, acute or progressive renal insufficiency, or hyperkalemia.
stanozolol Winstrol *Anabolic steroid* *Angioedema prophylactic* Preg. Risk Category: X Controlled Sub. Sched.: III	**tab:** 2 mg	*Prevention of hereditary angioedema* — **Adults:** initially, 2 mg PO tid. After response, slowly reduce dosage at 1- to 3-mo intervals to 2 mg/day PO. **Children < 6 yr:** 1 mg/day PO during attack only. **Children 6 to 12 yr:** up to 2 mg/day PO during attack only.	▪ Use cautiously in renal, cardiac, or hepatic disease; diabetes; migraine or other conditions aggravated by fluid retention; epilepsy; and in women of childbearing age unless pregnancy ruled out. ▪ Contraindicated in hypersensitivity to anabolic steroids; in males with breast cancer or prostate cancer; in nephrosis or nephrotic phase of nephritis; in women with breast cancer and with hypercalcemia; during pregnancy; and in breast-feeding patients.
stavudine (2, 3 dide-hydro-3-deoxythymidine, d4t) Zerit *Synthetic thymidine nucleoside analogue* *Antiviral* Preg. Risk Category: C	**cap:** 15, 20, 30, 40 mg	*Treatment of HIV-infected patients who have received prolonged zidovudine therapy* — **Adults ≥ 60 kg:** 40 mg PO q 12 hr. **Adults < 60 kg:** 30 mg PO q 12 hr.	▪ Use cautiously in impaired renal function or history of peripheral neuropathy and in pregnant women. ▪ Contraindicated in hypersensitivity to drug.

streptokinase
Kabikinase, Streptase
Plasminogen activator
Thrombolytic enzyme
Preg. Risk Category: C

inj: 250,000, 600,000, 750,000, 1,500,000 IU in vials for reconstitution

Arteriovenous cannula occlusion — **Adults:** 250,000 IU in 2 ml IV sol by IV pump infusion into each occluded limb of cannula over 25 to 35 min. Clamp off cannula for 2 hr. Then aspirate, flush, and reconnect.
Venous thrombosis, PE, arterial thrombosis and embolism — **Adults:** loading dose 250,000 IU IV over 30 min. Sustaining dose 100,000 IU/hr IV for 72 hr for DVT and 100,000 IU/hr over 24 to 72 hr for PE and arterial thrombosis or embolism.
Lysis of coronary artery thrombi — **Adults:** loading dose 20,000 IU bolus via coronary catheter, then 2,000 IU/min infusion over 60 min. Or, give as IV infusion. Usual adult dose 1.5 million IU IV over 60 min.

- Use cautiously when treating arterial embolism originating from left side of heart.
- Contraindicated in ulcerative wounds, active internal bleeding, recent CVA, recent trauma with possible internal injuries, visceral or intracranial malignant neoplasms, ulcerative colitis, diverticulitis, severe hypertension, acute or chronic hepatic or renal insufficiency, uncontrolled hypocoagulation, chronic pulmonary disease with cavitation, or subacute bacterial endocarditis or rheumatic valvular disease; recent cerebral embolism, thrombosis, hemorrhage; or severe allergic reaction to streptokinase.
- Also contraindicated within 10 days after intra-arterial diagnostic procedure or any surgery, including liver or kidney biopsy, lumbar puncture, thoracentesis, paracentesis, or extensive or multiple cutdowns.
- Should be used only by doctors with wide experience in thrombotic disease management, where clinical and lab monitoring can be performed.

streptozocin
Zanosar
Antibiotic antineoplastic nitrosurea
(cell cycle–phase nonspecific)
Antineoplastic
Preg. Risk Category: C

inj: 1-g vials

Metastatic islet cell carcinoma of pancreas — **Adults and children:** 500 mg/m² IV for 5 consecutive days q 6 wk until max benefit or toxicity observed. Or, 1,000 mg/m² at weekly intervals for 1st 2 wk. Max single dose 1,500 mg/m². Infuse diluted sol over ≥ 15 min.

- Use cautiously in renal disease.

DRUG/CLASS/ CATEGORY	DOSAGE FORMS	INDICATIONS/ DOSAGES	KEY PRECAUTIONS
strontium 89 (^{89}Sr) chloride Metastron *Radioisotope* *Radioisotope for bone pain* Preg. Risk Category: D	*inj:* 4 mCi/10 ml	*Relief of bone pain in patients with painful metastatic lesions* — **Adults:** 4 mCi by slow IV inj over 1 to 2 min.	• Use cautiously in patients with platelet counts < 60,000/mm³ or WBC counts < 2,400/mm³. • Contraindicated in hypersensitivity.
succimer Chemet *Heavy metal* *Chelating agent* Preg. Risk Category: C	*cap:* 100 mg	*Lead poisoning in children with blood lead levels > 45 mcg/dl* — **Children:** 10 mg/kg or 350 mg/m² q 8 hr for 5 days. Round dosage to nearest 100 mg (see chart). Then, decrease to q 12 hr for 2 wk. Weight (kg) Dose (mg) 8 to 15 100 16 to 23 200 24 to 34 300 35 to 44 400 > 45 500	• Use cautiously in compromised renal function. • Measure severity by initial blood lead level and by rate and degree of rebound of blood lead level. Use severity as guide for more frequent blood monitoring. • Contraindicated in hypersensitivity to drug.
succinylcholine chloride (suxamethonium chloride) Anectine, Anectine Flo-Pack, Quelicin, Scoline‡, Sucostrin *Depolarizing neuromuscular blocker* *Skeletal muscle relaxant* Preg. Risk Category: C	*inj:* 20, 50, 100 mg/ml; 100-mg, 500-mg, 1-g vial	*Adjunct to anesthesia to induce skeletal muscle relaxation; to facilitate intubation and assist with mechanical ventilation; to lessen muscle contractions in pharmacologically or electrically induced seizures* — Dosage depends on anesthetic used, individual needs, and response. Dosages listed are representative only. **Adults:** 25 to 75 mg IV, then 2.5 mg/min prn, or 2.5 mg/kg IM to max 150 mg IM in deltoid muscle. **Children:** 1 to 2 mg/kg IM or IV. Max IM dosage 150 mg. (Children may be less sensitive to succinylcholine than adults.)	• Use cautiously in elderly or debilitated patients; those receiving quinidine or cardiac glycoside therapy; those undergoing cesarean section; and in respiratory depression, severe burns or trauma, electrolyte imbalances, hyperkalemia, paraplegia, spinal neuraxis injury, CVA, degenerative or dystrophic neuromuscular disease, myasthenia gravis, myasthenic syndrome of lung or bronchiogenic cancer, dehydration, thyroid disorders, collagen diseases, porphyria, fractures, muscle spasms, eye surgery, pheochromocytoma, or impaired renal, pulmonary or hepatic function.

		▪ Contraindicated in hypersensitivity to drug, abnormally low plasma pseudocholinesterase, angle-closure glaucoma, malignant hyperthermia, or penetrating eye injuries.
sucralfate Carafate, SCF‡, Sulcrate† *Pepsin* *Antiulcer agent* Preg. Risk Category: B	*tab:* 1 g; *susp:* 1 g/10 ml	*Short-term (≤ 8 wk) treatment of duodenal ulcer —* **Adults:** 1 g PO qid 1 hr after meals and hs. *Maintenance therapy for duodenal ulcer —* **Adults:** 1 g PO bid.	▪ Use cautiously in chronic renal disease. ▪ No known contraindications.
sufentanil citrate Sufenta *Opioid* *Analgesic/adjunct to anesthesia/anesthetic* Preg. Risk Category: C Controlled Sub. Sched.: II	*inj:* 50 mcg/ml	*Adjunct to general anesthetic —* **Adults:** 1 to 8 mcg/kg IV administered with nitrous oxide and O₂; additional 10 to 25 mcg IV may be given prn when movement or vital sign changes indicate surgical stress or lightening of analgesia. *As primary anesthetic —* **Adults:** 8 to 30 mcg/kg IV administered with 100% O₂ and muscle relaxant; additional 10 to 50 mcg IV may be given prn when movement or vital sign changes indicate surgical stress or lightening of analgesia. **Children < 12 yr undergoing CV surgery:** 10 to 25 mcg/kg IV given with 100% O₂ and muscle relaxant. Additional doses up to 50 mcg IV may be given prn.	▪ Use cautiously in elderly or debilitated patients and in decreased respiratory reserve, head injuries, or renal, pulmonary or hepatic disease. ▪ Contraindicated in hypersensitivity to drug.
sulconazole nitrate Exelderm *Imidazole derivative* *Antifungal agent* Preg. Risk Category: C	*topical sol:* 1%; *cream:* 1%	*Tinea cruris, tinea corporis, tinea pedis, or tinea versicolor —* **Adults:** massage small amount into affected area daily to bid for 3 wk. Treat tinea pedis with cream bid for 4 wk.	▪ Use with caution in breast-feeding patients. ▪ Contraindicated in hypersensitivity to any drug component.

SULCONAZOLE NITRATE   237

DRUG/CLASS/ CATEGORY	DOSAGE FORMS	INDICATIONS/ DOSAGES	KEY PRECAUTIONS
sulfacetamide sodium 10% Bleph-10 Liquifilm Ophthalmic, Cetamide Ophthalmic, Ocu-Sul-10, Sodium Sulamyd 10% Ophthalmic, Sulf-10 Ophthalmic **sulfacetamide sodium 15%** Isopto Cetamide Ophthalmic, Ocu-Sul-15 **sulfacetamide sodium 30%** Ocu-Sul-30, Sodium Sulamyd 30% Ophthalmic *Sulfonamide* *Antibiotic* Preg. Risk Category: C	**ophth oint:** 10%; **ophth sol:** 10%; **sol:** 15%, 30%	*Inclusion conjunctivitis, corneal ulcers, chlamydial infection* — **Adults and children:** 1 to 2 drops 10% sol instilled into lower conjunctival sac q 2 to 3 hr during day; or 1 to 2 drops 15% sol instilled into lower conjunctival sac q 1 to 2 hr initially. Interval increased as condition responds; or 1 drop 30% sol instilled into lower conjunctival sac q 2 hr. 1.25 to 2.5 cm 10% oint applied into conjunctival sac qid and hs. Oint may be used at night along with drops during day.	• Contraindicated in hypersensitivity to sulfonamides. Not recommended for children < 2 mo.
sulfadiazine Coptint, Microsulfon *Sulfonamide* *Antibiotic* Preg. Risk Category: C (contraindicated at term)	**tab:** 500 mg	*Asymptomatic meningococcal carriers* — **Adults:** 1 g PO q 12 hr for 2 days. **Children 1 to 12 yr:** 500 mg PO q 12 hr for 2 days. **Children 2 to 12 mo:** 500 mg PO daily for 2 days. *Rheumatic fever prophylaxis, as alternative to penicillin* — **Children > 30 kg:** 1 g PO daily. **Children < 30 kg:** 500 mg PO daily. *Adjunct treatment in toxoplasmosis* — **Adults:** 2 to 8 g PO daily divided q 6 hr for 6 to 8 wk or until improvement occurs. Usually given with pyrimethamine. **Children:** 100 to 200 mg/kg PO daily divided q 6 hr (max 6 g daily) for 6 to 8 wk or until improvement occurs. Usually given with pyrimethamine.	• Use cautiously in impaired renal or hepatic function, bronchial asthma, multiple allergies, G6PD deficiency, or blood dyscrasia. • Contraindicated in hypersensitivity to sulfonamides, in porphyria, in infants < 2 mo (except in congenital toxoplasmosis), in pregnant women at term, and during breast-feeding.

sulfamethoxazole

Apo-Sulfamethoxazole†, Gantanol

Sulfonamide

Antibiotic

Preg. Risk Category: C (contraindicated at term)

tab: 500 mg; **oral susp:** 500 mg/5 ml

UTI and systemic infections — **Adults:** initially, 2 g PO, then 1 g PO bid or tid for severe infections. *C. trachomatis* — **Adults:** 1 g PO bid for 21 days. **Children and infants > 2 mo:** initially, 50 to 60 mg/kg PO, then 25 to 30 mg/kg bid. Max dosage 75 mg/kg/day.

- Use cautiously in renal or hepatic impairment, bronchial asthma, severe allergies, G6PD deficiency, or blood dyscrasia.
- Contraindicated in hypersensitivity to sulfonamides, in porphyria, in infants < 2 mo (except in congenital toxoplasmosis), in pregnant women at term, and during breast-feeding.

sulfasalazine (salazosulfapyridine, sulphasalazine)

Azulfidine, Azulfidine EN-Tabs, PMS Sulfasalazine E.C.†, EN-Tabs†‡, S.A.S.-Enteric

Sulfonamide

Antibiotic

Preg. Risk Category: B

tab: 500 mg; with or without enteric coating; **oral susp:** 250 mg/5 ml

Mild to moderate ulcerative colitis, adjunctive therapy in severe ulcerative colitis, Crohn's disease — **Adults:** initially, 3 to 4 g PO daily in evenly divided doses; usual maintenance dosage 2 g PO daily in divided doses q 6 hr. May start with 1 to 2 g, with gradual increase in dosage to minimize adverse effects. **Children > 2 yr:** initially, 40 to 60 mg/kg PO daily, divided into 3 to 6 doses; then 30 mg/kg daily in 4 doses.

- Use cautiously and in reduced dosages in impaired hepatic or renal function, severe allergy, bronchial asthma, and G6PD deficiency.
- Contraindicated in hypersensitivity to drug or its metabolites, porphyria, or intestinal and urinary obstruction and in infants < 2 yr.

sulfinpyrazone

Anturan†, Anturane

Uricosuric agent

Renal tubular-blocking agent

Preg. Risk Category: NR

tab: 100 mg; **cap:** 200 mg

Intermittent or chronic gouty arthritis — **Adults:** 200 to 400 mg PO bid 1st wk, then 400 mg PO bid. Max 800 mg daily.

- Use cautiously in healed peptic ulcer and in pregnant patients.
- Contraindicated in hypersensitivity to pyrazole derivatives (including oxyphenbutazone and phenylbutazone), blood dyscrasias, active peptic ulcer, or symptoms of GI inflammation or ulceration.

†Canadian ‡Australian

DRUG / CLASS / CATEGORY	DOSAGE FORMS	INDICATIONS / DOSAGES	KEY PRECAUTIONS
sulfisoxazole Gantrisin, Novo-Soxazole† **sulfisoxazole acetyl** Gantrisin Pediatric *Sulfonamide* *Antibiotic* Preg. Risk Category: C (contraindicated at term)	*tab*: 500 mg. *acetyl — liq*: 500 mg/5 ml	*UTI and systemic infections* — **Adults**: initially, 2 to 4 g PO, then 4 to 8 g/day divided in 4 to 6 doses. **Children > 2 mo**: initially, 75 mg/kg/day PO or 2 g/m² PO, then 150 mg/kg or 4 g/m² PO daily in divided doses q 6 hr. Max total dose 6 g/day. C. trachomatis — **Adults**: 500 mg PO for 10 to 21 days.	▪ Use oral form cautiously in impaired renal or hepatic function, severe allergies, bronchial asthma, or G6PD deficiency. ▪ Contraindicated in hypersensitivity to sulfonamides, in infants < 2 mo (except in congenital toxoplasmosis), in pregnant women at term, and during breast-feeding.
sulfisoxazole diolamine Gantrisin Ophthalmic Solution *Sulfonamide* *Antibiotic* Preg. Risk Category: C	*ophth sol*: 4%	*Conjunctivitis, corneal ulcers, and other superficial ocular infections; adjunct in systemic sulfonamide therapy of trachoma* — **Adults and children**: 2 to 3 drops instilled in conjunctival sac ≥ 3 times daily.	▪ Use with caution in severe dry eye. ▪ Contraindicated in hypersensitivity to drug or other sulfonamides, in infants < 2 mo, during pregnancy at full term, and in breast-feeding patients.
sulindac Aclin‡, Apo-Sulin‡, Clinoril, Novo-Sundac† *Nonsteroidal anti-inflammatory* *Nonnarcotic analgesic/anti-inflammatory* Preg. Risk Category: NR	*tab*: 100‡, 150, 200 mg	*Osteoarthritis, rheumatoid arthritis, ankylosing spondylitis* — **Adults**: initially, 150 mg PO bid; increase to 200 mg bid, prn. *Acute subacromial bursitis or supraspinatus tendinitis, acute gouty arthritis* — **Adults**: 200 mg PO bid for 7 to 14 days. Reduce dosage as symptoms subside.	▪ Use cautiously in history of ulcer or GI bleeding, renal dysfunction, compromised cardiac function, hypertension, or conditions predisposing to fluid retention. ▪ Contraindicated in hypersensitivity to drug and for patients in whom aspirin or NSAIDs trigger acute asthmatic attacks, urticaria, or rhinitis. ▪ Avoid use during pregnancy.

sumatriptan succinate
Imitrex
*Selective 5-hydroxytryptamine
receptor agonist
Antimigraine agent*
Preg. Risk Category: C

tab: 25, 50, 100 mg (base); **inj:** 6 mg/0.5 ml (12 mg/ml) in 0.5-ml pre-filled syringes and vials

Acute migraine attacks (with or without aura) — **Adults:** 6 mg SC. Max recommended dosage two 6-mg injections daily, with at least 1 hr in between. Or, initial dose of 25 to 100 mg PO and 2nd dose of up to 100 mg in 2 hr, prn. Further doses may be given q 2 hr, prn, to max oral dosage 300 mg/day.

- Use cautiously in patients at risk for CAD (such as postmenopausal women or males > 40 yr) or those with risk factors such as hypertension, hypercholesterolemia, obesity, diabetes, smoking, or family history. Also use cautiously in women of childbearing age and during pregnancy.
- Contraindicated in hypersensitivity to drug; in uncontrolled hypertension or ischemic heart disease (such as angina pectoris, Prinzmetal's angina, history of MI, or documented silent ischemia); in hemiplegic or basilar migraine; in patients taking ergotamine; and within 14 days of MAO therapy.

suprofen
Profenal
*Phenylalkanoic acid derivative
Nonsteroidal anti-inflammatory/
ophthalmic anti-inflammatory*
Preg. Risk Category: C

ophth sol: 1%

Inhibition of intraoperative miosis — **Adults:** 2 drops instilled into conjunctival sac q 4 hr on day before surgery. On day of surgery, 2 drops instilled 3 hr, 2 hr, and 1 hr before surgery.

- Use cautiously in hypersensitivity to other NSAIDs or aspirin.
- Use cautiously in bleeding disorders.
- Contraindicated in hypersensitivity to any component of formulation and in epithelial herpes simplex keratitis.
- Breast-feeding should be discontinued during administration.

t

DRUG/CLASS/CATEGORY	DOSAGE FORMS	INDICATIONS/DOSAGES	KEY PRECAUTIONS
tacrine hydrochloride Cognex *Cholinesterase inhibitor* *Psychotherapeutic* Preg. Risk Category: C	*cap:* 10, 20, 30, 40 mg	*Mild to moderate dementia of Alzheimer's type* — **Adults:** Initially, 10 mg PO qid. After 6 wk and if tolerated with no transaminase elevations, increase to 20 mg qid. After 6 wk, titrate to 30 mg qid. If still tolerated, increase to 40 mg qid after another 6 wk.	▪ Use cautiously in sick sinus syndrome, bradycardia, history of hepatic disease, renal disease, Parkinson's disease, asthma, prostatic hyperplasia, or other urinary outflow impairment and in patients at risk for peptic ulcer. ▪ Contraindicated in hypersensitivity to drug or acridine derivatives and in patients who previously developed drug-related jaundice.
tacrolimus Prograf *Bacteria-derived macrolide* *Immunosuppressant* Preg. Risk Category: C	*cap:* 1, 5 mg; *inj:* 5 mg/ml	*Prophylaxis of organ rejection in allogenic liver transplantation* — **Adults:** 0.05 to 0.1 mg/kg/day IV as cont inf ≥ 6 hr after transplantation. Initial PO dosage 0.15 to 0.3 mg/kg/day in 2 divided doses q 12 hr. Start 8 to 12 hr after stopping IV. Titrate per response. **Children:** 0.1 mg/kg/day IV, then 0.3 mg/kg/day PO on schedule similar to adults, adjusted prn.	▪ Use cautiously in impaired renal or hepatic function. ▪ Contraindicated in hypersensitivity to drug. IV form contraindicated in hypersensitivity to castor oil derivatives.
tamoxifen citrate Nolvadex, Nolvadex-D† ‡ *Nonsteroidal antiestrogen* *Antineoplastic* Preg. Risk Category: D	*tab:* 10, 20 mg; *tab (enteric-coated)*†: 10, 20 mg	*Advanced premenopausal and postmenopausal breast cancers* — **Adults:** 10 to 20 mg PO bid.	▪ Use cautiously in existing leukopenia or thrombocytopenia. ▪ Contraindicated in hypersensitivity to drug.
temazepam Restoril *Benzodiazepine* *Sedative-hypnotic* Preg. Risk Category: X Controlled Sub. Sched.: IV	*cap:* 7.5, 10‡, 15, 20‡, 30 mg	*Insomnia* — **Adults:** 7.5 to 30 mg PO hs. **Adults > 65 yr:** 7.5 mg PO hs.	▪ Use cautiously in impaired renal or hepatic function, chronic pulmonary insufficiency, severe or latent mental depression, suicide tendencies, or history of drug abuse. ▪ Contraindicated in hypersensitivity to drug or other benzodiazepines and during pregnancy.

teniposide (VM-26) Vumon *Podophyllotoxin (cell cycle–phase specific, G2 and late S phase)* *Antineoplastic* Preg. Risk Category: D	*inj:* 10 mg/ml	*Refractory childhood acute lymphoblastic leukemia* — **Children:** optimum dosage not established. In clinical trials, dosages ranged from 165 to 250 mg/m² IV once or twice weekly for 4 to 6 wk. Usually used in combination with other agents.	■ Contraindicated in hypersensitivity to drug or polyoxyethylated castor oil. Some clinicians may use despite patient history of hypersensitivity because therapeutic benefits outweigh risks. Treat such patients with antihistamines and corticosteroids before infusion begins and closely monitor during administration.
terazosin hydrochloride Hytrin *Selective alpha₁ blocker* *Antihypertensive* Preg. Risk Category: C	*tab:* 1, 2, 5, 10 mg	*Hypertension* — **Adults:** initially, 1 mg PO hs. Adjust dosage gradually based on response. Usual range 1 to 5 mg/day; max, 20 mg/day. *Symptomatic BPH* — **Adults:** initially, 1 mg PO hs. Increase in stepwise fashion to 2, 5, or 10 mg/day; most will need 10 mg/day.	■ Contraindicated in hypersensitivity to drug.
terbinafine hydrochloride Lamisil *Synthetic allylamine derivative* *Antifungal* Preg. Risk Category: B	*cream:* 1%	*Interdigital tinea pedis, tinea cruris, and tinea corporis* — **Adults:** cover affected and immediate surrounding area bid for at least 1 wk.	■ Contraindicated in hypersensitivity to drug.
terbutaline sulfate Brethaire, Brethine, Bricanyl, Bricanyl‡ *Adrenergic (beta₂ agonist)* *Bronchodilator* Preg. Risk Category: B	*tab:* 2.5, 5 mg; *aerosol inhaler:* 200 mcg/metered spray; *inj:* 1 mg/ml	*Bronchospasm in patients with reversible obstructive airway disease* — **Adults and children ≥ 12 yr:** dosage varies with form. *Aerosol inhaler* — 2 inhalations separated by 60-sec interval, repeated q 4 to 6 hr. *Inj* — 0.25 mg SC. May repeat in 15 to 30 min. prn. Max 0.5 mg in 4 hr. *Tab in adults* — 2.5 to 5 mg PO q 6 hr tid. Max 15 mg/day. *Tab in children 12 to 15 yr* — 2.5 mg PO q 6 hr tid during waking hours. Max 7.5 mg/day.	■ Use cautiously in CV disorders, hyperthyroidism, diabetes, or seizure disorders. ■ Contraindicated in hypersensitivity to drug or to sympathomimetic amines.

DRUG/CLASS/ CATEGORY	DOSAGE FORMS	INDICATIONS/ DOSAGES	KEY PRECAUTIONS
terconazole Terazol 3 Vaginal Suppositories, Terazol 7 Vaginal Cream *Triazole derivative* *Antifungal* Preg. Risk Category: C	*vag cream:* 0.4%, 0.8%; *vag supp:* 80 mg	*Vulvovaginal candidiasis* — **Adults:** 1 applicatorful of cream or 1 supp inserted into vagina hs. 0.4% cream used for 7 days; 0.8% cream or 80-mg supp for 3 days. Course repeated, prn, after reconfirmation by smear or culture.	• Contraindicated in sensitivity to terconazole or inactive ingredients in drug.
testolactone Teslac *Androgen* *Antineoplastic* Preg. Risk Category: C Controlled Sub. Sched.: III	*tab:* 50 mg	*Advanced postmenopausal breast cancer; advanced premenopausal breast cancer in women whose ovarian function has been terminated* — **Women:** 250 mg PO qid.	• Contraindicated in hypersensitivity to drug and in males with breast cancer.
testosterone Andro 100, Andronaq-50, Histerone, Tesamone 100 **testosterone cypionate** Depo-Testosterone, Testa-C **testosterone propionate** Malogen†, Testex **testosterone transdermal system** Androderm, Testoderm *Androgen* *Androgen replacement/antineoplastic* Preg. Risk Category: X Controlled Sub. Sched.: III	**testosterone — *inj (aqueous susp):*** 25, 50, 100 mg/ml. **cypionate — *inj (in oil):*** 50, 100, 200 mg/ml. **propionate — *inj (in oil):*** 25, 50, 100 mg/ml. **transderm system:** 2.5, 4, 6 mg/day	*Male hypogonadism* — **Adults:** 10 to 25 mg (testosterone or propionate) IM 2 to 3 times/wk or 50 to 400 mg (cypionate) IM q 2 to 4 wk. *Metastatic breast cancer in women 1 to 5 yr postmenopausal* — **Adults:** 100 mg IM 2 times weekly; 50 to 100 mg (propionate) IM 3 times weekly; or 200 to 400 mg (cypionate) IM q 2 to 4 wk. *Postpartum breast pain and engorgement* — **Adults:** 25 to 50 mg/day IM for 3 to 4 days. *Primary or hypogonadotropic hypogonadism in men* — **Adults:** (Testoderm) One 4-6-mg/day patch on scrotal area daily. Patch worn for 22 to 24 hr/day. **Adults:** (Androderm) 2 systems applied nightly. Apply to clean, dry skin on back, abdomen, upper arms, or thigh.	• Use cautiously in elderly patients and in renal, hepatic, or cardiac disease. • Avoid use in women of childbearing age until pregnancy ruled out. • Contraindicated in male patients with breast or prostate cancer; in hypercalcemia; in cardiac, hepatic, or renal dysfunction; and in pregnant or breast-feeding patients. Transdermal system contraindicated in women, in men with known or suspected breast or prostate cancer, and in hypersensitivity to drug.

tetanus immune globulin, human
Hyper-Tet
Immune serum
Tetanus prophylaxis agent
Preg. Risk Category: C

inj: 250-unit vial or syringe

Tetanus exposure — **Adults and children:** 250 units IM.
Tetanus treatment — **Adults and children:** single doses of 3,000 to 6,000 units IM have been used. Optimal dosage schedules not established.

- Use cautiously in history of systemic allergic reactions to human immunoglobulin preparations or in allergy to thimerosal.
- Contraindicated in thrombocytopenia or coagulation disorders that contraindicate IM injection unless benefits outweigh risks.

---

tetracycline hydrochloride
Achromycin V, Panmycin P‡, Robitet, Sumycin, Tetralean†
Tetracycline
Antibiotic
Preg. Risk Category: D

tab: 250, 500 mg; **cap:** 100, 250, 500 mg; **oral susp:** 125 mg/5 ml

Infections caused by susceptible organisms —
Adults: 250 to 500 mg PO q 6 hr. **Children > 8 yr:** 25 to 50 mg/kg/day PO, in divided doses q 6 hr.
C. trachomatis infections — **Adults:** 500 mg PO qid for 7 to 21 days.
Brucellosis — **Adults:** 500 mg PO q 6 hr for 3 wk with 1 g of streptomycin IM q 12 hr for 1st wk; once daily for 2nd wk.

- Use with extreme caution in impaired renal or hepatic function. Also use with extreme caution (if at all) during last half of pregnancy and in children < 9 yr.
- Contraindicated in hypersensitivity to tetracyclines.

---

tetracycline hydrochloride
Achromycin, Topicycline
Tetracycline
Antibiotic
Preg. Risk Category: B

oint: 3%; **topical sol:** 2.2 mg/ml

Acne vulgaris — **Adults and children > 11 yr:** rub sol into affected areas bid until skin thoroughly covered.
Treatment of superficial skin infections caused by susceptible bacteria — **Adults:** apply to affected area bid in morning and evening or tid.

- Use cautiously in hepatic or renal impairment.
- Contraindicated in hypersensitivity to drug.

---

tetrahydrozoline hydrochloride
Murine Plus, Optigene, Soothe, Tetrasine, Visine
Sympathomimetic
Vasoconstrictor/decongestant
Preg. Risk Category: C

ophth sol: 0.05%

Conjunctival congestion, irritation, and allergic conditions — **Adults and children > 2 yr:** 1 to 2 drops 0.05% sol instilled up to qid.

- Use cautiously in hyperthyroidism, heart disease, hypertension, or diabetes mellitus.
- Contraindicated in hypersensitivity to drug or any component and in angle-closure glaucoma or other serious eye diseases.

DRUG / CLASS / CATEGORY	DOSAGE FORMS	INDICATIONS / DOSAGES	KEY PRECAUTIONS
tetrahydrozoline hydrochloride Tyzine Drops, Tyzine Pediatric Drops *Sympathomimetic* *Vasoconstrictor/decongestant* Preg. Risk Category: C	**nasal sol:** 0.05%, 0.1%	*Nasal congestion* — **Adults and children > 6 yr:** 2 to 4 drops 0.1% sol into each nostril q 4 to 6 hr, prn. **Children 2 to 6 yr:** 2 to 3 drops 0.05% sol into each nostril q 4 to 6 hr, prn.	▪ Use cautiously in hyperthyroidism, hypertension, and diabetes mellitus. ▪ Contraindicated in hypersensitivity to drug and in angle-closure glaucoma or other serious eye diseases. Also contraindicated in children < 2 yr; 0.1% sol contraindicated in children < 6 yr.
theophylline *Immed-release liquids:* Accubron; *immed-release tab and cap:* Bronkodyl, Slo-Phyllin; *timed-release tab:* Theo-Dur; *timed-release cap:* Aerolate **theophylline sodium glycinate** Acet-Amt *Xanthine derivative* *Bronchodilator* Preg. Risk Category: C	**tab:** 100 to 300 mg; **tab (chew):** 100 to 500 mg; **cap:** 100, 200 mg; **cap (ext-release):** 50 to 300 mg; **elixir:** 27 mg/5 ml; **oral sol:** 27 mg, 50 mg/5 ml; **syrup:** 27 mg, 50 mg/5 ml; **dextrose 5% inj:** 200 to 800 mg in 50 to 1,000 ml. **sodium glycinate — elixir:** 110 mg/5 ml (equiv to 55 mg anhydrous theophylline/5 ml)	*Acute bronchospasm if not on drug* — for IV, loading dose 4.7 mg/kg IV slowly; then maint. **Adult (non-smoker):** 6 mg/kg PO, then 2–3 mg/kg q 6 hr for 2 doses. Maint.: 3 mg/kg q 8 hr. Or, 0.55 mg/kg/hr IV for 12 hr, then 0.39 mg/kg/hr IV. **Healthy adult smoker:** 6 mg/kg PO, then 3 mg/kg q 4 hr for 3 doses. Maint.: 3 mg/kg q 6 hr. Or, 0.79 mg/kg/hr IV for 12 hr, then 0.63 mg/kg/hr. **Adult with heart failure or liver disease:** 6 mg/kg PO, then 2 mg/kg q 8 hr for 2 doses. Maint.: 1–2 mg/kg q 12 hr. Or, 0.39 mg/kg/hr IV for 12 hr, then 0.08–0.16 mg/kg/hr. **9–16 yr:** 6 mg/kg PO, then 3 mg/kg q 4 hr for 3 doses. Maint.: 3 mg/kg q 6 hr. Or, 0.79 mg/kg/hr IV for 12 hr, then 0.63 mg/kg/hr. **6 mo–9 yr:** 6 mg/kg PO, then 4 mg/kg q 4 hr for 3 doses. Maint.: 4 mg/kg q 6 hr. Or, 0.95 mg/kg/hr IV for 12 hr; then 0.79 mg/kg/hr. *Chronic bronchospasm* — **Adult, child:** 16 mg/kg or 400 mg PO qd in 3–4 divided doses q 6–8 hr, or, 12 mg/kg or 400 mg PO qd in ext-release prep in 2–3 divided doses q 8 or 12 hr. Increase as tol q 2–3 day to max: **Over 16 yr:** 13 mg/kg or 900 mg PO qd. **12–16 yr:** 18 mg/kg PO qd. **9–12 yr:** 20 mg/kg PO qd. **Under 9 yr:** 24 mg/kg/day PO.	▪ Use cautiously in young children, infants < 1 yr, and neonates; in elderly patients; and in COPD, cardiac failure, cor pulmonale, renal or hepatic disease, peptic ulceration, hyperthyroidism, diabetes mellitus, glaucoma, severe hypoxemia, hypertension, compromised cardiac or circulatory function, angina, acute MI, or sulfite sensitivity. ▪ Contraindicated in hypersensitivity to xanthine compounds (caffeine, theobromine) and in active peptic ulcer or seizure disorders.

thiabendazole
Mintezol
Benzimidazole
Anthelmintic
Preg. Risk Category: C

tab (chew): 500 mg; **oral susp:** 500 mg/5 ml

Cutaneous infestations with larva migrans — **Adults and children:** 25 mg/kg PO bid for 2 to 5 days. Max 3 g/day. If lesions persist, repeat.
Roundworm, threadworm, whipworm — **Adults and children 13.6 to 70 kg:** 25 mg/kg PO bid daily for 2 days. **Adults and children > 70 kg:** 1.5 g q 12 hr for 2 days. Max 3 g/day.
Trichinosis — **Adults and children:** 25 mg/kg PO in 2 doses daily for 2 to 4 days.

- Use cautiously in hepatic or renal dysfunction, severe malnutrition, and anemia and in patients who are vomiting.
- Contraindicated in hypersensitivity to drug.

---

thiamine hydrochloride (vitamin B₁)
Betamin‡, Beta-Sol‡, Biamine,
Thiamilate
Water-soluble vitamin
Nutritional supplement
Preg. Risk Category: A

tab: 5, 10, 25, 50, 100, 250, 500 mg; **tab (enteric-coated):** 20 mg; **elixir †:** 250 mcg/5 ml; **inj:** 100, 200 mg/ml

Beriberi — **Adults:** 10 to 20 mg IM tid for 2 wk, then diet correction and multivitamin supplement containing 5 to 10 mg/day thiamine for 1 mo. **Children:** depending on severity, 10 to 50 mg/day IM for several wk with adequate diet.
Wernicke's encephalopathy — **Adults:** initially, 100 mg IV, followed by 50 to 100 mg/day IV or IM until patient eats balanced diet.

- Use with extreme caution when administering IV; use IV only when PO route not feasible.
- Contraindicated in hypersensitivity to thiamine products.

---

thioguanine (6-thioguanine, 6-TG)
Lanvist
Antimetabolite (cell cycle–phase specific, S phase)
Antineoplastic
Preg. Risk Category: D

tab (scored): 40 mg

Acute nonlymphocytic leukemia, chronic myelogenous leukemia — **Adults and children:** initially, 2 mg/kg/day PO (calculated to nearest 20 mg). If necessary, increase slowly to 3 mg/kg/day as tolerated.

- Use cautiously and with dosage modification in renal or hepatic dysfunction.
- Contraindicated when disease shows resistance to drug. Usually complete cross-resistance occurs between mercaptopurine and thioguanine.

DRUG / CLASS / CATEGORY	DOSAGE FORMS	INDICATIONS / DOSAGES	KEY PRECAUTIONS
thioridazine hydrochloride Aldazine†, Apo-Thioridazine†, Mellaril, Mellaril Concentrate, Novo-Ridazine†, PMS Thioridazine† *Phenothiazine (piperidine derivative)* *Antipsychotic* Preg. Risk Category: NR	**tab:** 10, 15, 25, 50, 100, 150, 200 mg; **oral susp:** 25, 100 mg/5 ml; **oral conc:** 30 mg/ml, 100 mg/ml (3% to 4.2% alcohol)	*Psychosis* — **Adults:** 50 to 100 mg PO tid, with gradual increases to 800 mg/day in divided doses, prn. Dosage varies. *Short-term treatment of moderate to marked depression with variable degrees of anxiety, treatment of multiple symptoms in geriatric patients* — **Adults:** 25 mg PO tid. Maintenance 20 to 200 mg/day. Max 200 mg/day. **Children 2 to 12 yr:** 0.5 to 3 mg/kg PO qd in divided doses.	■ Use cautiously in elderly or debilitated patients and in hepatic disease; CV disease; exposure to extreme heat or cold or to organophosphate insecticides; respiratory disorders; hypocalcemia; seizure disorder; or severe reactions to insulin or electroconvulsive therapy. ■ Contraindicated in hypersensitivity to drug and in coma, CNS depression, or severe hypertensive or hypotensive CV disease.
thiotepa (TESPA, triethylenethiophosphoramide, TSPA) Thioplex *Alkylating agent (cell cycle–phase nonspecific)* *Antineoplastic* Preg. Risk Category: D	**inj:** 15-mg vials	*Breast and ovarian cancers, lymphoma, Hodgkin's disease* — **Adults and children > 12 yr:** 0.3 to 0.4 mg/kg IV q 1 to 4 wk or 0.2 mg/kg for 4 to 5 days at 2- to 4-wk intervals.	■ Use cautiously in mild bone marrow suppression and renal or hepatic dysfunction. ■ Contraindicated in hypersensitivity to drug and in severe bone marrow, hepatic, or renal dysfunction. ■ Avoid use in pregnancy except when benefits outweigh risk of teratogenicity.
thiothixene Navane **thiothixene hydrochloride** Navane *Thioxanthene* *Antipsychotic* Preg. Risk Category: NR	**thiothixene — cap:** 1, 2, 5, 10, 20 mg. **hydrochloride — oral conc:** 5 mg/ml (7% alcohol); **inj:** 2, 5 mg/ml	*Mild to moderate psychosis* — **Adults:** 2 mg PO tid. Increase gradually to 15 mg/day. *Severe psychosis* — **Adults:** initially, 5 mg PO bid. Increase slowly to 20 to 30 mg/day. Max recommended 60 mg/day. Or, 4 mg IM bid or qid. Max 30 mg/day IM. PO should replace IM promptly.	■ Use with extreme caution in history of seizure disorder or in state of alcohol withdrawal. Use cautiously in elderly or debilitated patients and in CV disease, heat exposure, glaucoma, or prostatic hyperplasia. ■ Contraindicated in hypersensitivity to drug or in circulatory collapse, coma, CNS depression, or blood dyscrasia.

thyrotropin (thyroid-stimulating hormone, or TSH) Thytropar *Anterior pituitary hormone* *Thyrotropic hormone* Preg. Risk Category: C	***powder for inj:*** 10 IU-vial	*Diagnosis of thyroid cancer remnant with* [131] *after surgery —* **Adults:** 10 IU IM or SC for 3 to 7 days. *Differential diagnosis of primary and secondary hypothyroidism —* **Adults:** 10 IU IM or SC for 1 to 3 days. *In protein-bound iodine or* [131] *uptake determinations for differential diagnosis of subclinical hypothyroidism or low thyroid reserve —* **Adults:** 10 IU IM or SC.	▪ Use cautiously in angina pectoris, heart failure, hypopituitarism, and adrenocortical suppression. ▪ Contraindicated in hypersensitivity to drug, coronary thrombosis, or untreated Addison's disease.
ticarcillin disodium Ticar, Ticillin‡ *Extended-spectrum penicillin/ alpha-carboxypenicillin* *Antibiotic* Preg. Risk Category: B	***inj:*** 1, 3, 6 g; ***IV infusion:*** 3 g; ***pharm bulk pkg:*** 20, 30 g	*Severe systemic infections caused by susceptible organisms —* **Adults:** 18 g/day IV or IM, in divided doses q 4 to 6 hr. **Children:** 50 to 300 mg/kg/day IV or IM, in divided doses q 4 to 6 hr.	▪ Use cautiously in other drug allergies, especially to cephalosporins, and in impaired renal function, hemorrhagic conditions, hypokalemia, or sodium restrictions. ▪ Contraindicated in hypersensitivity to drug or other penicillins.
ticarcillin disodium/clavulanate potassium Timentin *Beta-lactamase inhibitor* *Antibiotic* Preg. Risk Category: B	***inj:*** 3 g ticarcillin and 100 mg clavulanic acid; ***pharm bulk pkg:*** 31 g	*Lower respiratory tract, urinary tract, bone and joint, and skin and skin-structure infections and septicemia when caused by beta-lactamase-producing strains of bacteria or by ticarcillin-susceptible organisms —* **Adults:** 3.1 g (3 g ticarcillin and 100 mg clavulanic acid) by IV infusion q 4 to 6 hr.	▪ Use cautiously in other drug allergies, especially to cephalosporins, and in impaired renal function, hemorrhagic conditions, hypokalemia, or sodium restrictions. ▪ Contraindicated in hypersensitivity to drug or other penicillins.
ticlopidine hydrochloride Ticlid *Platelet aggregation inhibitor* *Antithrombotic* Preg. Risk Category: B	***tab:*** 250 mg	*To reduce risk of thrombotic stroke in patients with history of stroke or with stroke precursors —* **Adults:** 250 mg PO bid with meals.	▪ Use cautiously and with close monitoring of CBC and WBC differential. ▪ Contraindicated in hypersensitivity to drug and in hematopoietic disorders (such as neutropenia, thrombocytopenia, or disorders of hemostasis), active pathologic bleeding from peptic ulceration or active intracranial bleeding, and severe hepatic impairment.

TICLOPIDINE HYDROCHLORIDE 249

DRUG/CLASS/CATEGORY	DOSAGE FORMS	INDICATIONS/DOSAGES	KEY PRECAUTIONS
timolol maleate Apo-Timol†, Blocadren *Beta-adrenergic blocker* *Antihypertensive/adjunct in MI/migraine headache prophylaxis* Preg. Risk Category: C	**tab:** 5, 10, 20 mg	*Hypertension* — **Adults:** 10 mg PO bid. Max 60 mg/day. Allow at least 7 days between dosage increases. *MI (long-term prophylaxis in patients who have survived acute phase)* — **Adults:** 10 mg PO bid. *Migraine headache prophylaxis* — **Adults:** 20 mg PO qd in 1 or divided doses bid. Increase prn to max 30 mg/day. Stop if no response after 6 to 8 wk at max dosage.	▪ Use cautiously in compensated heart failure, hepatic, renal, or respiratory disease; diabetes; and hyperthyroidism. ▪ Contraindicated in bronchial asthma, severe COPD, sinus bradycardia and heart block > first-degree, cardiogenic shock, overt heart failure, or hypersensitivity to drug.
timolol maleate Timoptic Solution, Timoptic-XE *Beta-adrenergic blocker* *Antiglaucoma agent* Preg. Risk Category: C	**ophth sol:** 0.25%, 0.5%; **ophth gel:** 0.25%, 0.5%	*Chronic open-angle, secondary, and aphakic glaucomas; ocular hypertension* — **Adults:** Initially, 1 drop 0.25% sol in each affected eye bid; maintenance dosage 1 drop daily. If no response, 1 drop 0.5% sol in each affected eye bid. If IOP controlled, reduce dosage to 1 drop daily. Alternatively, 1 drop gel in each affected eye qd.	▪ Use cautiously in nonallergic bronchospasm, chronic bronchitis, emphysema, diabetes, hyperthyroidism, or cerebrovascular insufficiency. ▪ Contraindicated in hypersensitivity to drug and in bronchial asthma, history of bronchial asthma or severe COPD, sinus bradycardia, 2nd- or 3rd-degree AV block, cardiac failure, and cardiogenic shock.
tioconazole Vagistat *Imidazole derivative* *Antifungal* Preg. Risk Category: C	**vag oint:** 6.5%	*Vulvovaginal candidiasis* — **Adults:** 1 applicatorful (about 4.6 g) inserted intravag hs 1 time only.	▪ Contraindicated in hypersensitivity to drug or other imidazole antifungal agents. ▪ Not known if drug excreted in breast milk; patient should temporarily stop breast-feeding during therapy.
tiopronin Thiola *Thiol compound* *Cystine-solubilizing agent* Preg. Risk Category: C	**tab:** 100 mg	*Prevention of urinary cysteine stone formation in severe homozygous cystinuria unresponsive to or intolerant of other therapies* — **Adults:** 800 mg PO daily, divided tid. **Children:** 15 mg/kg PO daily, divided tid. Maint dosage may be individualized.	▪ Contraindicated in history of agranulocytosis, aplastic anemia, or thrombocytopenia.

tobramycin
Aktob, Tobrex
Aminoglycoside
Antibiotic
Preg. Risk Category: B

ophth oint:
0.3%; *ophth sol:* 0.3%

External ocular infections caused by susceptible bacteria — **Adults and children:** in mild to moderate infections, 1 or 2 drops into affected eye q 4 hr, or thin strip (1 cm long) of oint q 8 to 12 hr. In severe infections, instill 2 drops into infected eye q 30 to 60 min until improvement; then reduce frequency. Or, thin strip of oint q 3 to 4 hr until improvement; then reduce frequency.

- Contraindicated in hypersensitivity to drug or other aminoglycosides.

tobramycin sulfate
Nebcin
Aminoglycoside
Antibiotic
Preg. Risk Category: D

multidose vials: 80 mg/2 ml, 20 mg/2 ml (ped); *premixed parenteral inj for IV infusion:* 60 or 80 mg in 0.9% NaCl sol

Serious infections caused by susceptible organisms — **Adults:** 3 mg/kg IM or IV daily divided q 8 hr. Up to 5 mg/kg daily divided q 6 to 8 hr for life-threatening infections; reduce to 3 mg/kg daily as soon as indicated. **Children:** 6 to 7.5 mg/kg IM or IV daily in 3 or 4 equally divided doses. **Neonates < 1 wk or premature infants:** up to 4 mg/kg/day IV or IM in 2 equal doses q 12 hr.

- Use cautiously in impaired renal function or neuromuscular disorders and in elderly patients.
- Contraindicated in hypersensitivity to drug or other aminoglycosides.

tocainide hydrochloride
Tonocard
Anesthetic
Ventricular antiarrhythmic
Preg. Risk Category: C

tab: 400, 600 mg

Suppression of symptomatic life-threatening ventricular arrhythmias — **Adults:** initially, 400 mg PO q 8 hr. Usual dosage 1,200 to 1,800 mg daily in 3 divided doses. May treat patients with renal or hepatic impairment with < 1,200 mg/day.

- Use cautiously in heart failure or diminished cardiac reserve and in hepatic or renal impairment.
- Contraindicated in hypersensitivity to lidocaine or other amide-type local anesthetics and in second- or third-degree AV block in absence of artificial pacemaker.

DRUG/CLASS/ CATEGORY	DOSAGE FORMS	INDICATIONS/ DOSAGES	KEY PRECAUTIONS
tolbutamide Apo-Tolbutamide, Mobenol†, Novo-Butamide†, Oramide†, Orinase *Sulfonylurea* *Antidiabetic* Preg. Risk Category: C	**tab:** 250, 500 mg	*Adjunct to diet to lower blood glucose in type 2 diabetes* — **Adults:** initially, 1 to 2 g PO daily as single dose or in divided doses bid to tid. Dosage adjusted, if necessary, to max 3 g daily; however, little benefit occurs with doses > 2 g daily. *To change from insulin to oral therapy* — **Adults:** if insulin dosage < 20 units daily, insulin stopped and oral therapy started at 1 to 2 g PO daily. If insulin dosage 20 to 40 units daily, insulin reduced by 30% to 50% and oral therapy started as above. If insulin dosage > 40 units daily, insulin reduced by 20% and oral therapy started as above. Further reductions based on response to oral therapy.	▪ Use cautiously in elderly, debilitated, or mal-nourished patients or in impaired hepatic or renal function or porphyria. ▪ Contraindicated in type 1 diabetes or diabetes adequately controlled by diet. Also contraindicated in type 2 diabetes complicated by fever, ketosis, acidosis, coma, or other acute complications such as major surgery, severe infection, or severe trauma; in hypersensitivity to drug or severe renal insufficiency; and during pregnancy or breast-feeding.
tolmetin sodium Tolectin 200, Tolectin 400, Tolectin 600, Tolectin DS *Nonsteroidal anti-inflammatory* *Nonnarcotic analgesic/ antipyretic/anti-inflammatory* Preg. Risk Category: C	**tab:** 200, 600 mg; **cap:** 400 mg	*Rheumatoid arthritis, osteoarthritis, juvenile rheuma-toid arthritis* — **Adults:** 400 mg PO tid. Max 1.8 g daily. **Children ≥ 2 yr:** initially, 20 mg/kg/day PO in divided doses (tid or qid), then maintenance dosage of 15 to 30 mg/kg PO daily in divided doses (tid or qid).	▪ Use cautiously in cardiac or renal disease, GI bleeding, history of peptic ulcer disease, hypertension, or conditions predisposing to fluid retention. ▪ Contraindicated in hypersensitivity to drug, in lactation, or when aspirin or NSAIDs trigger acute asthmatic attacks, urticaria, or rhinitis.
tolnaftate Aftate for Athlete's Foot, Dr. Scholl's Athlete's Foot Powder, Fungatin, Genaspor, NP-27, Tinactin *Antifungal* *Topical anti-infective* Preg. Risk Category: C	**aerosol liq:** 1% (36% alcohol); **aerosol powder:** 1% (14% alcohol); **cream:** 1%; **gel:** 1%; **powder:** 1%; **pump**	*Superficial fungal infections of skin; infections due to common pathogenic fungi; tinea pedis* — **Adults and children:** apply ¼" to ½" ribbon of cream or 2 to 3 drops of sol to cover area; same amount of cream or 2 to 3 drops of sol to cover toes and interdigital webs of 1 foot; or gel, powder, or spray to cover affected area. Apply and massage gently into skin bid for 2 to 6 wk.	▪ Contraindicated in hypersensitivity to drug.

	spray liq: 1% (36% alcohol); topical sol: 1%	
topotecan hydrochloride Hycamtin *Semi-synthetic camptothecin derivative* *Antineoplastic* Preg. Risk Category: D	*inj:* 4 mg single-dose vial	*Metastatic carcinoma of ovary after failure of initial or subsequent chemotherapy* — **Adults:** 1.5 mg/m² IV infusion over 30 min daily for 5 days, starting on day 1 of 21-day cycle. Give minimum 4 cycles.	▪ Contraindicated in hypersensitivity to drug or any component, in severe bone marrow depression, and in pregnant or breast-feeding patients. ▪ For creatinine clearance of 20 to 39 ml/min, decrease dosage to 0.75 mg/m². If severe neutropenia occurs, reduce dosage by 0.25 mg/m² for subsequent courses.
torsemide Demadex *Loop diuretic* *Diuretic/antihypertensive* Preg. Risk Category: B	*inj:* 10 mg/ml; *tab:* 5, 10, 20, 100 mg	*Diuresis in patients with heart failure* — **Adults:** 10 to 20 mg/day PO or IV. If response inadequate, double dose until response obtained. Max 200 mg/day. *Diuresis in patients with chronic renal failure* — **Adults:** initially, 20 mg/day PO or IV. If response inadequate, double dose until response obtained. Max 200 mg/day. *Hypertension* — **Adults:** 5 mg/day PO. Increase to 10 mg prn. If response inadequate, add another antihypertensive.	▪ Use cautiously in hepatic disease and associated cirrhosis and ascites; sudden changes in fluid and electrolyte balance may trigger hepatic coma in these patients. ▪ Contraindicated in anuria or hypersensitivity to drug or other sulfonylurea derivatives.
tramadol hydrochloride Ultram *Synthetic derivative* *Analgesic* Preg. Risk Category: C	*tab:* 50 mg	*Moderate to moderately severe pain* — **Adults:** 50 to 100 mg PO q 4 to 6 hr, prn. Max 400 mg/day. In patients > 75 yr, max 300 mg/day in divided doses.	▪ Use cautiously in risk for seizures or respiratory depression; in increased ICP or head injury, acute abdominal conditions, or renal or hepatic impairment; and in physical dependence on opioids. ▪ Contraindicated in hypersensitivity to drug or in acute intoxication from alcohol, hypnotics, centrally acting analgesics, opioids, or psychotropic drugs.

DRUG/CLASS/ CATEGORY	DOSAGE FORMS	INDICATIONS/ DOSAGES	KEY PRECAUTIONS
trandolapril Mavik *ACE inhibitor* *Antihypertensive* Preg. Risk Category: C (D in 2nd and 3rd trimesters)	*tab:* 1, 2, 4 mg	*Hypertension* — **Adults:** for patients not receiving diuretics, initially 1 mg for nonblack patient and 2 mg for black patient PO daily. If control not adequate, can increase dosage at ≥ 1-wk intervals. Maint dosage 2 to 4 mg/day. Some patients receiving 4 mg/day may need bid doses. For patient receiving diuretic, initial dose 0.5 mg/day PO. Dosage per BP response.	▪ Use cautiously in impaired renal function, heart failure, or renal artery stenosis. ▪ Contraindicated in hypersensitivity to drug and in history of angioedema related to previous treatment with ACE inhibitor. ▪ Not recommended for use in pregnant or breast-feeding women.
trazodone hydrochloride Desyrel, Trazon, Trialodine *Triazolopyridine derivative* *Antidepressant* Preg. Risk Category: C	*tab:* 50, 100, 150, 300 mg	*Depression* — **Adults:** initially, 150 mg PO daily in divided doses; increased by 50 mg/day q 3 to 4 days, prn. Average dosage 150 to 400 mg/day. Max daily dosage for inpatients 600 mg; for outpatients, 400 mg.	▪ Use cautiously in cardiac disease and in risk for suicide. ▪ Contraindicated during initial recovery phase of MI or in hypersensitivity to drug.
tretinoin Vesanoid *Retinoid* *Antineoplastic* Preg. Risk Category: D	*cap:* 10 mg	Induction of remission in patients with acute promyelocytic leukemia (APL), French-American-British (FAB) classification M3 (including M3 variant), when anthracycline chemotherapy contraindicated or unsuccessful — **Adults and children ≥ 1 yr:** 45 mg/m²/day PO in 2 even doses. Discontinue 30 days after complete remission or after 90 days of treatment, whichever is first.	▪ Use with extreme caution: Patients with APL are at high risk and can have severe reactions. Must be given under supervision of doctor with experience managing such patients and in facility able to monitor drug tolerance and protect and maintain patient compromised by toxicity. ▪ Contraindicated in known hypersensitivity to retinoids. Don't give to patients sensitive to parabens. ▪ Not recommended in pregnant or breast-feeding patients.
tretinoin (vitamin A acid, retinoic acid) Renova, Retin-A, StieVAA†	*cream:* 0.025%, 0.05%, 0.1%;	*Acne vulgaris* — **Adults and children:** clean affected area and lightly apply daily hs. *Adjunct therapy to skin care and sun avoidance pro-*	▪ Use cautiously in eczema. ▪ Contraindicated in hypersensitivity to any tretinoin component.

Vitamin A derivative Antiacne agent Preg. Risk Category: C	gel: 0.025%, 0.01%; sol: 0.05%	gram — **Adults:** apply to affected area daily hs.	

| **triamcinolone**
Aristocort, Atolone, Kenacort
triamcinolone acetonide
Azmacort, Kenalog-10, Triamonide 40, Trilog
Glucocorticoid
Anti-inflammatory/antiasthmatic
Preg. Risk Category: C | **triamcino-
lone — tab:** 1,
2, 4, 8 mg.
**acetonide —
inhal aerosol:**
100 mcg/metered spray;
inj (susp): 3,
10, 40 mg/ml | *Severe inflammation or immunosuppression* —
Adults: 4 to 48 mg PO daily in divided doses; 40 mg IM weekly; 1 mg into lesions; 2.5 to 40 mg into joints or soft tissue.
Persistent asthma — **Adults:** Azmacort 2 inhal tid or qid. Max 16 inhal daily. Total daily dosage may be given bid for maint. **Children 6 to 12 yr:** Azmacort 1 to 2 inhal tid or qid. Max 12 inhal daily. | • Use cautiously in GI ulcer, renal disease, hypertension, osteoporosis, diabetes mellitus, hypothyroidism, cirrhosis, diverticulitis, nonspecific ulcerative colitis, recent intestinal anastomoses, thromboembolic disorders, seizures, myasthenia gravis, heart failure, tuberculosis, ocular herpes simplex, emotional instability, or psychotic tendencies. Use Azmacort cautiously in TB, untreated fungal, bacterial or systemic viral infections or ocular herpes simplex.
• Contraindicated in hypersensitivity to any component of formulation or in systemic fungal infections. Azmacort contraindicated for hypersensitivity to any component of formulation, in status asthmaticus, and in patients receiving systemic corticosteroids.
• Breast-feeding not recommended. |

| **triamcinolone
acetonide**
Aristocort, Flutex, Kenalog, Kenalone‡, Triacet
Glucocorticoid
Anti-inflammatory
Preg. Risk Category: C | **aerosol:** 0.2
mg/2-sec spray;
cream: 0.02‡,
0.025, 0.1,
0.5%; **lotion:**
0.025, 0.1; **oint:**
0.02‡, 0.025,
0.1, 0.5%;
paste: 0.1%;
sol: 0.1% | *Inflammation associated with coricosteroid-responsive dermatoses*—**Adults and children:** clean area, apply aerosol, cream, lotion, or ointment sparingly bid to qid.
Inflammation associated with oral lesions — **Adults and children:** apply paste hs and bid to tid, prn, preferably after meals. Apply small amount without rubbing, and press to lesion in mouth until thin film develops. | • Contraindicated in hypersensitivity to drug. |

DRUG/CLASS/CATEGORY	DOSAGE FORMS	INDICATIONS/DOSAGES	KEY PRECAUTIONS
triamcinolone acetonide Nasacort *Glucocorticoid* *Anti-inflammatory* Preg. Risk Category: C	**nasal aerosol:** 55 mcg/metered spray	*Relief of symptoms of seasonal or perennial allergic rhinitis* — **Adults and children ≥ 12 yr:** initially, 2 sprays (110 mcg) in each nostril once daily. Increased prn up to 440 mcg qd as one dose or in divided doses to qid. After desired effect, decrease to as little as 1 spray (55 mcg) in each nostril qd.	▪ Use cautiously in breast-feeding patients; in patients with respiratory tract TB; untreated fungal, bacterial, or systemic viral infections or ocular herpes simplex; recent nasal septal ulcers, surgery, or trauma; and in those already receiving systemic corticosteroids. ▪ Contraindicated in hypersensitivity to drug.
triamterene Dyrenium, Dytac‡ *Potassium-sparing diuretic* *Diuretic* Preg. Risk Category: B	**tab:** 50†, 100 mg; **cap:** 50, 100 mg	*Edema* — **Adults:** initially, 100 mg PO bid after meals. Max total dosage 300 mg/day	▪ Use cautiously in impaired hepatic function or diabetes mellitus and in elderly or debilitated patients. ▪ Contraindicated in anuria, severe or progressive renal disease or dysfunction, severe hepatic disease, or hyperkalemia.
triazolam Apo-Triazo†, Halcion *Benzodiazepine* *Sedative-hypnotic* Preg. Risk Category: X Controlled Sub. Sched.: IV	**tab:** 0.125, 0.25 mg	*Insomnia* — **Adults:** 0.125 to 0.5 mg PO hs. **Adults > 65 yr:** 0.125 mg PO hs; increased, prn, to 0.25 mg PO hs.	▪ Use cautiously in breast-feeding patients and in impaired hepatic or renal function, chronic pulmonary insufficiency, sleep apnea, mental depression, suicidal tendencies, or history of drug abuse. ▪ Contraindicated in hypersensitivity to benzodiazepines and in pregnant patients.
trientine hydrochloride Syprine *Chelating agent* *Heavy metal antagonist* Preg. Risk Category: C	**cap:** 250 mg	*Wilson's disease in patients intolerant of penicillamine* — **Adults:** 750 to 1,250 mg PO qd in 2, 3, or 4 divided doses. May then increase dosage up to 2,000 mg qd. **Children ≤ 12 yr:** 500 to 750 mg PO daily in 2, 3, or 4 divided doses. May increase up to 1,500 mg daily. Long-term maint dosage determined q 6 to 12 mo based on serum copper analysis.	▪ Use with caution in breast-feeding patients and children. ▪ Contraindicated in hypersensitivity to drug and in cystinuria, rheumatoid arthritis, or biliary cirrhosis.

trifluoperazine hydrochloride

Apo-Trifluoperazine†, Calmazine‡, Solazine†, Stelazine, Terfluzine†

Phenothiazine (piperazine derivative)

Antipsychotic

Preg. Risk Category: NR

tab (reg and film-coated): 1, 2, 5, 10 mg; **oral conc:** 10 mg/ml; **inj:** 2 mg/ml

Anxiety states — **Adults:** 1 to 2 mg PO bid. Max 6 mg/day. Don't give > 12 wk.

Schizophrenia and other psychotic disorders — **Adults:** 2 to 5 mg PO bid, gradually increased until response. Or 1 to 2 mg deep IM q 4 to 6 hr, prn. More than 6 mg IM in 24 hr rarely required. **6 to 12 yr (hospitalized or under close supervision):** 1 mg PO qd or bid; may increase gradually to 15 mg daily.

- Use cautiously in elderly or debilitated patients and in CV disease, exposure to extreme heat, seizure disorder, glaucoma, or prostatic hyperplasia.
- Contraindicated in hypersensitivity to phenothiazines or in coma, CNS depression, bone marrow suppression, or liver damage.

trifluridine

Viroptic Ophthalmic Solution 1%

Fluorinated pyrimidine nucleoside

Antiviral

Preg. Risk Category: C

ophth sol: 1%

Primary keratoconjunctivitis and recurrent epithelial keratitis caused by herpes simplex virus, types I and II — **Adults:** 1 drop of sol into affected eye q 2 hr while patient awake to max 9 drops/day until corneal ulcer reepithelialization occurs; then 1 drop q 4 hr (min 5 drops/day) for another 7 days.

- Contraindicated in hypersensitivity to drug.
- Consider using other form of therapy if no improvement after 7 days, treatment or if reepithelialization not complete after 14 days, treatment. Shouldn't be used > 21 days continuously.

trihexyphenidyl hydrochloride

Aparkane†, Apo-Trihex†, Artane, Novohexidyl†, Trihexane

Anticholinergic

Antiparkinsonian agent

Preg. Risk Category: NR

tab: 2, 5 mg; **cap (sust-release):** 5 mg; **elixir:** 2 mg/5 ml

All forms of parkinsonism, drug-induced parkinsonism, and adjunctive treatment to levodopa in parkinsonism management — **Adults:** 1 mg PO 1st day, 2 mg 2nd day; then increased in 2-mg increments q 3 to 5 days until total of 6 to 10 mg/day. Usually given tid with meals, sometimes given qid (last dose hs) or switched to sust-release form bid. Postencephalitic parkinsonism may require 12 to 15 mg total daily dosage.

- Use cautiously in glaucoma; cardiac; hepatic, or renal disorders; obstructive disease of GI or genitourinary tracts; and prostatic hyperplasia.
- Contraindicated in hypersensitivity to drug.

trilostane

Modrastane

Synthetic steroid

Glucocorticoid suppressant

Preg. Risk Category: X

cap: 30, 60 mg

Adrenocortical hyperfunction in Cushing's syndrome — **Adults:** 30 mg PO qid initially. May increase at intervals of 3 to 4 days to max 480 mg/day. Most patients respond to doses < 360 mg/day.

- Use cautiously in patients receiving drugs that suppress adrenal function.
- Contraindicated in severe renal or hepatic disease.

DRUG/CLASS/ CATEGORY	DOSAGE FORMS	INDICATIONS/ DOSAGES	KEY PRECAUTIONS
trimethoprim Proloprim, Trimpex, Triprim‡ *Synthetic folate antagonist* *Antibiotic* Preg. Risk Category: C	**tab:** 100, 200 mg	*Uncomplicated UTI caused by susceptible organisms —* **Adults:** 200 mg PO daily as single dose or in divided doses q 12 hr for 10 days. Not recommended in children < 12 yr.	▪ Use cautiously in impaired hepatic or renal function or in folate deficiency. Decrease dosage in severely impaired renal function. Not recommended when creatinine clearance < 15 ml/min. ▪ Contraindicated in hypersensitivity to drug and in documented megaloblastic anemia caused by folate deficiency.
trimipramine maleate Apo-Trimip†, Surmontil *Tricyclic antidepressant* *Antidepressant/antianxiety agent* Preg. Risk Category: C	**tab:** 25 mg; **cap:** 25, 50, 100 mg	*Depression —* **Adults:** 75 to 100 mg PO daily in divided doses, increased to 200 to 300 mg/day. Dosages > 300 mg/day not recommended in hospitalized patients; ≤ 200 mg in outpatients. Total dosage requirement may be given hs. **Elderly and adolescent patients:** initially, 50 mg/day, gradually increased to 100 mg/day.	▪ Use with extreme caution in CV disease, history of urine retention or angle-closure glaucoma, increased IOP, hyperthyroidism, impaired hepatic function, or history of seizures; in patients receiving thyroid medications, guanethidine, or similar agents; and in elderly and debilitated patients. ▪ Contraindicated during acute recovery of MI, in hypersensitivity to drug, and within 14 days of MAO inhibitor therapy.
triprolidine hydrochloride Actidil, Alleract, Myidyl *Alkylamine antihistamine derivative* *Antihistamine (H₁-receptor antagonist)* Preg. Risk Category: C	**tab:** 2.5 mg; **syrup:** 1.25 mg/5 ml	*Colds and allergy symptoms —* **Adults and children ≥ 12 yr:** 2.5 mg PO q 4 to 6 hr. Max 10 mg/day. **6 to 12 yr:** 1.25 mg PO q 4 to 6 hr. Max 5 mg/day. **4 to 6 yr:** 0.938 mg PO q 4 to 6 hr. Max 3.744 mg/day. **2 to 4 yr:** 0.625 mg PO q 4 to 6 hr. Max 2.5 mg/day. **4 mo to 2 yr:** 0.313 mg PO q 4 to 6 hr. Max 1.252 mg/day.	▪ Use with extreme caution in increased IOP, angle-closure glaucoma, hyperthyroidism, CV disease, hypertension, bronchial asthma, prostatic hyperplasia, bladder-neck obstruction, and stenosing peptic ulcerations and in children < 12 yr. ▪ Contraindicated in hypersensitivity to drug, in acute asthma, and in neonates, premature infants, and breast-feeding patients.

troglitazone
Rezulin
PPAR gamma activator
Antidiabetic
Preg. Risk Category: B

tab: 200, 400 mg

Adjunct to diet and insulin therapy in type 2 diabetes if hyperglycemia inadequately controlled with insulin > 30 units/day as multiple injections — **Adults:** for patients on insulin, continue with current insulin dose and begin therapy with 200 mg/day PO, with meal. May increase after 2 to 4 wk. Usual daily dose 400 mg; max 600 mg/day. Insulin dose may be decreased 10% to 25% when fasting glucose < 120 mg/dl in patients on troglitazone and insulin.

- Use cautiously in hepatic disease and in heart failure with class III or IV status.
- Contraindicated in known hypersensitivity to drug.
- Use in pregnancy only if benefit justifies potential risk to fetus. Insulin preferred antidiabetic agent in pregnancy.
- Not for use in breast-feeding women.
- Safety and efficacy in children not established.

---

tromethamine
Tham
Sodium-free organic amine
Systemic alkalinizer
Preg. Risk Category: C

inj: 18 g/500 ml

Metabolic acidosis associated with cardiac bypass surgery or cardiac arrest — **Adults:** dosage depends on bicarbonate deficit. Calculate as follows: Each ml of 0.3 M tromethamine sol required = weight in kg × bicarbonate deficit (mEq/L). Additional therapy based on serial determinations of existing bicarbonate deficit. Administer over ≥ 1 hr; individual doses shouldn't exceed 500 mg/kg.
Acidosis during bypass surgery: avg dose of 9 ml/kg (2.7 mEq/kg or 0.32 g/kg); total single dose of 500 ml (150 mEq or 18 g) adequate for most adults; not to exceed 500 mg/kg over period of < 1 hr.
Cardiac arrest: 3.6 to 10.8 g (111 to 333 ml) inj into large peripheral vein.

- Use cautiously in renal disease and poor urine output.
- Contraindicated in anuria, uremia, or chronic respiratory acidosis or during pregnancy (except in acute, life-threatening situations).

---

tubocurarine chloride
Tubarine†
Nondepolarizing neuromuscular blocker
Skeletal muscle relaxant
Preg. Risk Category: C

inj: 3 mg (20 units)/ml; 10 mg/ml‡

Adjunct to anesthesia to induce skeletal muscle relaxation; to facilitate intubation, orthopedic manipulations — dosage depends on anesthetic used, individual needs, and response. Dosages listed are representative; must be adjusted. **Adults:** 1.1 unit/kg or 0.165 mg/kg IV slowly over 60 to 90 sec. Average dose initially 40 to 60 units IV. May give 20 to 30 units in 3 to 5 min. For longer procedures, give 20 units prn.

- Use cautiously in elderly or debilitated patients and in hepatic or pulmonary impairment, hypothermia, respiratory depression, myasthenia gravis, myasthenic syndrome of lung cancer or bronchogenic carcinoma, dehydration, thyroid disorders, collagen diseases, porphyria, electrolyte disturbances,

(continued)

TUBOCURARINE CHLORIDE   259

DRUG / CLASS / CATEGORY	DOSAGE FORMS	INDICATIONS / DOSAGES	KEY PRECAUTIONS
tubocurarine chloride *(continued)*		*To assist with mechanical ventilation* — **Adults and children:** initially, 0.0165 mg/kg IV (average: 1 mg or 7 units); adjust subsequent doses to patient response. *To lessen muscle contractions in pharmacologically or electrically induced seizures* — **Adults and children:** 1.1 mg/kg or 0.165 mg/kg over 60 to 90 sec. Initial dose 20 units (3 mg) less than calculated dose. *Diagnosis of myasthenia gravis* — **Adults:** 4 to 33 mcg/kg as single IV dose.	fractures, and muscle spasms. Use large doses cautiously in patients undergoing cesarean section. ■ Contraindicated in hypersensitivity to drug or when histamine release hazardous (asthmatic patients).
u			
uracil mustard Uracil Mustard Capsules *Alkylating agent (cell cycle–phase nonspecific)* *Antineoplastic* Preg. Risk Category: D	*cap:* 1 mg	*Chronic lymphocytic and myelocytic leukemia, Hodgkin's disease* — **Adults:** 0.15 mg/kg PO as single dose weekly for 4 wk. If response occurs, continue weekly administration. Or, 1 to 2 mg PO qd for 3 mo or until desired response or toxicity; maint 1 mg qd for 3 out of 4 wk until optimum response or relapse; or 3 to 5 mg PO for 7 days, not to exceed total dosage of 0.5 mg/kg, then 1 mg qd until response, then 1 mg PO for 3 to 4 wk. **Children:** 0.3 mg/kg PO as single dose weekly for 4 wk. If response occurs, continue weekly administration.	■ Use with caution in sensitivity to aspirin or tartrazine. ■ Contraindicated in hypersensitivity to drug and in aplastic anemia, thrombocytopenia, or leukopenia.
urea (carbamide) Ureaphil *Carbonic acid salt* *Osmotic diuretic* Preg. Risk Category: C	*inj:* 40 g/150 ml	*Elevated ICP or IOP* — **Adults:** 1 to 1.5 g/kg as 30% soln by slow IV infusion over 1 to 2½ hr. Rate should not exceed 4 ml/min. **Children:** 0.5 to 1.5 g/kg by slow IV infusion (rate not to exceed 4 ml/min) or 35 g/m² in 24 hr. Children < 2 yr may re-	■ Use cautiously in cardiac disease or hepatic or renal impairment and during pregnancy and breast-feeding. ■ Contraindicated in severely impaired renal function, marked dehydration, frank hepatic

		ceive as little as 0.1 g/kg by slow IV infusion.	failure, active intracranial bleeding, and sickle cell disease with CNS involvement.

urokinase
Abbokinase, Abbokinase Open-Cath, Ukidan‡
Thrombolytic enzyme
Thrombolytic
Preg. Risk Category: B

inj: 5,000 units (IU) per unit-dose vial; 9,000 IU per unit-dose vial; 250,000-IU vial

Lysis of acute massive PE or PE accompanied by unstable hemodynamics — **Adults:** for IV infusion only by constant infusion pump. Priming dose: 4,400 IU/kg with 0.9% NaCl or D₅W sol admixture over 10 min. Then 4,400 IU/kg/hr for 12 hr.

Coronary artery thrombosis — **Adults:** after bolus dose of heparin from 2,500 to 10,000 units, infuse 6,000 IU/min of urokinase into occluded artery for up to 2 hr. Avg total dosage 500,000 IU. Initiate within 6 hr of symptoms. Follow with IV infusion of heparin, then oral anticoagulants.

Venous catheter occlusion — **Adults:** 5,000 IU/ml sol into occluded line, then after 5 min, aspirate. Repeat aspiration attempts q 5 min for 30 min. If not patent, cap line and leave for 30 to 60 minutes before aspirating again. May require 2nd instillation.

- Contraindicated in active internal bleeding, history of CVA, aneurysm, AVM, known bleeding diathesis, recent trauma with possible internal injuries, visceral or intracranial malignancy, pregnancy and 1st 10 days postpartum, ulcerative colitis, diverticulitis, severe hypertension, hemostatic defects, uncontrolled hypocoagulation, chronic pulmonary disease with cavitation, subacute bacterial endocarditis or rheumatic valvular disease, and recent cerebral embolism, thrombosis, or hemorrhage.
- Also contraindicated within 10 days after intra-arterial diagnostic procedure or any surgery (liver or kidney biopsy, lumbar puncture, thoracentesis, paracentesis, or extensive or multiple cutdowns) or within 2 mo after intracranial or intraspinal surgery.
- Should be used only by doctors with extensive experience in thrombotic disease management in facilities where clinical and lab monitoring can be performed.

ursodiol
Actigall
Bile acid
Gallstone solubilizing agent
Preg. Risk Category: B

cap: 300 mg

Dissolution of gallstones < 20 mm diameter when surgery precluded — **Adults:** 8 to 10 mg/kg PO daily in 2 or 3 divided doses.

- Use with caution in breast-feeding women.
- Contraindicated in hypersensitivity to drug or other bile acids and in chronic hepatic disease, unremitting acute cholecystitis, cholangitis, biliary obstruction, gallstone-induced pancreatitis, or biliary fistula.

V

DRUG/CLASS/CATEGORY	DOSAGE FORMS	INDICATIONS/DOSAGES	KEY PRECAUTIONS
valacyclovir hydrochloride Valtrex *Synthetic purine nucleoside Antiviral* Preg. Risk Category: B	**tab:** 500 mg	*Herpes zoster infection (shingles)* — **Adults:** 1 g PO tid for 7 days. Adjust for impaired renal function based on creatinine clearance. *For first episode of genital herpes* — **Adults:** 1 g PO bid for 10 days. If creatinine clearance ≥ 30 ml/min, 1 g PO q 12 hr; for 10 to 29 ml/min, 1 g PO q 24 hr; for < 10 ml/min, 500 mg PO q 24 hr. *Recurrent genital herpes* — **Adults:** 500 mg PO bid for 5 days, given at first sign.	▪ Use cautiously in renal impairment, elderly patients, those receiving other nephrotoxic drugs, and breast-feeding patients. ▪ Contraindicated in hypersensitivity or intolerance to valacyclovir, acyclovir, or any component of formulation. Not recommended in immunocompromised patients. Thrombotic thrombocytopenic purpura and hemolytic uremic syndrome have occurred, resulting in death in some patients with advanced HIV infection; also in bone marrow transplant and renal transplant recipients participating in clinical trials. ▪ Use in pregnant patients only if benefits outweigh risks. Manufacturer maintains ongoing registry of women exposed to drug during pregnancy. Health care providers encouraged to report such exposures to registrar at 1-800-722-9292, ext 58465. ▪ Safety and efficacy in children not established.
valproate sodium Depakene Syrup, Epilim‡, Myproic Acid Syrup **valproic acid** Depakene, Myproic Acid **divalproex sodium** Depakote, Depakote Sprinkle, Epival†, Valcote‡	**valproate sodium — syrup:** 250 mg/ml. **valproic acid — tab (enteric-coated):** 200, 500 mg‡; **crush tab:** 100 mg‡; **cap:** 250 mg‡;	*Simple and complex absence seizures, mixed seizure types* — **Adults and children:** 15 mg/kg PO daily, divided bid or tid; increase by 5 to 10 mg/kg daily q wk to max 60 mg/kg qd. *Mania (delayed-release capsules)* — **Adults and children:** 750 mg qd in divided doses. Adjust per response; max 60 mg/kg/day. *Prophylaxis for migraine (Depakote only)* — **Adults:** initially, 250 mg PO bid. Some patients may need up	▪ Contraindicated in hepatic disease, significant hepatic dysfunction, and hypersensitivity to drug.

Drug	Forms	Indications & Dosage	Considerations
Carboxylic acid derivative *Anticonvulsant* Preg. Risk Category: D	mg; *syrup:* 200 mg/5 ml‡. **divalproex sodium — *cap* (delayed-release):** 125 mg; *tab (enteric-coated):* 125, 250, 500 mg	to 1,000 mg/day.	
valsartan Diovan *Angiotensin II antagonist* *Antihypertensive* Preg. Risk Category: C (D in 2nd and 3rd trimesters)	*cap:* 80, 160 mg	*Hypertension* — **Adults:** initially, 80 mg PO qd. Expect BP reduction in 2 to 4 wk. For additional effect, increase to 160 or 320 mg daily, or add diuretic. (Adding diuretic has greater effect than increases over 80 mg.) Usual dosage range: 80 to 320 mg daily.	▪ Use cautiously in renal or hepatic disease. ▪ Contraindicated in known hypersensitivity to drug and in breast-feeding patients. ▪ Can cause fetal or neonatal morbidity and death if given to pregnant woman in second or third trimester. ▪ Safety and efficacy in children not established.
vancomycin hydrochloride Lyphocin, Vancocin, Vancoled *Glycopeptide* *Antibiotic* Preg. Risk Category: C	*cap:* 125, 250 mg; *powder for oral sol:* 1-, 10-g bottles; *powder for inj:* 500-mg, 1-g vials; *pharm bulk pkg:* 5, 10 g; *IV infusion (frozen):* 500 mg in 100 ml D₅W	*Serious infections when other antibiotics ineffective or contraindicated* — **Adults:** 1 to 1.5 g IV q 12 hr. **Children:** 10 mg/kg IV q 6 hr. **Neonates and young infants:** 15 mg/kg IV loading dose, then 10 mg/kg IV q 12 hr if < 1 wk old, and 10 mg/kg IV q 8 hr if > 1 wk but < 1 mo. *Antibiotic-associated pseudomembranous and staphylococcal enterocolitis* — **Adults:** 125 to 500 mg PO q 6 hr for 7 to 10 days. **Children:** 40 mg/kg PO qd, in divided doses q 6 hr for 7 to 10 days. Max 2 g/day. *Endocarditis prophylaxis for dental procedures* — **Adults:** 1 g IV slowly over 1 hr, starting 1 hr before procedure. **Children:** > 27 kg, adult dose; < 27 kg, 20 mg/kg.	▪ Use cautiously in patients receiving other neurotoxic, nephrotoxic, or ototoxic drugs; in patients > 60 yr; and in impaired hepatic or renal function, preexisting hearing loss, or allergies to other antibiotics. ▪ Contraindicated in hypersensitivity to drug.

DRUG/CLASS/CATEGORY	DOSAGE FORMS	INDICATIONS/DOSAGES	KEY PRECAUTIONS
varicella-zoster immune globulin (VZIG) *Immune serum* *Varicella-zoster prophylaxis agent* Preg. Risk Category: C	**inj:** 10% to 18% sol of globulin fraction human plasma containing 125 units varicella-zoster virus antibody (volume approx 1.25 ml)	*Passive immunization of susceptible immunodeficient patients after exposure to varicella (chickenpox or herpes zoster) —* **Adults and children > 40 kg:** 625 units IM. **Children 30.1 to 40 kg:** 500 units IM. **Children 20.1 to 30 kg:** 375 units IM. **Children 10.1 to 20 kg:** 250 units IM. **Children ≤ 10 kg:** 125 units IM.	▪ Use cautiously in breast-feeding patients. ▪ Contraindicated in history of severe reaction to human immune serum globulin or thrombocytopenia.
vasopressin (ADH) Pitressin *Posterior pituitary hormone* *Antidiuretic hormone/hemostatic* Preg. Risk Category: C	**inj:** 0.5-ml and 1-ml ampules, 20 units/ml	*Nonnephrogenic, nonpsychogenic diabetes insipidus —* **Adults:** 5 to 10 units IM or SC bid to qid, prn; or intranasally in individualized dosages, based on response. **Children:** 2.5 to 10 units IM or SC bid to qid, prn; or intranasally in individualized doses.	▪ Use cautiously in children, elderly or pregnant patients, preop and postop polyuric patients, and in seizure disorders, migraine headache, asthma, CV disease, heart failure, renal disease, goiter with cardiac complications, arteriosclerosis, and fluid overload. ▪ Contraindicated in chronic nephritis accompanied by nitrogen retention.
vecuronium bromide Norcuron *Nondepolarizing neuromuscular blocker* *Skeletal muscle relaxant* Preg. Risk Category: C	**inj:** 10-, 20-mg vials	*Adjunct to general anesthesia to facilitate ET intubation and to provide skeletal muscle relaxation during surgery or mechanical ventilation —* dosage depends on anesthetic used, individual needs, and response. Dosages listed are representative and must be adjusted. **Adults and children > 9 yr:** initially, 0.08 to 0.1 mg/kg IV bolus. Give maintenance doses of 0.01 to 0.015 mg/kg within 25 to 40 min of initial dose during prolonged surgical procedures. May give mainte-	▪ Use cautiously in elderly patients; in altered circulation caused by CV disease and edematous states; in hepatic disease, severe obesity, bronchogenic carcinoma, electrolyte disturbances, and neuromuscular disease. ▪ Contraindicated in hypersensitivity to bromides.

		nance doses q 12 to 15 min in patients receiving balanced anesthesia. Or, may give by continuous IV infusion of 1 mcg/kg/min 20 to 40 min after initial dose. **Children < 9 yr:** may require slightly higher initial dose; also may need supplementation slightly more often than adults.	
venlafaxine hydrochloride Effexor *Serotonin, norepinephrine, dopamine reuptake inhibitor* Antidepressant Preg. Risk Category: C	**tab:** 25, 37.5, 50, 75, 100 mg	*Depression* — **Adults:** initially, 75 mg PO daily, in 2 or 3 divided doses with food. Increase prn by 75 mg/day at intervals of ≥ 4 days. For moderate depression, usual max 225 mg/day; certain severely depressed patients may receive 375 mg/day.	▪ Use cautiously in renal or hepatic impairment, diseases or conditions that could affect hemodynamic responses or metabolism, and in history of mania or seizures. ▪ Contraindicated in hypersensitivity to drug or within 14 days of MAO inhibitor therapy.
verapamil Apo-Verap†, Calan, Isoptin, Novo-Veramil†, Nu-Verap† **verapamil hydrochloride** Calan, Calan SR, Isoptin, Isoptin SR, Verelan *Calcium channel blocker* Antianginal/antihypertensive/ antiarrhythmic Preg. Risk Category: C	**verapamil** — **tab:** 40, 80, 120 mg. **hydrochloride** — **tab:** 40, 80, 120, 160 mg; **tab (ext-release):** 120, 180, 240, 360 mg; **cap (ext-release):** 120, 160, 180, 240 mg; **inj:** 2.5 mg/ml	*Vasospastic angina and classic chronic, stable angina pectoris; chronic atrial fibrillation* — **Adults:** 80 to 120 mg PO tid. Increase q wk prn. Max 480 mg qd. *Supraventricular arrhythmias* — **Adults:** 0.075 to 0.15 mg/kg by IV push over 2 min. 0.15 mg/kg in 30 min if no response. **Children < 1 yr:** 0.1 to 0.2 mg/kg IV over 2 min. **Children 1 to 15 yr:** 0.1 to 0.3 mg/kg IV over 2 min. For children, may repeat in 30 min. *Hypertension* — **Adults:** 80 mg PO tid. Max 480 mg. Or, 120 to 240 mg ext-release tab PO qd in morning. May add ½ tab daily.	▪ Use cautiously in elderly patients, increased ICP, and hepatic or renal disease. ▪ Contraindicated in hypersensitivity to drug, severe left ventricular dysfunction, cardiogenic shock, second- or third-degree AV block or sick sinus syndrome except in with functioning pacemaker, atrial flutter or fibrillation and accessory bypass tract syndrome, severe heart failure (unless secondary to verapamil therapy), and severe hypotension. IV form contraindicated in ventricular tachycardia and in patients receiving IV beta-adrenergic blockers.

VERAPAMIL HYDROCHLORIDE **265**

DRUG / CLASS / CATEGORY	DOSAGE FORMS	INDICATIONS / DOSAGES	KEY PRECAUTIONS
vidarabine Vira-A *Purine nucleoside* *Antiviral* Preg. Risk Category: C	*ophth oint:* 3% in 3.5-g tube (equiv to 2.8% vidarabine)	*Acute keratoconjunctivitis, superficial keratitis, and recurrent epithelial keratitis caused by herpes simplex* — **Adults and children:** 1 cm oint into lower conjunctival sac 5 times daily at 3-hr intervals.	▪ Use cautiously and with close monitoring when given with steroids. Vidarabine continued for several days after steroid therapy. ▪ Contraindicated in hypersensitivity to drug.
vinblastine sulfate (VLB) Alkaban-AQ, Velban, Velbet‡, Velsar *Vinca alkaloid* *Antineoplastic* Preg. Risk Category: D	*inj:* 10-mg vials (lyoph powder), 1 mg/ml in 10-ml vials	*Breast or testicular cancer, Hodgkin's disease and malignant lymphoma* — **Adults:** 3.7 mg/m² IV q 1 to 2 wk. Max 18.5 mg/m² IV q wk per response. Don't repeat if WBC < 4,000/mm³. **Children:** 2.5 mg/m² IV q wk. Increase by 1.25 mg/m² until WBC < 3,000/mm³ or tumor response seen. Max 12.5 mg/m² IV q wk.	▪ Use cautiously in hepatic dysfunction. ▪ Contraindicated in severe leukopenia or bacterial infection.
vincristine sulfate (VCR) Oncovin, Vincasar PFS *Vinca alkaloid* *Antineoplastic* Preg. Risk Category: D	*inj:* 1 mg/ml in 1-ml, 2-, 5-ml multidose vials; 1 mg/ml in 1-, 2-, 5-ml preserv-free vials	*Acute lymphoblastic and other leukemias, Hodgkin's disease* — **Adults:** 1.4 mg/m² IV weekly. Max weekly dosage 2 mg. **Children > 10 kg:** 2 mg/m² IV weekly. **Children ≤ 10 kg or with BSA < 1 m²:** initially 0.05 mg/kg IV weekly.	▪ Use cautiously in hepatic dysfunction, neuromuscular disease, or infection. ▪ Contraindicated in hypersensitivity to drug or in demyelinating form of Charcot-Marie-Tooth syndrome. Don't give to patients concurrently receiving radiation therapy through ports that include liver.
vinorelbine tartrate Navelbine *Vinca alkaloid* *Antineoplastic* Preg. Risk Category: D	*inj:* 10 mg/ml, 50 mg/5 ml	*Alone or with cisplatin for 1st-line treatment of ambulatory patients with nonresectable advanced non-small-cell lung cancer (NSCLC); alone or with cisplatin in stage IV of NSCLC; with cisplatin in stage III of NSCLC* — **Adults:** 30 mg/m² IV weekly. In combination treatment, same dosage used with 120 mg/m² cisplatin, on days 1 and 29, then q 6 wk.	▪ Use with extreme caution if bone marrow may have been compromised by previous exposure to radiation therapy or chemotherapy or if bone marrow still recovering from chemotherapy. ▪ Use cautiously in hepatic impairment. ▪ Contraindicated in pretreatment granulocyte counts < 1,000 cells/mm³.

vitamin A (retinol)

Acon, Aquasol A, Del-Vi-A

Fat-soluble vitamin

Vitamin

Preg. Risk Category: C

tab: 10,000 IU; **cap:** 10,000, 25,000, 50,000 IU; **drops:** 30 ml with dropper (50,000 IU/0.1 ml); **inj:** 2-ml vials (50,000 IU/ml with 0.5% chlorobutanol, polysorbate 80, butylated hydroxyanisol and butylated hydroxytoluene)

RDA — Note: RDAs converted to retinol equivalents (RE). One RE has activity of 1 mcg all-*trans* retinol, 6 mcg beta carotene. **Neonates and infants < 1 yr:** 375 mcg RE or 1,250 IU. **Children 1 to 3 yr:** 400 mcg RE or 1,330 IU. **Children 4 to 6 yr:** 500 mcg RE or 1,665 IU. **Children 7 to 10 yr:** 700 mcg RE or 2,330 IU. **Males > 11 yr:** 1,000 mcg RE or 2,665 IU. **Females > 11 yr:** 800 mcg RE or 2,665 IU. **Pregnant women:** 800 mcg RE or 2,665 IU. **Breast-feeding women (1st 6 mo):** 1,300 mcg RE or 4,330 IU. **Breast-feeding women (2nd 6 mo):** 1,200 mcg RE or 4,000 IU.

Severe vitamin A deficiency — **Adults and children > 8 yr:** 100,000 IU IM or 100,000 to 500,000 IU PO for 3 days, then 50,000 IU IM or PO for 2 wk; then 10,000 to 20,000 IU PO for 2 mo. Follow with adequate dietary nutrition and RDA vitamin A supplements. **Infants < 1 yr:** 7,500 to 15,000 IU IM daily for 10 days. **Children 1 to 8 yr:** 17,500 to 35,000 IU IM daily for 10 days.

Maintenance dosage to prevent recurrence of vitamin A deficiency — **Children 1 to 8 yr:** 5,000 to 10,000 IU PO daily for 2 mo, then adequate dietary nutrition and RDA vitamin A supplements.

- Use cautiously in pregnant patients, avoiding doses exceeding RDA.
- Contraindicated orally in malabsorption syndrome; if malabsorption due to inadequate bile secretion, oral route may be used with concurrent administration of bile salts (dehydrocholic acid). Also contraindicated in hypervitaminosis A and hypersensitivity to any ingredient in product. IV route contraindicated except for special water-miscible forms intended for infusion with large parenteral volumes. IV push of vitamin A of any type contraindicated.

vitamin C (ascorbic acid)

Ascorbicap, Cevi-Bid, Flavettes‡, Redoxon†

Water-soluble vitamin

Vitamin

Preg. Risk Category: C

tab: 25, 50, 100, 250, 500, 1,000 mg; **tab (chew):** 50, 100, 250, 500, 1,000 mg; **tab (effery):** 1,000 mg sugar-free; **tab (timed-release):** 500,

RDA — **Neonates and infants < 6 mo:** 30 mg. **Infants 6 mo to 1 yr:** 35 mg. **Children 1 to 3 yr:** 40 mg. **Children 4 to 10 yr:** 45 mg. **Children 11 to 14 yr:** 50 mg. **Adults and children ≥ 15 yr:** 60 mg. **Pregnant women:** 70 mg. **Breast-feeding women (1st 6 mo):** 95 mg. **Breast-feeding women (2nd 6 mo):** 90 mg.

Frank and subclinical scurvy — **Adults:** depending on severity, 300 mg to 1 g PO, SC, IM, or IV daily, then 70 to 150 mg daily for maintenance. **Children:** depending on severity, 100 to 300 mg PO, SC, IM, or IV

- Use cautiously in renal insufficiency.

(continued)

VITAMIN C   267

DRUG/CLASS/ CATEGORY	DOSAGE FORMS	INDICATIONS/ DOSAGES	KEY PRECAUTIONS
vitamin C *(continued)*	1,000, 1,500 mg; *cap (timed-release):* 500 mg; *crystals:* 100, 500 g (4 g/tsp); *lozenges:* 60 mg; *oral liq.:* 50 ml (35 mg/0.6 ml); *oral sol.:* 60, 100 mg/ml; *powder:* 100, 500 g (4 g/tsp); *syrup:* 20 mg/ml in 120 ml, 480 ml; 500 mg/5 ml in 5, 120, 480 ml; *inj:* 100, 250, 500 mg/ml	daily, then ≥ 30 mg daily for maintenance. **Premature infants:** 75 to 100 mg PO, IM, IV, or SC daily. *Extensive burns —* **Adults:** 300 to 500 mg SC, IM, or IV daily for 7 to 10 days. 1 to 2 g daily for extensive burns. **Children:** 100 to 200 mg PO, SC, IM, or IV daily.	
vitamin E (tocopherol) Amino-Opti-E, Aquasol E, E-200 I.U. Softgels, E Vitamin Succinate, Vita-Plus E Softgels *Fat-soluble vitamin* *Vitamin* Preg. Risk Category: NR	*tab (chew):* 200, 400 I.U. *cap:* 200, 400, 500, 600, 1,000 IU and 330, 147, 73.5 mg; *oral sol.:* 50 mg/ml	*RDA — Note:* RDAs converted to alpha-tocopherol equivalents (α-TE). One α-TE equals 1 mg D-alpha tocopherol or 1.49 IU. **Neonates and infants < 6 mo:** 3 α-TE or 4 IU. **Infants 6 mo to 1 yr:** 4 α-TE or 6 IU. **Children 1 to 3 yr:** 6 α-TE or 9 IU. **Children 4 to 10 yr:** 7 α-TE or 10 IU. **Males ≥ 11 yr:** 10 α-TE or 15 IU. **Females ≥ 11 yr:** 8 α-TE or 12 IU. **Pregnant women:** 10 α-TE or 15 IU. **Breast-feeding women (1st 6 mo):** 12 α-TE or 18 IU. **Breast-feeding women (2nd 6 mo):** 11 α-TE or 16 IU.	• Use cautiously in liver or gallbladder disease.

Vitamin E deficiency in premature neonates and in patients with impaired fat absorption — **Adults:** depending on severity, 60 to 75 IU PO daily. **Children:** 1 IU/kg daily.

w–x–y

warfarin sodium
Coumadin, Panwarfin, Sofarin,
Warfilone Sodium†
Coumarin derivative
Anticoagulant
Preg. Risk Category: X

tab: 1, 2, 2.5, 4, 5, 7.5, 10 mg

Pulmonary embolism with DVT, MI, rheumatic heart disease with heart valve damage, prosthetic heart valves, chronic atrial fibrillation — **Adults:** 2 to 5 mg PO daily for 2 to 4 days, then dosage based on daily PT and INR. Usual maintenance dosage 2 to 10 mg PO daily.

- Use cautiously in diverticulitis, colitis, mild or moderate hypertension, mild or moderate hepatic or renal disease, with drainage tubes in any orifice; with regional or lumbar block anesthesia; in any condition that increases risk of hemorrhage; and in breast-feeding patients.
- Contraindicated in known hypersensitivity to drug; pregnancy, threatened abortion, eclampsia, or preeclampsia; blood dyscrasias or hemorrhagic tendencies; recent surgery involving large open areas, eye, brain, or spinal cord; recent prostatectomy; major regional lumbar block anesthesia; spinal puncture, diagnostic or therapeutic invasive procedures; bleeding from GI, GU, or respiratory tracts; aneurysm; cerebrovascular hemorrhage; severe or malignant hypertension; severe renal or hepatic disease; subacute bacterial endocarditis, pericarditis, or pericardial effusion; history of warfarin-induced necrosis; unsupervised patients with senility, alcoholism, or psychosis; or if lab facilities for coagulation testing inadequate.

Z

DRUG/CLASS/CATEGORY	DOSAGE FORMS	INDICATIONS/DOSAGES	KEY PRECAUTIONS
zafirlukast Accolate *Antileukotriene* *Anti-inflammatory* Preg. Risk Category: B	**tab:** 20 mg	*Prophylaxis and chronic treatment of asthma —* **Adults and children ≥ 12 yr:** 20 mg PO bid 1 hr before or 2 hr after meals.	▪ Use cautiously in hepatic impairment and in elderly patients. Use in pregnant patients only if clearly needed. Safety and efficacy in children < 12 yr not established. ▪ Not for use in reversing bronchospasm in acute asthma attacks or in breast-feeding patients. ▪ Contraindicated in known hypersensitivity.
zalcitabine (dideoxycytidine, ddC) Hivid *Nucleoside analogue* *Antiviral* Preg. Risk Category: C	**tab:** 0.375, 0.75 mg	*Monotherapy for treatment of advanced HIV disease in patients who can't tolerate zidovudine or who have disease progression while receiving zidovudine —* **Adults and children ≥ 13 yr:** 0.75 mg PO q 8 hr. *Combination therapy with zidovudine for treatment of advanced HIV disease (CD4+ count ≤ 300 cells/mm³) —* **Adults and children ≥ 13 yr:** 0.75 mg PO q 8 hr given concomitantly with zidovudine 200 mg PO q 8 hr.	▪ Use cautiously in renal impairment, hepatic failure, history of pancreatitis, baseline cardiomyopathy, or history of heart failure and peripheral neuropathy. ▪ Contraindicated in hypersensitivity to drug or any component of formulation.
zidovudine (azidothymidine, AZT) Apo-Zidovudine†, Novo-AZT†, Retrovir *Thymidine analogue* *Antiviral* Preg. Risk Category: C	**cap:** 100 mg; **tab:** 300 mg; **syrup:** 50 mg/5 ml; **inj:** 10 mg/ml	*Symptomatic HIV infection, including AIDS —* **Adults and children ≥ 12 yr:** 100 mg PO q 4 hr around the clock or 300 mg (1 tab) PO q 12 hr; IV infusion 1 mg/kg (infuse over 1 hr) q 4 hr for total of 6 mg/kg/day. **Children 3 mo to 12 yr:** 180 mg/m² PO q 6 hr (720 mg/m²/day), ≤ 200 mg q 6 hr. *Asymptomatic HIV infection —* **Adults and children ≥ 12 yr:** 100 mg PO q 4 hr while awake (500 mg daily); IV infusion 1 mg/kg (infuse over 1 hr) q 4 hr while awake for total 5 mg/kg/day. **Children 3 mo to 12 yr:**	▪ Use cautiously and with close monitoring in advanced symptomatic HIV infection; in severe bone marrow depression, hepatomegaly, hepatitis, or other risk factors for liver disease; and in renal insufficiency. ▪ Contraindicated in hypersensitivity to drug.

180 mg/m² PO q 6 hr (720 mg/m²/day), not to exceed 200 mg q 6 hr.
To reduce risk of HIV transmission from infected mother with baseline CD4+ lymphocyte count > 200 cells/mm³ to fetus — **Adults:** 100 mg PO 5 times daily given initially between 14 and 34 wks' gestation and continued throughout pregnancy. During labor, give loading dose of 2 mg/kg IV over 1 hr, followed by continuous IV infusion of 1 mg/kg/hr until umbilical cord clamped. **Neonates:** 2 mg/kg PO (syrup) q 6 hr for 6 wk, starting within 12 hr after birth. Or, 1.5 mg/kg IV (infuse over 30 min) q 6 hr.

---

zileuton
Zyflo
Antileukotriene
Anti-inflammatory
Preg. Risk Category: C

tab: 600 mg

Prophylaxis and chronic treatment of asthma — **Adults and children ≥ 12 yr:** 600 mg PO qid.

- Use cautiously in hepatic impairment and in history of heavy alcohol use.
- Not indicated for reversing bronchospasm in acute asthma attacks.
- Contraindicated in known hypersensitivity to drug and in active liver disease or transaminase elevations at least 3 times upper limit of normal.
- Use in pregnant patients only if benefit outweighs potential risk to fetus.
- Don't give to breast-feeding patients.
- Safety and efficacy in children < 12 yr not established.

---

zolpidem tartrate
Ambien
Imidazopyridine
Hypnotic
Preg. Risk Category: B
Controlled Sub. Sched.: IV

tab: 5, 10 mg

Short-term management of insomnia — **Adults:** 10 mg PO immediately before bedtime. In elderly or debilitated patients and in hepatic insufficiency, 5 mg PO immediately before bedtime. Max 10 mg daily.

- Use cautiously in conditions that could affect metabolism or hemodynamic response and in decreased respiratory drive, depression, or history of alcohol or drug abuse.

Appendix 1

Components of a properly written prescription

A properly written prescription (shown on the right) should include:

- the date of the prescription
- the patient's full name
- the patient's address
- the drug name
- the dosage form (if more than one form exists)
- the amount of each dose
- the administration route
- the administration schedule or time
- the total amount of the drug to be dispensed
- the number of times the prescription can be refilled
- the prescriber's signature and credentials.

Lakeview Hospital
2000 N. Main Street
Lewistown, N.J. 00265

PATIENT'S
NAME: *William R. Weaver*
ADDRESS: *1000 Limerick Lane*
Dresher, N.J. 00265

ADDRESSOPLATE OR COMPLETE ABOVE

DATE: *9/15/98*

This Rx NOT VALID For Schedule Drugs.

Synthroid 0.2mg P.O. daily

Disp: #30

John Jackson, MD

Refill _3_

IN ORDER FOR A BRAND NAME PRODUCT TO BE DISPENSED, THE PRE-
SCRIBER MUST HANDWRITE, "BRAND NECESSARY" OR "BRAND MEDICAL-
LY NECESSARY" IN THE SPACE ABOVE.

Pharmacy will dispense a generic equivalent (under the formulary system) unless
the particular drug is encircled.
PRESCRIBER'S PRINTED NAME ___*John Jackson, MD*___

Pharmacologic abbreviations to avoid

The Joint Commission on Accreditation of Healthcare Organizations mandates that every health care facility develop a list of approved abbreviations for staff use. Certain abbreviations should be avoided whenever possible, however, because they can be misunderstood easily, especially when handwritten. Here's a list of abbreviations to avoid.

Abbreviation	Intended meaning	Misinterpretation	Correction
Apothecaries' symbols			
℥	fluidounce	Frequently misinterpreted	Use metric equivalents.
ℨ	fluidram	Frequently misinterpreted	Use metric equivalents.
♏	minim	Frequently misinterpreted	Use metric equivalents.
Drug names			
MTX	methotrexate	mustargen	Use complete spelling.
CPZ	Compazine (prochlorperazine)	chlorpromazine	Use complete spelling.
HCl	hydrochloric acid	potassium chloride (*H* may be misinterpreted as *K*.)	Use complete spelling.
MgSO₄	morphine sulfate	magnesium sulfate ($MgSO_4$)	Use complete spelling.
DIG	digoxin	digitoxin	Use complete spelling.
MVI	Multivitamins without fat-soluble vitamins	Multivitamins with fat-soluble vitamins	Use complete spelling.

(continued)

Pharmacologic abbreviations to avoid (continued)

Abbreviation	Intended meaning	Misinterpretation	Correction
Drug names (continued)			
HCTZ	hydrochlorothiazide	hydrocortisone (HCT)	Use complete spelling.
ara-a	vidarabine	cytarabine (ara-C)	Use complete spelling.
Dosage directions			
Au	auris uterque (each ear)	Frequently misinterpreted as OU (oculus uterque, each eye)	Write it out.
µg	microgram	Frequently misinterpreted as mg	Use mcg.
OD	once daily	Frequently misinterpreted as OD (oculus dexter, right eye)	Don't abbreviate daily. Write it out.
OJ	orange juice	Frequently misinterpreted as OD (oculus dexter, right eye) or OS (oculus sinister, left eye)	Write it out.
t̄id	once daily	Misinterpreted as tid (three times daily)	Write it out.
per os	orally	os frequently misinterpreted as OS (oculus sinister, left eye)	Use PO, by mouth, or orally.
q.d.	every day	Period after the q misinterpreted as i, incorrectly indicating qid (4 times a day)	Write it out.

hs	nightly or at bedtime	Misinterpreted as *qh* (every hour)	Use *h.s.* or *nightly.*
qod	every other day	Misinterpreted as *qd* (daily) or *qid* (4 times a day)	Use *q other day* or *every other day.*
SubQ	subcutaneous	*q* misinterpreted as *every*, may lead to misinterpretations in abbreviations to follow (Ex: An S.Q. heparin dose meant to be given 2 hours before surgery may be given every 2 hours instead.)	Use *subcut*, or write out *subcutaneous.*
u	unit	Misinterpreted as a *0* or *4*	Write it out.

Appendix 3

Therapeutic classifications of selected drugs

The following is a list of commonly prescribed drugs, organized by their clinical use or therapeutic classification.

Acidifiers and alkalinizers
- ammonium chloride
- sodium bicarbonate
- sodium lactate
- tromethamine

Adrenergic blockers (sympatholytics)
- dihydroergotamine mesylate
- ergotamine tartrate
- methysergide maleate

Adrenergics (sympathomimetics)
- dobutamine hydrochloride
- dopamine hydrochloride
- metaraminol bitartrate
- norepinephrine bitartrate
- phenylephrine hydrochloride
- pseudoephedrine hydrochloride

- neomycin sulfate
- tobramycin sulfate

Androgens and anabolic steroids
- danazol
- fluoxymesterone
- methyltestosterone
- nandrolone decanoate
- nandrolone phenpropionate
- stanozolol
- testosterone
- testosterone cypionate
- testosterone propionate
- testosterone transdermal system

Antacids, adsorbents, and antiflatulents
- aluminum carbonate
- aluminum hydroxide

Antianxiety drugs
- alprazolam
- buspirone hydrochloride
- chlordiazepoxide
- chlordiazepoxide hydrochloride
- clorazepate dipotassium
- diazepam
- hydroxyzine embonate
- hydroxyzine hydrochloride
- hydroxyzine pamoate
- lorazepam
- meprobamate
- midazolam hydrochloride
- oxazepam

Antiarrhythmics
- amiodarone hydrochloride
- atropine sulfate
- bretylium tosylate
- disopyramide

Anticholinergics
- dicyclomine hydrochloride
- glycopyrrolate
- hyoscyamine
- hyoscyamine sulfate
- propantheline bromide
- scopolamine
- scopolamine butylbromide

Anticoagulants
- dalteparin sodium
- danaparoid sodium
- enoxaparin sodium
- heparin calcium
- heparin sodium
- warfarin sodium

Anticonvulsants
- carbamazepine
- clonazepam
- divalproex sodium

- pseudoephedrine sulfate

Alkylating drugs
- busulfan
- carboplatin
- carmustine
- chlorambucil
- cisplatin
- cyclophosphamide
- ifosfamide
- lomustine
- melphalan
- streptozocin
- thiotepa
- uracil mustard

Amebicides and antiprotozoals
- atovaquone
- metronidazole
- metronidazole hydrochloride
- paromomycin sulfate
- pentamidine isethionate

Aminoglycosides
- amikacin sulfate
- gentamicin sulfate

- aluminum phosphate
- calcium carbonate
- magaldrate
- magnesium oxide
- simethicone

Anthelmintics
- mebendazole
- pyrantel pamoate
- thiabendazole

Antianginals
- amlodipine besylate
- amyl nitrite
- bepridil hydrochloride
- diltiazem hydrochloride
- isosorbide dinitrate
- isosorbide mononitrate
- nadolol
- nicardipine
- nifedipine
- nitroglycerin
- propranolol hydrochloride
- verapamil
- verapamil hydrochloride

- disopyramide phosphate
- esmolol hydrochloride
- flecainide acetate
- ibutilide fumarate
- lidocaine hydrochloride
- mexiletine hydrochloride
- moricizine hydrochloride
- procainamide hydrochloride
- propafenone hydrochloride
- quinidine gluconate
- quinidine sulfate
- sotalol
- tocainide hydrochloride

Antibiotic antineoplastic drugs
- bleomycin sulfate
- dactinomycin
- daunorubicin hydrochloride
- doxorubicin hydrochloride
- idarubicin hydrochloride
- mitomycin
- pentostatin
- plicamycin

- ethosuximide
- fosphenytoin sodium
- gabapentin
- lamotrigine
- magnesium sulfate
- mephobarbital
- phenobarbital
- phenobarbital sodium
- phensuximide
- phenytoin
- phenytoin sodium
- phenytoin sodium (extended)
- primidone
- valproate sodium
- valproic acid

Antidepressants
- amitriptyline hydrochloride
- amitriptyline pamoate
- amoxapine
- bupropion hydrochloride
- clomipramine hydrochloride
- desipramine hydrochloride
- doxepin hydrochloride
- fluoxetine hydrochloride

(continued)

Antidepressants *(continued)*
- imipramine hydrochloride
- imipramine pamoate
- maprotiline hydrochloride
- mirtazapine
- nefazodone hydrochloride
- paroxetine hydrochloride
- protriptyline hydrochloride
- sertraline hydrochloride
- trazodone hydrochloride
- trimipramine maleate
- venlafaxine hydrochloride

Antidiabetic drugs and glucagon
- acarbose
- glimepiride
- glipizide
- glucagon
- glyburide
- insulin
- metformin hydrochloride
- tolbutamide
- troglitazone

- itraconazole
- ketoconazole
- nystatin

Antigout drugs
- allopurinol
- colchicine
- probenecid
- sulfinpyrazone

Antihistamines
- astemizole
- brompheniramine maleate
- cetirizine hydrochloride
- chlorpheniramine maleate
- clemastine fumarate
- diphenhydramine hydrochloride
- fexofenadine hydrochloride
- loratadine
- promethazine hydrochloride
- promethazine theoclate
- triprolidine hydrochloride

- nisoldipine
- nitroprusside sodium
- penbutolol sulfate
- phentolamine mesylate
- pindolol
- prazosin hydrochloride
- propranolol hydrochloride
- quinapril hydrochloride
- ramipril
- reserpine
- terazosin hydrochloride
- timolol maleate
- trandolapril
- valsartan
- verapamil hydrochloride

Antilipemics
- atorvastatin
- cholestyramine
- colestipol hydrochloride
- fluvastatin sodium
- gemfibrozil
- lovastatin
- niacin
- pravastatin sodium

- bicalutamide
- estramustine phosphate sodium
- flutamide
- leuprolide acetate
- megestrol acetate
- tamoxifen citrate
- testolactone

Antiparkinsonian drugs
- amantadine hydrochloride
- benztropine mesylate
- biperiden hydrochloride
- biperiden lactate
- carbidopa-levodopa
- levodopa
- pergolide mesylate
- selegiline hydrochloride
- trihexyphenidyl hydrochloride

Antipsychotics
- chlorpromazine hydrochloride
- clozapine
- fluphenazine decanoate

Antidiarrheals
- attapulgite
- bismuth subsalicylate
- kaolin and pectin mixtures
- loperamide
- octreotide acetate
- opium tincture
- opium tincture, camphorated

Antiemetics
- dimenhydrinate
- dronabinol
- granisetron hydrochloride
- meclizine hydrochloride
- metoclopramide hydrochloride
- ondansetron hydrochloride
- prochlorperazine
- prochlorperazine edisylate
- prochlorperazine maleate
- promethazine hydrochloride

Antifungals
- amphotericin B
- fluconazole
- flucytosine
- griseofulvin microsize
- griseofulvin ultramicrosize

Antihypertensives
- acebutolol
- acebutolol hydrochloride
- amlodipine besylate
- atenolol
- benazepril hydrochloride
- betaxolol hydrochloride
- captopril
- carteolol
- clonidine
- clonidine hydrochloride
- diltiazem hydrochloride
- doxazosin mesylate
- enalapril maleate
- felodipine
- fosinopril sodium
- guanethidine monosulfate
- hydralazine hydrochloride
- isradipine
- labetalol hydrochloride
- lisinopril
- losartan potassium
- methyldopa
- methyldopate hydrochloride
- metoprolol succinate
- metoprolol tartrate
- moexipril hydrochloride
- simvastatin

Antimalarials
- chloroquine hydrochloride
- chloroquine phosphate
- chloroquine sulfate
- hydroxychloroquine sulfate
- mefloquine hydrochloride
- primaquine phosphate
- pyrimethamine
- pyrimethamine with sulfadoxine

Antimetabolites
- cladribine
- cytarabine
- fludarabine phosphate
- fluorouracil
- hydroxyurea
- mercaptopurine
- methotrexate
- methotrexate sodium
- thioguanine

Antineoplastics that alter hormone balance
- anastrozole

- fluphenazine enanthate
- fluphenazine hydrochloride
- haloperidol
- haloperidol decanoate
- haloperidol lactate
- loxapine hydrochloride
- loxapine succinate
- mesoridazine besylate
- molindone hydrochloride
- olanzapine
- perphenazine
- pimozide
- prochlorperazine
- promazine hydrochloride
- risperidone
- thioridazine hydrochloride
- thiothixene
- thiothixene hydrochloride
- trifluoperazine hydrochloride

Antituberculars and antileprotics
- capreomycin sulfate
- clofazimine
- dapsone
- ethambutol hydrochloride

(continued)

Antituberculars and antileprotics *(continued)*

- isoniazid
- pyrazinamide
- rifabutin
- rifampin

Antiulcer drugs

- cimetidine
- famotidine
- lansoprazole
- misoprostol
- nizatidine
- omeprazole
- ranitidine hydrochloride
- sucralfate

Antivirals

- acyclovir sodium
- amantadine hydrochloride
- cidofovir
- didanosine
- famciclovir
- foscarnet sodium
- ganciclovir

- levamisole hydrochloride
- sargramostim

Blood derivatives

- albumin 5%
- albumin 25%
- antihemophilic factor
- anti-inhibitor coagulant complex
- antithrombin III, human
- factor IX (human)
- factor IX complex
- plasma protein fraction

Bronchodilators

- albuterol
- albuterol sulfate
- aminophylline
- epinephrine
- epinephrine bitartrate
- epinephrine hydrochloride
- ipratropium bromide
- isoetharine hydrochloride
- isoetharine mesylate
- isoproterenol

- cephalexin monohydrate
- cephapirin sodium
- cephradine
- loracarbef

Cholinergics (parasympathomimetics)

- ambenonium chloride
- bethanechol chloride
- neostigmine methylsulfate

CNS stimulants

- amphetamine sulfate
- caffeine
- dextroamphetamine sulfate
- methamphetamine hydrochloride
- methylphenidate hydrochloride
- pemoline
- phentermine hydrochloride

Corticosteroids

- betamethasone
- betamethasone acetate and

- triamcinolone acetonide

Digestive enzymes and gallstone solubilizers

- monoctanoin
- pancreatin
- pancrelipase
- ursodiol

Diuretics

- acetazolamide
- acetazolamide sodium
- amiloride hydrochloride
- bumetanide
- chlorothiazide
- chlorothiazide sodium
- chlorthalidone
- ethacrynic acid
- furosemide
- hydrochlorothiazide
- indapamide
- mannitol
- methazolamide
- metolazone
- spironolactone

- indinavir sulfate
- lamivudine
- nevirapine
- ribavirin
- rimantadine hydrochloride
- ritonavir
- saquinavir mesylate
- stavudine
- valacyclovir hydrochloride
- zalcitabine
- zidovudine

Biological response modifiers

- aldesleukin
- epoetin alfa
- filgrastim
- interferon alfa-2a, recombinant
- interferon alfa-2b, recombinant
- interferon alfa-n3
- interferon beta-1a
- interferon beta-1b, recombinant
- interferon gamma-1b

- isoproterenol hydrochloride
- isoproterenol sulfate
- metaproterenol sulfate
- oxtriphylline
- pirbuterol
- salmeterol xinafoate
- terbutaline sulfate
- theophylline
- theophylline sodium glycinate

Cephalosporins

- cefaclor
- cefazolin sodium
- cefixime
- cefonicid sodium
- cefoperazone sodium
- cefotaxime sodium
- cefotetan disodium
- cefoxitin sodium
- ceftazidime
- ceftibuten
- ceftizoxime sodium
- ceftriaxone sodium
- cefuroxime axetil
- cefuroxime sodium
- cephalexin hydrochloride

- betamethasone sodium phosphate
- betamethasone sodium phosphate
- cortisone acetate
- dexamethasone
- dexamethasone acetate
- dexamethasone sodium phosphate
- fludrocortisone acetate
- hydrocortisone
- hydrocortisone acetate
- hydrocortisone sodium phosphate
- hydrocortisone sodium succinate
- methylprednisolone
- methylprednisolone acetate
- methylprednisolone sodium succinate
- prednisolone
- prednisolone sodium phosphate
- prednisolone tebutate
- prednisone
- triamcinolone

- torsemide
- triamterene
- urea

Electrolytes and replacement solutions

- calcium acetate
- calcium carbonate
- calcium chloride
- calcium citrate
- calcium glubionate
- calcium gluceptate
- calcium gluconate
- calcium lacate
- calcium phosphate, dibasic
- calcium phosphate, tribasic
- dextran, low-molecular-weight
- dextran, high-molecular-weight
- hetastarch
- magnesium chloride
- magnesium sulfate
- potassium acetate
- potassium bicarbonate
- potassium chloride

(continued)

Electrolytes and replacement solutions (continued)

- potassium gluconate
- Ringer's injection
- Ringer's injection, lactated
- sodium chloride

Estrogens and progestins

- diethylstilbestrol
- diethylstilbestrol diphosphate
- esterified estrogens
- estradiol
- estradiol cypionate
- estradiol valerate
- estrogens, conjugated
- estropipate
- ethinyl estradiol
- ethinyl estradiol and desogestrel
- ethinyl estradiol and ethynodiol diacetate
- ethinyl estradiol and levonorgestrel
- ethinyl estradiol and norethindrone

Fluoroquinolones

- ciprofloxacin
- levofloxacin
- lomefloxacin hydrochloride
- norfloxacin
- ofloxacin
- sparfloxacin

Gold salts

- auranofin
- aurothioglucose
- gold sodium thiomalate

Gonadotropins

- gonadorelin acetate
- histrelin acetate
- menotropins
- nafarelin acetate

Hematinics

- ferrous fumarate
- ferrous gluconate
- ferrous sulfate
- ferrous sulfate, dried
- iron dextran

- muromonab-CD3
- mycophenolate mofetil
- tacrolimus

Inotropics

- amrinone lactate
- digoxin
- milrinone lactate

Laxatives

- bisacodyl
- calcium polycarbophil
- docusate calcium
- docusate sodium
- glycerin
- lactulose
- magnesium citrate
- magnesium hydroxide
- magnesium sulfate
- methylcellulose
- polyethylene glycol and electrolyte solution
- psyllium
- senna
- sodium phosphates

Macrolide anti-infectives

- azithromycin
- clarithromycin
- dirithromycin
- erythromycin base
- erythromycin estolate
- erythromycin ethylsuccinate
- erythromycin lactobionate
- erythromycin stearate

Miotics

- acetylcholine chloride
- carbachol (intraocular)
- carbachol (topical)
- demecarium bromide
- echothiophate iodide
- physostigmine sulfate
- pilocarpine
- pilocarpine hydrochloride
- pilocarpine nitrate

Miscellaneous antagonists and antidotes

- activated charcoal
- aminocaproic acid

- ethinyl estradiol and norethin-drone acetate
- ethinyl estradiol and norgesti-mate
- ethinyl estradiol and norgestrel
- ethinyl estradiol, norethindrone acetate, and ferrous fumarate
- mestranol and norethindrone
- mestranol and norethynodrel
- hydroxyprogesterone caproate
- levonorgestrel
- medroxyprogesterone acetate
- norethindrone
- norethindrone acetate
- norgestrel
- progesterone

Expectants and antitus-sives
- benzonatate
- dextromethorphan hydrobro-mide
- guaifenesin

- polysaccharide iron complex

Immune serums
- cytomegalovirus immune globulin, intravenous
- hepatitis B immune globulin, human
- immune globulin intramuscular
- immune globulin intravenous
- rabies immune globulin, human
- respiratory syncytial virus immune globulin intravenous, human
- Rh₀ (D) immune globulin, human
- Rh₀ (D) immune globulin intravenous, human
- tetanus immune globulin, human
- varicella-zoster immune globulin

Immunosuppressants
- azathioprine
- cyclosporine

Local anti-infectives
- acyclovir
- amphotericin B
- bacitracin
- butoconazole nitrate
- clindamycin phosphate
- clotrimazole
- econazole nitrate
- erythromycin
- gentamicin sulfate
- ketoconazole
- metronidazole (topical)
- miconazole nitrate
- mupirocin
- naftifine
- neomycin sulfate
- nitrofurazone
- nystatin
- oxiconazole nitrate
- silver sulfadiazine
- sulconazole nitrate
- terbinafine hydrochloride
- terconazole
- tetracycline hydrochloride
- tioconazole
- tolnaftate

- deferoxamine mesylate
- digoxin immune FAB
- dimercaprol
- disulfiram
- d-penicillamine
- edetate calcium disodium
- edetate disodium
- flumazenil
- ipecac syrup
- naloxone hydrochloride
- naltrexone hydrochloride
- pralidoxime chloride
- protamine sulfate
- sodium polystyrene sulfonate
- succimer
- trientine hydrochloride

Miscellaneous anti-infectives
- aztreonam
- chloramphenicol
- clindamycin hydrochloride
- clindamycin palmitate hydrochloride

(continued)

THERAPEUTIC CLASSIFICATIONS OF SELECTED DRUGS   283

Miscellaneous anti-infectives
(continued)

- clindamycin phosphate
- fosfomycin tromethamine
- imipenem/cilastatin sodium
- meropenem
- methenamine hippurate
- methenamine mandelate
- nitrofurantoin macrocrystals
- nitrofurantoin microcrystals
- polymyxin B sulfate
- trimethoprim
- vancomycin hydrochloride

Miscellaneous antineoplastic drugs

- altretamine
- amifostine
- asparaginase
- docetaxel
- etoposide
- etoposide phosphate
- gemcitabine hydrochloride

- nicotine polacrilex
- nicotine transdermal system
- sumatriptan succinate
- tacrine hydrochloride

Miscellaneous ophthalmics

- apraclonidine hydrochloride
- betaxolol hydrochloride
- botulinum toxin type A
- carteolol hydrochloride
- dipivefrin
- dorzolamide hydrochloride
- fluorescein sodium
- isosorbide
- latanoprost
- levobunolol hydrochloride
- lodoxamide tromethamine
- metipranolol hydrochloride
- timolol maleate

Miscellaneous respiratory drugs

- buprenorphine hydrochloride
- butorphanol tartrate
- codeine phosphate
- codeine sulfate
- fentanyl citrate
- fentanyl transdermal system
- fentanyl transmucosal
- hydromorphone hydrochloride
- meperidine hydrochloride
- methadone hydrochloride
- morphine hydrochloride
- morphine sulfate
- morphine tartrate
- oxycodone hydrochloride
- oxycodone pectinate
- oxymorphone hydrochloride
- pentazocine hydrochloride
- pentazocine hydrochloride and naloxone hydrochloride
- pentazocine lactate
- propoxyphene hydrochloride
- propoxyphene napsylate

Nonnarcotic analgesics and antipyretics

- choline magnesium trisalicylate
- choline salicylate
- diflunisal
- salsalate

Nonsteroidal anti-inflammatory drugs

- diclofenac sodium
- diclofenac potassium
- fenoprofen calcium
- flurbiprofen
- ibuprofen
- indomethacin
- indomethacin sodium trihydrate
- ketoprofen
- ketorolac tromethamine
- meclofenamate
- nabumetone
- naproxen

- irinotecan hydrochloride
- mitotane
- mitoxantrone hydrochloride
- paclitaxel
- procarbazine hydrochloride
- teniposide
- topotecan hydrochloride
- tretinoin
- vinblastine sulfate
- vincristine sulfate
- vinorelbine tartrate

Miscellaneous cardiovascular drugs
- alprostadil
- dipyridamole
- isoxsuprine hydrochloride
- pentoxifylline
- ticlopidine hydrochloride

Miscellaneous CNS drugs
- donepezil hydrochloride
- fluvoxamine maleate
- lithium carbonate
- lithium citrate

- acetylcysteine
- alpha proteinase inhibitor (human)
- beclomethasone dipropionate
- beractant
- cromolyn sodium
- dexamethasone sodium phosphate inhalation
- dornase alfa
- flunisolide
- nedocromil sodium
- triamcinolone acetonide
- zafirlukast
- zileuton

Mydriatics
- atropine sulfate
- cyclopentolate hydrochloride
- homatropine hydrobromide
- phenylephrine hydrochloride
- scopolamine hydrobromide

Narcotic and opioid analgesics
- alfentanil hydrochloride

- sufentanil
- tramadol hydrochloride

Nasal drugs
- azelastine hydrochloride
- beclomethasone dipropionate
- budesonide
- dexamethasone sodium phosphate
- ephedrine sulfate
- epinephrine hydrochloride
- flunisolide
- fluticasone propionate
- naphazoline hydrochloride
- oxymetazoline hydrochloride
- phenylephrine hydrochloride
- triamcinolone acetonide

Neuromuscular blockers
- atracurium besylate
- pancuronium bromide
- rocuronium bromide
- succinylcholine chloride
- tubocurarine chloride
- vecuronium bromide

- naproxen sodium
- piroxicam
- sulindac
- tolmetin sodium

Ophthalmic anti-infectives
- bacitracin
- ciprofloxacin hydrochloride
- erythromycin
- gentamicin sulfate
- ofloxacin 0.3%
- polymyxin B sulfate
- silver nitrate 1%
- sulfacetamide sodium 10%
- sulfacetamide sodium 15%
- sulfacetamide sodium 30%
- sulfisoxazole diolamine
- tobramycin
- trifluridine
- vidarabine

Ophthalmic anti-inflammatory drugs
- dexamethasone

(continued)

Ophthalmic anti-inflammatory drugs *(continued)*

- dexamethasone sodium phosphate
- diclofenac sodium 0.1%
- flurbiprofen sodium
- ketorolac tromethamine
- prednisolone acetate (suspension)
- prednisolone sodium phosphate (solution)
- rimexolone
- suprofen

Ophthalmic vasoconstrictors

- naphazoline hydrochloride
- oxymetazoline hydrochloride
- tetrahydrozoline hydrochloride

Otics

- acetic acid
- carbamide peroxide
- chloramphenicol

- dicloxacillin sodium
- mezlocillin sodium
- nafcillin sodium
- oxacillin sodium
- penicillin G benzathine
- penicillin G potassium
- penicillin G procaine
- penicillin G sodium
- penicillin V
- penicillin V potassium
- piperacillin sodium
- piperacillin sodium and tazobactam sodium
- ticarcillin disodium
- ticarcillin disodium/clavulanate potassium

Pituitary hormones

- corticotropin
- cosyntropin
- desmopressin acetate
- somatrem
- somatropin
- vasopressin

Sulfonamides

- co-trimoxazole
- sulfadiazine
- sulfamethoxazole
- sulfisoxazole
- sulfisoxazole acetyl

Tetracyclines

- demeclocycline hydrochloride
- doxycycline calcium
- doxycycline hyclate
- doxycycline hydrochloride
- doxycycline monohydrate
- minocycline hydrochloride
- oxytetracycline hydrochloride
- tetracycline hydrochloride

Thrombolytic enzymes

- alteplase
- anistreplase
- reteplase, recombinant
- streptokinase
- urokinase

- diflorasone diacetate
- fluocinolone acetonide
- fluocinonide
- flurandrenolide
- fluticasone propionate
- hydrocortisone
- hydrocortisone acetate
- hydrocortisone butyrate
- hydrocortisone valerate
- mometasone furoate
- triamcinolone acetonide

Vitamins and minerals

- cyanocobalamin
- folic acid
- leucovorin calcium
- niacin
- niacinamide
- phytonadione
- pyridoxine hydrochloride
- riboflavin
- sodium fluoride
- sodium fluoride, topical
- thiamine hydrochloride
- vitamin A

Oxytocics
- carboprost tromethamine
- dinoprostone
- oxytocin, synthetic injection
- oxytocin, synthetic nasal solution

Parathyroid-like drugs
- calcifediol
- calcitonin (human)
- calcitonin (salmon)
- calcitriol
- dihydrotachysterol
- etidronate disodium

Penicillins
- amoxicillin/clavulanate potassium
- amoxicillin trihydrate
- ampicillin
- ampicillin sodium
- ampicillin trihydrate
- ampicillin sodium/sulbactam sodium
- bacampicillin hydrochloride
- cloxacillin sodium

Scabicides and pediculicides
- lindane
- permethrin
- pyrethrins

Sedative-hypnotics
- chloral hydrate
- flurazepam hydrochloride
- pentobarbital
- pentobarbital sodium
- quazepam
- secobarbital sodium
- temazepam
- triazolam
- zolpidem tartrate

Skeletal muscle relaxants
- baclofen
- carisoprodol
- cyclobenzaprine hydrochloride
- dantrolene sodium
- methocarbamol

Spasmolytics
- oxybutynin chloride

Thyroid hormone antagonists
- methimazole
- potassium iodide
- potassium iodide, saturated solution
- strong iodine solution
- propylthiouracil
- radioactive iodine (sodium iodide) [131]

Thyroid hormones
- levothyroxine sodium
- liothyronine sodium
- thyrotropin

Topical corticosteroids
- amcinonide
- betamethasone dipropionate
- betamethasone valerate
- clobetasol propionate
- desonide
- desoximetasone
- dexamethasone
- dexamethasone sodium phosphate

- vitamin C
- vitamin E

Uncategorized drugs
- abciximab
- acetohydroxamic acid
- alendronate sodium
- alprostadil
- aminoglutethimide
- aprotinin
- calcipotriene
- cisapride
- clomiphene citrate
- cysteamine bitartrate
- etretinate
- finasteride
- gallium nitrate
- imiglucerase
- isotretinoin
- levocarnitine
- levomethadyl acetate hydrochloride
- mesalamine
- mesna

(continued)

Uncategorized drugs

(continued)

- methoxsalen
- nimodipine
- olsalazine sodium
- pamidronate disodium
- pilocarpine hydrochloride
- riluzole
- ritodrine hydrochloride
- strontium 89 (^{89}SR) chloride
- sulfasalazine
- tiopronin
- tretinoin
- trilostane

Appendix 4

Unlabeled and unusual uses of drugs

This chart lists unusual or unlabeled uses for certain drugs. The uses described do not necessarily reflect the same dosage, administration, route, or schedule as those of the approved drug indications. Thorough research regarding unlabeled or unusual uses is recommended before prescribing the drug.

Drug	Unlabeled or unusual use	Drug	Unlabeled or unusual use
acetazolamide	Increases ventilatory drive in COPD	captopril	Diagnosis of anatomic renal artery stenosis
acetylcysteine	Attenuates loss of vasodilatory response to nitroglycerin	carbamazepine	Treatment of diabetes insipidus
albuterol	Treatment of hyperkalemia	chloroquine	Treatment of hypercalcemia associated with sarcoidosis
amantadine	Treatment of certain aspects of fatigue in multiple sclerosis	chlorothiazide	Prevention of calcium-containing renal calculi
amiloride	Treatment of lithium-induced polyuria without increasing lithium levels	cholestyramine	Treatment of pruritus in primary biliary cirrhosis
amyl nitrite	Prevention of penile tumescence	cimetidine	Treatment of androgenic alopecia in women
aspirin	Primary prevention of colorectal cancer	cisapride	Treatment of esophagitis in patients with fibrosis
atenolol	Treatment of mild to moderate alcohol withdrawal	cystic	
		clonidine	Treatment of opiate withdrawal
baclofen	Treatment of ACE inhibitor–induced cough	colchicine	Treatment of hepatic cirrhosis
bethanechol	Treatment of stuttering	cromolyn	Treatment of decubitus ulcers
bleomycin	Treatment of malignant pleural effusions	cyanocobalamin	Placebo in various disease states (for example, chronic fatigue syndrome)
bromocriptine	Treatment of cocaine addiction		

(continued)

Unlabeled and unusual uses of drugs *(continued)*

Drug	Unlabeled or unusual use	Drug	Unlabeled or unusual use
dapsone	Treatment of brown recluse spider bite	naloxone	Diagnosis of adrenal insufficiency
demeclocycline	Treatment of SIADH secretion	naltrexone	Treatment of chorea of Huntington's disease
desipramine	Treatment of cocaine withdrawal	niacin	Treatment of hypercholesterolemia
dihydroergotamine	Prophylaxis of thromboembolic disorders	nifedipine	Inhibits premature labor
diltiazem	Prevention, with other drugs, of renal transplant rejection	nortriptyline	Treatment of enuresis
		octreotide	Treatment of bleeding esophageal varices
divalproex	Treatment of intractable hiccups	ondansetron	Treatment of panic attacks
doxepin	Treatment of postprandial hypoglycemia	pemoline	Treatment of narcolepsy
enalapril	Treatment of postrenal transplant erythrocytosis	pentoxifylline	Treatment of recurrent aphthous stomatitis
		pergolide	Treatment of acromegaly
erythromycin	Treatment of gastroparesis	phenytoin	Treatment of cardiac arrhythmia due to digitalis intoxication
estrogens, conjugated	Treatment of uremic bleeding		
flecainide	Treatment of neuropathic pain	prazosin	Treatment of benign prostatic hypertrophy
flumazenil	Treatment of hepatic encephalopathy	probenecid	Differentiate parkinsonism from unipolar depression
gabapentin	Treatment of neuropathic pain		
haloperidol	Treatment of emesis	propantheline	Treatment of acne vulgaris
hydralazine	Treatment of anorexia and cachexia	sulindac	Prevention of fetal complications through reduced amniotic fluid index
hydroxyurea	Treatment of sickle cell anemia		
indomethacin	Treatment of nephrotic syndrome	terbutaline	Prevention and inhibition of premature labor
ketoconazole	Treatment of prostate cancer	tetracycline	Treatment of peptic ulcer caused by *Helicobacter pylori*
lamivudine	Treatment of hepatitis B		

lithium	Treatment of bradycardia
medroxyprogesterone	Prevention of Wernicke's encephalopathy in
	acute alcohol withdrawal
mesna	Treatment of tinnitus
methylphenidate	Treatment of black hairy tongue
mexiletine	Treatment of trigeminal neuralgia
midodrine	Prophylaxis for cluster headache

lithium	Treatment of herpes simplex (topical use)	theophylline	Treatment of bradycardia
medroxyprogesterone	Stimulates appetite	thiamine	Prevention of Wernicke's encephalopathy in acute alcohol withdrawal
mesna	Mucolytic agent	tocainide	Treatment of tinnitus
methylphenidate	Treatment of neurocardiogenic syncope	tretinoin	Treatment of black hairy tongue
mexiletine	Treatment of diabetic neuropathy	valproic acid	Treatment of trigeminal neuralgia
midodrine	Treatment of female stress urinary incontinence	verapamil	Prophylaxis for cluster headache
misoprostol	Treatment of cervical ripening and induction of labor		

Index